T0177627

.

OXFORD HANDBOOK OF

Head and Neck Anatomy

Published and forthcoming Oxford Handbooks

OXFORD HANDBOOK OF
Head and Neck Anatomy

FIRST EDITION

Daniel R. van Gijn (Author)

Specialist Registrar Oral and Maxillofacial Surgery
Royal Surrey County Hospital, Guildford, UK

WITH

Jonathan Dunne (Co-author)

Consultant Plastic and Reconstructive Surgeon
Charing Cross Hospital
Imperial College Healthcare NHS Trust, London, UK

CONSULTANT EDITORS

Susan Standring

Emeritus Professor of Anatomy, Department of Anatomy
King's College London, UK

Simon Eccles

Consultant in Craniofacial Plastic and Reconstructive Surgery
Chelsea and Westminster Hospital NHS Foundation Trust,
London, UK

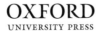

OXFORD
UNIVERSITY PRESS

OXFORD
UNIVERSITY PRESS

Great Clarendon Street, Oxford, OX2 6DP,
United Kingdom

Oxford University Press is a department of the University of Oxford.
It furthers the University's objective of excellence in research, scholarship,
and education by publishing worldwide. Oxford is a registered trade mark of
Oxford University Press in the UK and in certain other countries

© Oxford University Press 2022

The moral rights of the authors have been asserted

First Edition Published in 2022

Published in the United States of America by Oxford University Press
198 Madison Avenue, New York, NY 10016, United States of America

British Library Cataloguing in Publication Data
Data available

Library of Congress Control Number: 2021945504

ISBN 978–0–19–876783–1

DOI: 10.1093/med/9780198767831.001.0001

Printed and bound in China by
C&C Offset Printing Co., Ltd.

To my darling Polly and dear son, Wilfred

Foreword by Carrie Newlands

Daniel is to be commended for his combination of enthusiasm, dedication and artistic talent, which has given us this wonderful book. Anatomy is the backbone of much of a surgeon's working day; we need to have its intricacies, vagaries, and three-dimensional complexity at our fingertips in order for us to do our jobs well and to deserve the trust our patients place in us.

Artistry and surgery go hand in hand and Daniel's exquisite drawings in this highly practical book make anatomy easy to understand with clarity and elegance. Each picture paints a thousand words and thus, this first edition is both detailed and portable.

The etymology of anatomical terms and the historical tit-bits accompanying many anatomical eponyms serve to add another layer to the book's readability. Likewise, the inclusion of operative considerations bridges the frequent gap between anatomical facts and surgical relevance.

A sound grounding in anatomy is still quite rightly required at undergraduate level in medicine and dentistry and often serves to kindle an early interest in many a future surgical career. I have no doubt that this addition to the bookshelf will help many students to find head and neck anatomy less of a terrifying prospect by sheer dint of its simplicity.

The *Oxford Handbook of Head and Neck Anatomy* will be particularly welcomed by those of us in head and neck surgical specialities at all stages of our careers, and members of many medical specialities will find the artistry and accessibility of this excellent resource to be invaluable.

Carrie Newlands
Consultant Oral and Maxillofacial Surgeon
Guildford, UK
Chair, UK OMFS FRCS Examination Board

Foreword by Alice Roberts

If you want head and neck anatomy distilled down to its essence—this is it.

The head and neck are so densely packed with anatomical structures, it's easy to get bogged down in unnecessary details while missing others that are more clinically relevant. Written by an experienced clinician, this book is laid out in a masterfully succinct and logical way, with clear, engineering-style diagrams that help the reader to conceptualize the three-dimensional jigsaw puzzle of head and neck anatomy. Along the way, there are nuggets of etymological delight that are historically fascinating—but also make the elaborate terminology more understandable and memorable. Covered as well are those much beloved TLAs—the three letter abbreviations that litter the clinical landscape of anatomy.

This book will be useful to undergraduates learning anatomy for the first time, but also for trainees specializing in those anatomical areas above the clavicle—who will look back and wish they'd had this text at medical school.

Armed with this powerful tome, the pterygopalatine fossa will never again hold such terror, the infamous infratemporal fossa will be laid bare, and the lacrimal lake of despond will dry up. And with this map in hand, a safari in tiger country will be much, much less dangerous.

Professor Alice Roberts
Anatomist, author & broadcaster
Professor of Public Engagement in Science, University of Birmingham

Preface

One day I will find the right words and they will be simple.

Jack Kerouac

The idea for this book began while a medically qualified dental student, embarking (again) on the seemingly Herculean task of learning head and neck anatomy—under the watchful eye and tutelage of Professor Susan Standring. The book is aimed at medical and dental undergraduates facing similar struggles—as well as dentists, ENT, oral and maxillofacial or plastic surgeons, anaesthetists, and radiologists with a particular interest in the pathology of the head and neck.

The principle of the book is to provide a succinct yet comprehensive pocket guide to the elegant and three-dimensional anatomy of the head and neck, accompanied by simple-to-use schematic line diagrams. It intends to distil conceptually difficult regions of the head and neck into their respective 'bare bones'—constructing a skeleton on which the flesh can be subsequently added, in a format that can be reproduced (and hopefully remembered) on the operating theatre whiteboard or in a notebook in the outpatient clinic or ward environment.

Anatomy, like medicine, has a specific language. A language monopolized by Latin. As with any language, understanding the meaning of a word helps to glean its purpose—and perhaps provide a glimpse into its etymological or eponymous past. How can regional anatomy that includes references to the winged helmet of Hermes, a goat, and a wandering vagrant not help but spark inspiration and stimulate excitatory synapses?

The science of anatomy (from ἀνατομή meaning 'to cut up') underpins pathology ('the study of suffering') which in turn provides the link to medicine and its subsequent inquiry into disease. We are all anatomists at heart: a strong foundation in anatomy promotes clinical 'common sense', acumen, and surgical confidence—allowing you to interpret the problem and to propose a solution on anatomical grounds.

My personal appreciation of the anatomy of the head and neck significantly improved over the course of writing, researching and illustrating this book. I have tried to balance bullet points and prose and to provide easy-to-negotiate illustrations that are intended to simplify complicated anatomical relationships. As a reader and 'learner', you will have your own areas of difficulty and confusion and I welcome your suggestions as to how to improve the text and figures.

Whether you are from a dental, medical, or surgical background, I hope this book gives you the enthusiasm to continue to explore the anatomy, surgery, and pathology that makes a career in a head and neck specialty so rewarding.

Daniel R. van Gijn

Acknowledgement

Professor Patricia Collins
Chapter 15: Embryology of the head and neck
Professor of Anatomy, Anglo-European College of Chiropractic, Bournemouth, UK

Miss Lisa Pitkin
Chapter 8: The Larynx
ENT and Head and Neck surgeon, Royal Surrey County Hospital, UK

Contents

Symbols and abbreviations

➔	cross-reference
a.	artery
AICA	anterior inferior cerebellar artery
ACF	anterior cranial fossa
CCA	common carotid artery
CNS	central nervous system
CSF	cerebrospinal fluid
CT	computed tomography
DCR	dacrocystorhinostomy
ECA	external carotid artery
EJV	external jugular vein
ENT	ear, nose, and throat
f.	foramen
ICA	internal carotid artery
ICP	intercuspal position
IJV	internal jugular vein
IMF	intermaxillary fixation
LPS	levator palpebrae superioris
m.	muscle

MCF	middle cranial fossa
MPL	medial palpebral ligament
n.	nerve
NOE	naso-orbito-ethmoidal
ORIF	open reduction internal fixation
PCF	posterior cranial fossa
PICA	posterior inferior cerebellar artery
RAPD	relative afferent pupillary defect
ROOF	retro-orbicularis oculi fat
RSTL	relaxed skin tension line
SOOF	suborbicularis oculi fat
SCC	squamous cell carcinoma
SCM	sternocleidomastoid
SMAS	superficial muscular aponeurotic system
SOF	superior orbital fissure
TMJ	temporomandibular joint
v.	vein

Symbols and abbreviations

The skull

Introduction

The human skull is the skeleton of the head and is considered along with the mandible. It consists of paired bones and unpaired midline bones that contribute to the muscular attachments for mastication and facial expression, a bony foundation for the upper aerodigestive tract, and support and housing for those structures susceptible to trauma—the special sensory organs and brain.

The skull without the mandible is termed the *cranium* and consists of the *neurocranium* (skull vault) and *viscerocranium* (facial skeleton). The precise number of bones, rather surprisingly, varies depending on the source—with some including the hyoid and ossicles and others discounting paired bones (➲ Fig. 1.1b, p. 5 and Fig. 1.2b, p. 7).

The *calvaria* consists of the cranium without the facial skeleton and cranial base. It consists of the frontal, parietal, and occipital bones and is completed laterally by the greater wings of the sphenoid and the temporal bones. It comprises an external layer or 'table' and internal table with a middle cancellous, diploic bone between. Fractures may involve either in isolation or both, with varying clinical consequences.

There is significant variety in the thickness of the bones of the skull, with those areas covered by muscle thinner than those without, with obvious sequelae following trauma. The boundaries of these more vulnerable areas are the strong vertical and horizontal buttresses of the face that are the prime focus of reconstruction and restoration for the facial trauma surgeon.

The sutures found between adjoining bones of the skull are fibrous joints that allow for the growth of the developing skull and brain. The premature fusion of sutures prevents the normal expansion of the skull perpendicular to the stenosed suture and results in a multitude of *craniosynostoses*, classified according to the suture or sutures involved. Joints found between the bones of the skull base are cartilaginous, the most important perhaps being the synchondrosis between the sphenoid and occipital bones, which fuses at approximately 18 years of age and allow the forensic physician to attribute an age to a cadaver or isolated bones with a reasonable degree of confidence and window of accuracy.

While the base of the skull and its primary cartilaginous joints separate the neurocranium from the viscerocranium, synovial joints separate the cranium from the mandible and the skull from the cervical spine by way of the temporomandibular and atlanto-occipital joints, respectively.

Frontal view

The upper third of the skull is principally formed by the frontal bones and exaggerated at the superciliary ridges of the superior orbit and smooth glabellar region centrally. The paired maxillary bones form the middle third, creating the circumference of the piriform aperture between them, and are separated from the frontal and temporal bones by the zygoma laterally on each side (Fig. 1.1a). They house the maxillary sinuses and meet in the midline inferiorly to form the upper jaw and most of the hard palate at the intermaxillary suture. The mandible forms the lower third of the frontal view (Fig. 1.1b).

Key features

Supraorbital foramen
- May be a notch or a foramen in the frontal bone. Lies above the orbit at the junction of the medial and lateral two-thirds of the superior orbital rim.
- Transmits the supraorbital nerve (V_1) and supraorbital artery from the ophthalmic artery.

Optic canal
- Bound by the lesser wing of the sphenoid bone.
- Transmits the optic nerve and ophthalmic artery (from ICA).

Superior orbital fissure
- Between the greater and lesser wings of the sphenoid.
- Transmits the oculomotor, trochlear, and abducens nerves, the ophthalmic division of the trigeminal nerve (V_1), and the superior and inferior ophthalmic veins.

Inferior orbital fissure
- Bound by the greater wing of the sphenoid, the maxilla, and the orbital process of the palatine bone.
- Transmits the maxillary division of the trigeminal nerve (V_2), the infraorbital vessels, and the zygomatic nerve.

Zygomaticofacial foramen
- Malar part of the zygomatic bone (malar meaning 'cheek'—the most prominent part).
- Transmits the zygomaticofacial nerve of V_2

Infraorbital foramen
- Found 7 mm below the inferior orbital rim of the maxilla, approximately in the mid-pupillary line.
- Transmits the infraorbital (V_2) nerve and vessels.

Mental foramen
- Located between the first and second premolars, midway between the upper and lower mandibular border.
- Transmits the mental nerve and vessels, which are continuations of the inferior alveolar neurovascular bundle.

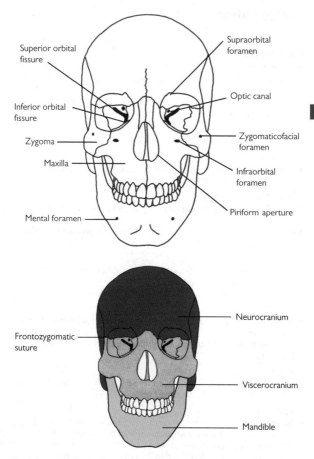

Fig. 1.1 (a) Skull, frontal view. (b) Neurocranium, viscerocranium, and mandible, frontal view.

Reproduced courtesy of Daniel R. van Gijn.

Lateral view

See Fig. 1.2.

Key features

Temporal fossa
- Lies between the temporal line and zygomatic arch. Filled by the temporalis muscle.
- Communicates with the infratemporal fossa via the space between the zygoma and skull.

Infratemporal fossa
- The irregular space posterior to the maxilla.

Zygomatic arch
- Formed by the temporal process of the zygomatic bone and the zygomatic process of the temporal bone.

External acoustic meatus
- The elliptical opening circumscribed by the tympanic part of the temporal bone.
- Communicates with the auricle *in vivo* by the cartilaginous part of the external acoustic meatus.

Mastoid process
- Inferior projection of the temporal bone, posterior to the external acoustic meatus.
- Attachment of sternocleidomastoid (SCM) muscle.

Styloid process
- A slender anteroinferior projection of the temporal bone, deep to the plane of the mastoid process.
- Has several important anatomical relationships and muscular and ligamentous attachments.

Pterion
- Confluence of temporal, parietal, sphenoid, and frontal bones (Fig. 1.2a).
- Landmark for the middle meningeal vessels.

Temporal lines
- Superior and inferior arches traversing the parietal bone between the supramastoid crest and zygomatic process of the frontal bone.
- Temporalis fascia is attached to the superior temporal line and the upper limit of temporalis muscle to the inferior temporal line.

Supramastoid crest
- Extension of the posterior root of the zygomatic arch above the external acoustic meatus.
- Marks the common origin of the superior and inferior temporal lines.

Suprameatal triangle
- Lies between the posterosuperior edge of the external acoustic meatus and the root of the zygomatic arch.
- Marks the site of the mastoid antrum.

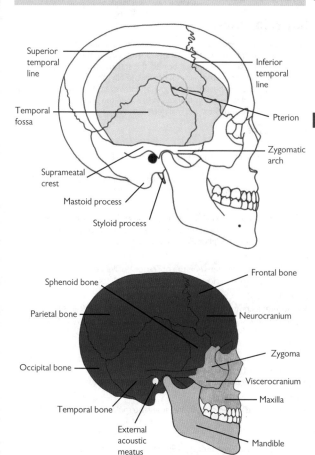

Fig. 1.2 (a) Skull, lateral view. (b) Neurocranium, viscerocranium, and mandible, lateral view.

Reproduced courtesy of Daniel R. van Gijn.

Superior view

Ordinarily ovoid, wider posteriorly than anteriorly, and maximally broad at the parietal eminences. When viewed from above, the skull provides a deceptively simple view of four bones: the squamous part of the frontal bone anteriorly, the paired parietal bones laterally, and the squamous part of the occipital bone posteriorly (Fig. 1.3). However, the activity occurring at their boundaries results in marked variation in the size and shape of the skull along a spectrum from normality to pathology.

Key features

Sagittal suture
- Runs in the midline, connecting the two parietal bones and links the bregma to the lambda.
- The sagittal suture and the anterior fontanelle and lambda posteriorly resemble an arrow, hence its name.

Coronal suture
- The articulation between the frontal bone and paired parietal bones.
- The lateral extents are at the pterion, where the coronal suture meets the greater wing of sphenoid and the squamous temporal bone.

Lambdoidal suture
- Marks the junction between the posterior borders of the parietal bones and the antero-superior border of the occipital bone.

Bregma
- The intersection of the coronal and sagittal sutures indicates the position of the anterior fontanelle of the fetus and neonate, at the head of the '*sagitta*' or arrow.

Lambda
- Represents the position of the posterior fontanelle; usually closes 2 to 3 months after birth.
- At the intersection of the sagittal and lambdoidal sutures.

Vertex
- Highest point of the skull, found along the middle third of the sagittal suture.

Temporal lines
- Superior and inferior temporal lines to which the temporalis fascia and temporalis muscle, respectively, are attached.
- Clearer on the lateral view, an extension of the supramastoid crest.

Parietal foramina
- Situated a few centimetres in front of the lambda, the parietal foramina on either side of the sagittal suture transmit emissary veins between the superior sagittal sinus and veins of the scalp.

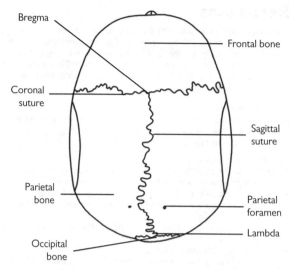

Fig. 1.3 Skull, superior view.
Reproduced courtesy of Daniel R. van Gijn.

Etymology

- *Pterion*—from the Greek *pteron* meaning 'wing'; in the context of the positioning of the winged helmet of Hermes, provides one charming explanation for the origin of the word. Pterodactyl and pterygoid ('wing-like') are other examples with a common stem.
- *Sagittal*—meaning 'shaped like an arrow' from the modern Latin *sagitta* (arrow). The mythological centaur archer of the constellation Sagittarius also derives his name from the same prefix.
- *Bregma*—meaning top or front part of the head.
- *Lambda*—referring to the shape of the Greek letter of that name.
- *Styloid*—from the Greek meaning 'pillar' (consider also stylus).
- *Mastoid*—resembling a female breast, from the Greek *mastoeides* (consider also mastectomy).

Frontal bone

The frontal bone is the cockleshell-shaped expanse of bone contributing to the anterior part of the anterior cranial fossa, the anterior parts of the temporal fossae bilaterally, and the roofs of the orbits inferiorly (Fig. 1.4). The horizontal orbital plates are interrupted by the U-shaped ethmoidal notch. The frontal bone is traditionally considered according to its squamous, orbital, and nasal parts (Fig. 1.5b).

Squamous part

Represents the main smooth convex external surface of the frontal bone, covered by frontalis, and a concave internal surface bearing impressions for the gyri of the frontal lobes and grooves that house the meningeal vessels.

Features

- *Metopic suture*—an occasional persistent suture between the two embryological components of the frontal bone (Fig. 1.6).
- *Superciliary ridges*—the arching elevations between the frontal eminences superiorly and supraorbital margins inferiorly. Converge at the glabella (Fig. 1.5a).
- *Glabella*—the smooth midline communication between the superciliary ridges.
- *Supraorbital notch/foramen*—lies above the superior rim of the orbit at junction of its medial and lateral two-thirds. Transmits the supraorbital neurovascular bundle.
- *Frontal eminence (boss)*—most convex part of the frontal bone, lying approximately 4 cm above the lateral margins of the superciliary ridges.
- *Zygomatic process*—lateral extent of the supraorbital rim, articulating with the frontal process of the zygomatic bone.
- *Temporal line*—posterosuperiorly arching line from the zygomatic process, which divides into the superior and inferior temporal lines and continues across the parietal bone.
- *Sagittal sulcus*—midline groove on the internal surface which houses the anterior part of the superior sagittal sinus.
- *Frontal crest*—the inferior convergence of the sagittal sulcus. Gives attachment to the falx cerebri (with the sulcus and posterior crista galli).
- *Foramen caecum*—a blind-ending foramen, formed by articulation between the lower end of the frontal crest notch and the ethmoid bone.

Nasal part

The serrated area between the supraorbital margins inferior to the level of the zygomatic arch, converging as the midline nasal spine.

Features

- *Nasion*—at the frontonasal suture (the point of intersection between the frontal and nasal bones).
- *Nasal notch*—articulates with the nasal and lacrimal bones and the frontal process of the maxilla.
- *Nasal spine*—the triangular central extension of the nasal notch, articulates with the perpendicular plate of the ethmoid posteriorly and the nasal bones anteriorly. Its grooved surfaces contribute to the roof of the left and right nasal cavities.

Orbital part

The orbital plates are two smooth, horizontal, triangular concavities separated by the ethmoidal notch. They form the majority of the roof of each orbit inferiorly and the floor of the anterior cranial fossa superiorly.

Features

- *Trochlear fovea*—site of attachment of the fibrocartilaginous trochlea (pulley) that acutely changes the direction and pull of the superior oblique muscle.
- *Lacrimal fossa*—anterolateral depression housing the orbital part of the lacrimal gland.
- *Frontal sinuses*—large triangular-shaped sinuses extending superolaterally and deep to the superciliary ridges. Variable in shape and separated from one another by an off-centre bony septum.
- *Supraorbital margin*—provides attachment for the orbital septum which suspends the superior tarsal plate.

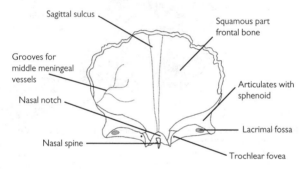

Fig. 1.4 Frontal bone, internal aspect.

Reproduced courtesy of Daniel R. van Gijn.

Superciliary ridges

The superciliary ridge was particularly prominent in the species *Homo neanderthalensis* of which La Chapelle-aux-Saints (the 'Old Man') is an impressive example.

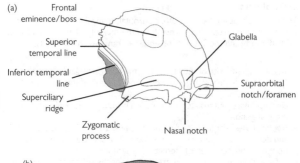

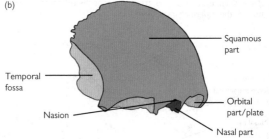

Fig. 1.5 (a) Features of the frontal bone, right anterolateral view. (b) Parts of the frontal bone, right anterolateral view.

Reproduced courtesy of Daniel R. van Gijn.

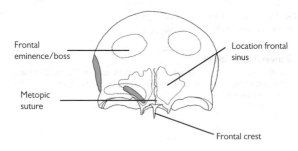

Fig. 1.6 Features of the frontal bone.

Reproduced courtesy of Daniel R. van Gijn.

Frontal bone fracture and frontal sinus involvement

It takes considerable force to fracture the frontal bone and injury is therefore often associated with additional maxillofacial fractures. The proportion of frontal bone occupied by frontal sinus means that this structure is at risk in injuries involving this area. The following structures must also be assessed with a high index of suspicion for injury given their proximity to the zone of injury:

- *Supraorbital nerve*—forehead paraesthesia.
- *Frontal lobes of brain* and associated dura—altered Glasgow Coma Scale score and cerebrospinal fluid (CSF) rhinorrhoea.
- *Superior sagittal sinus*—altered Glasgow Coma Scale score and increased intracranial pressure.
- *Frontonasal duct*—outflow tract between frontal sinus and ethmoid sinus/nasal cavity. Difficult to exclude; usually presents months later with mucocele or mucopyocele.
- *Orbital roof and orbit*—proptosis, abnormal extraocular muscle function, damage to globe.

Frontal sinus fractures can be classified according to the extent of the injury, which will guide the subsequent management options:

- Anterior wall.
- Posterior wall.
- Involvement of frontal recess ± frontonasal duct.

The management principles are essentially to render the sinus 'safe', restore cosmesis, and prevent complications. The treatment options range from observation to obliteration or cranialization of the frontal sinus with autologous abdominal fat.

Percivall Pott and his puffy tumour

Sir Percivall Pott was an eighteenth-century English surgeon synonymous with the foundation of 'orthopedy'. Integral in recognizing the role of environmental pathogens in carcinogenesis, Pott's name is also ascribed to and associated with the following maladies:

- *Pott's spine*—arthritic tuberculosis of the spine.
- *Pott's puffy tumour*—frontal bone osteomyelitis with associated subperiosteal abscess secondary to frontal trauma, sinusitis, or iatrogenic causes. Presents as a swelling of the forehead. May result in cortical venous thrombosis via communicating diploic veins.
- *Squamous cell carcinoma of the scrotum*—Pott recognized the higher incidence in chimney sweeps; first occupational link to cancer.

Sir Harold Delf Gillies (1882–1960)

A New Zealand-born, London-based surgeon considered as the father of modern plastic surgeon due to his pioneering work on injured servicemen during the First World War, at Queen Mary's Hospital, Sidcup, England. In the context of the zygoma, the *Gillies lift* is a 'closed' technique used to elevate the zygomatic arch via an incision placed in the temporal hairline and through the superficial temporal fascia and temporalis muscle fascia. An instrument is then passed inferiorly (taking advantage of the insertion of temporalis onto the coronoid process) beyond and deep to the zygomatic arch where it can be elevated. This dissection plane avoids injury to the temporal branch of the facial nerve.

Zygomatic bone

The paired zygomatic bones, forming most of the skeleton of the cheeks and the lateral walls of the orbits, have important articulations that are key to understanding the assessment and management of a patient with facial trauma. Each zygomatic bone has facial (lateral), orbital and temporal surfaces, which have respective projections, features, and articulations (Fig. 1.7a).

Lateral (facial) surface

Convex, producing the prominence of the cheek, and covered from superficial to deep by the zygomatic muscles and fibres of orbicularis oculi. Displays four borders: anterior superior, anterior inferior, posterior superior, and posterior inferior (Fig. 1.7b).

Features
- *Frontal process*—the thick vertical projection that articulates with the zygomatic process of the frontal bone superiorly.
- *Temporal process*—extends backwards and articulates with the zygomatic process of the temporal bone.
- *Infraorbital process*—a triangular projection along the infraorbital margin providing attachment for levator labii superioris.
- *Zygomaticofacial foramen*—pierces the lateral surface and may be single, double, or absent; transmits the vessels and nerves of the same name.
- *Oblique ridge*—a faint line below the zygomaticofacial foramen providing attachment for zygomaticus minor anteriorly and zygomaticus major posteriorly.
- *Anterior superior border*—inferolateral margin of the orbit.
- *Anterior inferior border*—articulates with the maxilla.
- *Posterior superior border*—forms a defined sinusoidal border continuous with the zygomatic process of the frontal bone and the superior border of the arch proper. The temporalis fascia is attached along its length.
- *Posterior inferior border*—inferior edge of the zygomatic arch proper. Serves as attachment for masseter muscle.

Orbital surface

The concave, smooth surface of the zygomatic bone that contributes to the lateral wall and inferior rim of each orbit (Fig. 1.8).

Features
- *Zygomatico-orbital foramen*—leads to a Y-shaped canal that traverses the zygomatic bone from its orbital to its facial and temporal surfaces and carries the zygomaticofacial and zygomaticotemporal neurovascular bundles via its superior and inferior arms, respectively.
- *Whitnall's tubercle*—found approximately 1 cm inferior to the zygomaticofrontal suture. Gives attachment to the lateral palpebral ligament, the check ligament of lateral rectus, Lockwood's ligament, and the aponeurosis of levator palpebrae superioris.
- *Infraorbital process*.
- *Orbital process*—the serrated posterior edge which articulates with the greater wing of the sphenoid.

Temporal surface

Features

Represents the posterior aspect of the orbital surface. The posteromedial border articulates with the greater wing of the sphenoid bone.

- Deeply concave and contributes to the formation of the anterior wall of the temporal fossa and (partial) lateral wall of the infratemporal fossa.
- Anteriorly, articulates with the zygomatic process of the maxillary bone. Pierced by the zygomaticotemporal foramen near the base of the frontal process (Fig. 1.8).
- *Posteromedial border*—articulates with the lateral border of the orbital surface of the greater wing of the sphenoid and the maxilla inferiorly. Occasionally interrupted by a notch accommodating the lateral extent of the inferior orbital fissure.

Zygomatic fracture

The zygomatic complex forms one of the major buttresses of the face and gives the cheek its prominence. The arch of the zygoma may be fractured in isolation, with trismus (coronoid and temporalis muscle impingement) and deformity but preservation at its articulations, or as a complex, involving one or more of its articulations resulting in respective palpable steps among other symptoms:

- Zygomaticofrontal/sphenozygomatic sutures (frontal process).
- Zygomaticomaxillary suture (infraorbital process).
- Zygomaticotemporal (temporal process) suture.

Additional structures at risk

- *Infraorbital nerve*—cheek and upper lip paraesthesia.
- Superior and lateral walls of the maxillary sinus—epistaxis and blood in the sinus on imaging.
- *Lateral palpebral ligament*—Whitnall's tubercle may be displaced inferiorly giving rise to a downward palpebral slant.
- *Lockwood's suspensory ligament*—combined with the above-mentioned mechanism may result in displacement of the globe (hypoglobus) and orbital contents.
- Extraocular muscle dysfunction—causing diplopia.

Surgical treatment

The aims of surgical management are to examine the zygomatic complex and its respective articulations, restore alignment, and prevent/improve complications. Broadly speaking, surgical management may be open or closed and involve one to three/four-point fixation with or without the need to address the orbital floor, via the lower eyelid, maxillary vestibule, superolateral orbital rim, or existing lacerations.

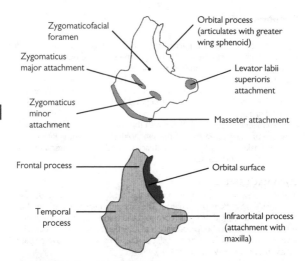

Fig. 1.7 (a) Parts of the right zygomatic bone, lateral view. (b) Right zygomatic bone, external/facial surface.
Reproduced courtesy of Daniel R. van Gijn.

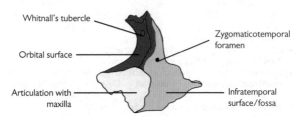

Fig. 1.8 Right zygomatic bone, medial surface.
Reproduced courtesy of Daniel R. van Gijn.

Occipital bone

A large, unpaired bone with a concave internal surface that forms much of the posterior cranial fossa and a convex external surface that articulates with the first cervical vertebra (atlas) via the occipital condyles. Its distinguishing feature is the large ovoid foramen magnum, which transmits the medulla oblongata and meninges, vertebral and spinal vessels, and the spinal accessory nerves. Like the midpoint on the face of a compass, it divides the occipital bone into four parts: paired condylar (lateral/west and east), basilar (anterior/north), and squamous (posterior/south) parts (Fig. 1.9a).

Lateral part

The lateral parts of the occipital bone are the anterolateral projections either side of the foramen magnum, which consist of the condylar part proper and jugular processes (Fig. 1.9b).

External surface features

- *Occipital condyles*—convex kidney-shaped processes separated by the foramen magnum. Articulate with the superior facets of the atlas inferiorly via their hyaline cartilage-covered surfaces.
- *Hypoglossal canal*—obliquely pierces the base of each condylar process; transmits the hypoglossal nerve and the meningeal branch of the ascending pharyngeal artery.
- *Condyloid fossa* (and canal)—receives the posterior aspect of the superior facet of the atlas when the neck is extended. A canal occasionally appears at its base and allows communication between the sigmoid sinus and a suboccipital venous plexus.
- *Jugular process*—the quadrilateral part lateral to the condyles.
- *Jugular notch*—the anterior free concave border of the jugular process. Forms the posterior aspect of the jugular foramen. Transmits the internal jugular vein (IJV) as a continuation of the sigmoid sinus.

Internal surface features

- *Jugular tubercle*—projects anteromedially from the foramen magnum. There is an oblique groove over the posterior aspect for cranial nerves IX, X, and XI.

Basilar part

The thick area anterior to the foramen magnum. Articulates with the petrous part of the temporal bones laterally and the sphenoid bone at its quadrilateral anterior surface via a primary cartilaginous joint.

External surface features

- *Pharyngeal tubercle*—a midline projection 1 cm anterior to the foramen magnum. The site of attachment of the midline pharyngeal raphe and the apex of the superior pharyngeal constrictor muscle.
- Rectus capitis anterior, longus capitis and the anterior atlanto-occipital membrane are all attached to the basiocciput.

Internal surface features

- *Clivus*—a sloped gutter from the foramen magnum superiorly, proceeding 'uphill' towards the posterior clinoid processes and bridges the basiocciput and sphenoid. The basilar artery, pons, and medulla oblongata lie on the clivus.
- *Groove for inferior petrosal sinus*—superior to the articulation between the petrous temporal bone and basiocciput.

Squamous part

The largest component of the occipital bone, posterior to the foramen magnum. Articulates with the temporal and parietal bones (Fig. 1.9b).

External surface features

- *External occipital protuberance*—approximately midway between the foramen magnum and lambda (the superior angle).
- *Inion*—most prominent point of the external occipital protuberance.
- *Highest nuchal lines*—arch bilaterally from the external occipital protuberance. The galea aponeurotica gains attachment medially and the occipital component of occipitofrontalis laterally.
- *Superior nuchal lines*—the boundary between the scalp and neck; arch bilaterally from the external occipital protuberance (inferior to the highest nuchal line).
- *Median nuchal line*—a ridge running between the lambda and the foramen magnum. Attachment for ligamentum nuchae.
- *Inferior nuchal lines*—arch bilaterally from midpoint of median nuchal line.
- *Planum occipital and nuchale*—part of the squamous occipital bone superior and inferior to the highest nuchal lines, respectively.

Internal surface features

Concave and can be divided into four fossae by the cruciate eminence. The two superior triangular areas house the occipital lobes; the inferior pair accommodate the cerebellar hemispheres (Fig. 1.10).

- *Cruciate eminence*—the horizontal element houses the transverse sinus and provides attachment for the falx cerebelli. The vertical component contains the posterior part of the superior sagittal sinus and provides attachment for the falx cerebri.
- *Internal occipital protuberance*—the point of confluence of the cruciate eminences.
- *Internal occipital crest*—the internal equivalent of the median nuchal line. Runs from the internal occipital protuberance to the foramen magnum.
- *Vermian fossa*—the triangular hollow where the internal occipital crest splays at the posterior margin of the foramen magnum. Houses the vermis of the cerebellum.
- *Torcular herophili*—the confluence of the sinuses. Creates a depression adjacent to the internal occipital protuberance.

Spheno-occipital synchondrosis

The spheno-occipital synchondrosis is a primary cartilaginous joint and growth centre between the sphenoid and occipital bones. It plays a key role in cranial base growth—in particular, the final shape of the cranial base and its relationship with the maxillae and mandible. The development and timing of fusion of the spheno-occipital synchondrosis as an estimate of age for forensic purposes are topics for continuing research..

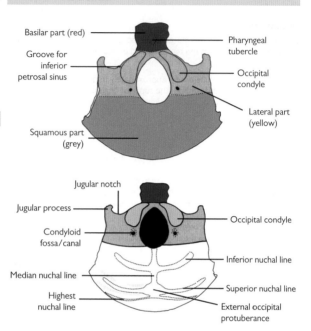

Fig. 1.9 Occipital bone, inferior view.
Reproduced courtesy of Daniel R. van Gijn.

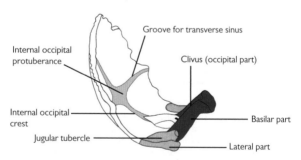

Fig. 1.10 Occipital bone, right lateral/oblique view.
Reproduced courtesy of Daniel R. van Gijn.

Temporal bone

The paired temporal bones at the side of the skull separate the middle from the posterior cranial fossae. Each bone articulates with the greater wing of the sphenoid bone anteriorly, the occipital bone posteriorly, and the parietal bone superiorly. The temporal bone can be described according to its squamous, petrous, mastoid, tympanic, and styloid parts (Fig. 1.11a).

Squamous part

The squamous temporal is thin and translucent (the site of temporal craniotomy): its thickness is compensated for by the temporalis muscle. It consists of a convex external surface that forms the base of the temporal fossa, and a concave internal surface that is divided by the petrous temporal bone into an upper *cerebral* surface and lower *cerebellar* surface. It bears impressions of the gyri of the temporal lobes and grooves that house the anterior and posterior middle meningeal vessels.

External features

- *Groove for middle temporal artery*—runs posterosuperiorly.
- *Supramastoid crest (spine of Henle)*—extension of the posterior root of the zygomatic arch, above the external acoustic meatus (Fig. 1.11b).
- *Suprameatal triangle (MacEwen)*—between the posterior root of the zygomatic process and the posterior wall of the external acoustic meatus. An important landmark in mastoidectomy because the mastoid antrum lies 15–20 mm deep to this point.

Zygomatic process

A thin piece of bone projecting anteriorly from the squama by anterior and posterior bony roots. It articulates with the zygomatic bone via its anterior serrated edge.

- *Anterior root*—broad and continuous with the articular eminence, the anterior boundary of the mandibular fossa.
- *Posterior root*—continuous with the temporal line and supramastoid crest, extending laterally above the external acoustic meatus to blend with the superior border of the zygomatic process.
- *Superior border*—long and fine. Provides attachment for temporalis fascia.
- *Inferior border*—thicker and shorter than the superior part. Gives origin to some fibres of masseter.

Mandibular fossa

- Bound by the articular eminence anteriorly and the postglenoid tubercle posteriorly.
- Divided by Glaser's squamotympanic fissure into an articular surface anterolaterally and a non-articular surface posteromedially.
- Separated by the descending tegmen tympani separates this fissure into petrotympanic and petrosquamous components (Fig. 1.12).
- The canal of Huguier in the medial petrotympanic part transmits the chorda tympani, the anterior ligament of the malleus, and the tympanic branch of the maxillary artery.

Petrous part

The pyramidal petrous part of the temporal bone, between the sphenoid and occipital bones, separates the middle and posterior cranial fossae. It houses the vestibular and auditory apparatus and is traversed by the internal carotid artery (ICA) and facial nerve. It has an pronounced apex and anterior, posterior and inferior surfaces (Fig. 1.13).

Apex

- *Apex*—anteromedial limit of the petrous temporal bone. Angled between the posterior border of the greater wing of the sphenoid and the basilar part of the occipital bone. Contains the anterior opening of the carotid canal. Limits the foramen lacerum posterolaterally
- *Petrosphenoidal* (Gruber's) ligament—runs between the apex and the posterior clinoid process.
- *Sulcus tubae*—groove for the pharyngotympanic (auditory, Eustachian) tube. Between the posterolateral margin of the greater wing of the sphenoid and the petrous temporal bone.

Anterior surface

Forms the posterior border of the middle cranial fossa and is joined to the squamous temporal bone via the petrosquamous suture (Fig. 1.14).
- *Trigeminal impression*—houses the trigeminal ganglion within its dural pouch (Meckel's cave).
- *Arcuate eminence*—central. Upward bulge caused by the underlying superior semicircular canal.
- *Tegmen tympani*—thin plate of bone forming the roof of the mastoid antrum, extending forwards above the tympanic cavity and the canal for tensor tympani. Its anterior edge extends inferiorly as a flange that divides the squamotympanic fissure into the petrosquamous fissure in front and petrotympanic fissure behind.
- *Hiatuses for greater and lesser petrosal nerves*—medial and lateral to the trigeminal impression, respectively.

Posterior surface features

Almost vertical in plane, forming the anterior part of the posterior cranial fossa (Fig. 1.14).
- *Internal acoustic meatus*—transmits the facial and vestibulocochlear nerves and the auditory branch of the basilar artery.
- *Aquaductus vestibule (vestibular aqueduct)*—posterior to the internal acoustic meatus. Contains the endolymphatic duct. Closely related to the posterior and lateral semicircular canals.
- *Subarcuate fossa*—inferior to the arcuate eminence and superoposterior to the internal acoustic meatus. Transmits a small vein and a projection of dura.

Inferior surface

Irregular and wedged between the posterior border of the greater wing of the sphenoid laterally and the basiocciput medially. Forms part of the base of the skull. It contains several important structures, from anterior to posterior these are: (Fig. 1.15):
- *Rough quadrangular surface*—deep to the petrous apex, the site of attachment of levator veli palatini and the pharyngotympanic (Eustachian) tube, which sits in the sulcus tubae. The pharyngotympanic tube is also attached to the posterior border of the greater wing of the sphenoid,

- *Carotid canal*—transmits the ICA (surrounded by a plexus of sympathetic nerves).
- *Cochlear aqueduct*—at the apex of a triangular depression; transmits a vein from the cochlea to the IJV.
- *Jugular fossa*—houses the bulb of the IJV.
- *Inferior tympanic canaliculus*—between the carotid canal and jugular fossa; transmits the tympanic branch of IX.
- *Mastoid canaliculus*—one or more foramina on the lateral wall of the jugular fossa that transmit the auricular branch of X.
- *Jugular surface*—quadrangular area posterior to the jugular fossa; articulates with the jugular process of the occipital bone.
- *Vaginal process*—lamina of bone projecting inferiorly from the tympanic plate and jugular surface. Splits to enclose the styloid process. Provides attachment for parotidomasseteric fascia.
- *Styloid process*—prominent downward process of variable length (usually absent in carelessly handled cadaveric skulls). Provides attachment for three muscles and two ligaments (styloglossus, stylopharyngeus, stylohyoid, the stylomandibular ligament and stylohyoid ligaments).
- *Stylomastoid foramen*—between the styloid and mastoid processes; transmits VII at the start of its extracranial course.
- *Tympanomastoid fissure*—fissure between the mastoid process and tympanic part; transmits the auricular branch of X.

Eagle's syndrome

Watt Weems Eagle (1898–1980)—American otolaryngologist

Eagle's syndrome is an array of signs and symptoms arising as a result of either an elongated styloid process or a calcified stylohyoid ligament (calcification may extend along its entire length). Symptoms arise as a result of compression from adjacent structures:

- Otalgia.
- Dysphagia.
- Tinnitus.
- Unilateral facial pain.

Compression of the ICA may result in dissection and subsequent transient ischaemic attack or stroke.

Johan Glaser (1629–1675) Swiss anatomist.

Pierre Charles Huguier (1804–1873) French surgeon and gynaecologist. Known predominantly for his work on genitourinary disease.

Friedrich Gustav Jacob Henle (1809–1885) German anatomist and pathologist. Several eponymous structures, including the loop of Henle.

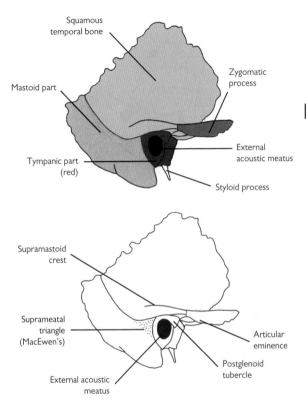

Fig. 1.11 (a) Right temporal bone parts, lateral view. (b)Right temporal bone features, lateral view.

Reproduced courtesy of Daniel R. van Gijn.

Mastoid part

Situated most posteriorly. Has an external and internal surface and superior and posterior borders. It articulates superiorly with the mastoid or posteroinferior angle of the parietal bone and posteriorly with the occipital bone. Evidence of the squamomastoid suture can occasionally be seen inferior to the squamomastoid crest and posterior to the suprameatal triangle.

External surface

- *Mastoid foramen/canal*—the largest of numerous foramina perforating the outer surface. Transmits a vein to the transverse sinus and a small branch of the occipital artery that supplied the dura mater (Fig. 1.15).
- *Mastoid process*—variable in size but palpable. Muscles attached (from above downwards) are SCM, splenius capitis, and longissimus capitis.

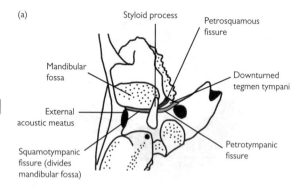

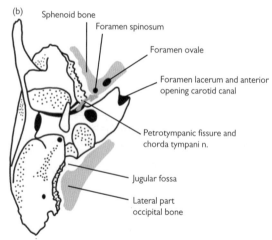

Fig. 1.12 (a) The mandibular fossa and squamotympanic fissure, inferior view of temporal bone. (b) The relations of the right temporal bone, inferior view.
Reproduced courtesy of Daniel R. van Gijn.

- *Mastoid (digastric) notch*—on the medial aspect of the mastoid process. Posterior belly of digastric is attached.
- *Occipital groove*—medial to the mastoid notch, occupied by the occipital artery.

Internal surface

- *Sigmoid sulcus*—a prominent S-shaped groove *en route* to the jugular fossa and continuous with corresponding grooves on the petrous temporal and occipital bones.

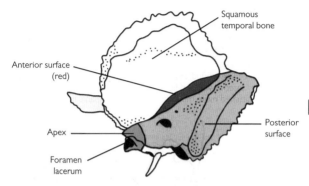

Fig. 1.13 The petrous part of the right temporal bone, internal view.
Reproduced courtesy of Daniel R. van Gijn.

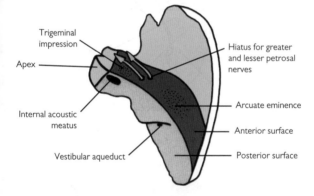

Fig. 1.14 Right petrous temporal bone, superior view.
Reproduced courtesy of Daniel R. van Gijn.

Tympanic part

A thin plate of bone furled firmly between the squamous part anteriorly and mastoid part posteriorly. Contains the external acoustic meatus, and has anterior and posterior surfaces and superior, inferior, and lateral borders. It is separated from the mastoid part posteriorly by the tympanomastoid fissure and from the squamous part anterosuperiorly by the squamotympanic fissure. Its inferior process is a thin descending bony projection that splits to engulf the styloid as the vaginal process. Its free lateral border is rough and provides attachment for the cartilaginous part of the external acoustic meatus (Fig. 1.16).

Anterior surface
- Smooth and quadrilateral, forming the posterior element of the mandibular fossa.
- Intimately related to the parotid gland.

Posterior surface
- U-shaped, curling around and inferior to the external acoustic meatus, forming its anterior wall and floor, and part of its posterior wall.
- A groove situated more medially houses the tympanic membrane.

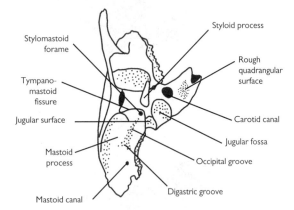

Styloid process

Stylomastoid forame

Tympano-mastoid fissure

Rough quadrangular surface

Jugular surface

Carotid canal

Mastoid process

Jugular fossa

Occipital groove

Mastoid canal

Digastric groove

Fig. 1.15 The right temporal bone, inferior view.
Reproduced courtesy of Daniel R. van Gijn.

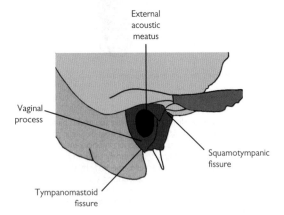

External acoustic meatus

Vaginal process

Squamotympanic fissure

Tympanomastoid fissure

Fig. 1.16 Right tympanic part (red) of the temporal bone, lateral view.
Reproduced courtesy of Daniel R. van Gijn.

Parietal bone

The paired parietal bones are irregularly quadrilateral in shape and form the mainstay of the roof and sides of the cranial vault. Each has an external convex and internal concave surface, four borders and four angles (or corners) (Fig. 1.17).

External surface

Features
- *Parietal tuber*—prominent convexity above the temporal lines indicating the centre of ossification.
- *Temporal lines*—paired superior and inferior arching lines to which the temporal fascia and temporalis muscle, respectively are attached.
- *Parietal foramen*—situated posteriorly, close to the sagittal border. Inconsistent in presence and size. When present, transmits an emissary vein to the superior sagittal sinus.

Internal surface

Features
- *Surface impressions*—multiple grooves corresponding to the cerebral gyri and housing branches of the middle meningeal vessels (Fig. 1.18).
- *Groove for transverse sinus*—inner surface of the posteroinferior or mastoid angle.
- *Sagittal sulcus*—a groove near the superior border. When paired with its contralateral fellow, houses the superior sagittal sinus and provides attachment for the falx cerebri.
- *Granular foveolae*—depressions, more numerous in the elderly skull, that house arachnoid granulations.

Borders and angles
- *Frontal border*—serrated, bevelled, and articulates with the frontal bone to form one-half of the coronal suture.
- *Sagittal border*—articulates with the contralateral parietal bone at the sagittal suture.
- *Inferior border*—articulates with (from anterior to posterior) the greater wing of the sphenoid, the squamous temporal bone, and the mastoid part of the temporal bone.
- *Occipital border*—articulates with the occipital bone, forming one-half of the lambdoidal suture.
- *Anterosuperior angle*—approximately 90° at the bregma, where the sagittal and coronal sutures meet, marking the site of the anterior fontanelle in the neonatal skull
- *Anteroinferior angle*—acute and wedged between the frontal bone and the greater wing of the sphenoid.
- *Posterosuperior angle*—meeting of the sagittal and lambdoid sutures, which marks the site of the posterior fontanelle in the neonatal skull.
- *Posteroinferior (mastoid) angle*—articulates with the occipital bone and mastoid part of the temporal bone at the asterion.

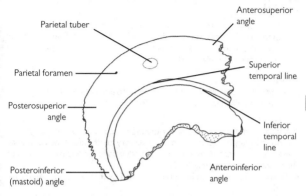

Fig. 1.17 The parietal bone, lateral (external) view.
Reproduced courtesy of Daniel R. van Gijn.

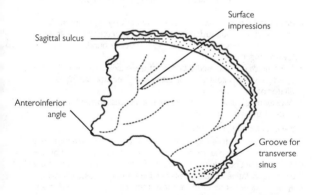

Fig. 1.18 The right parietal bone, internal view.
Reproduced courtesy of Daniel R. van Gijn.

Maxilla

The paired maxillae are the pneumatized pyramidal bones of the midface and upper jaw. Each has a body and alveolar, palatine, frontal, and zygomatic processes that contribute to the formation of the oral, nasal, and orbital cavities, respectively (Fig. 1.19).

Body

The body of the maxilla contains the maxillary paranasal sinus (of Highmore) and can be subdivided according to its four surfaces:

Anterior surface

A broad surface made concave by the zygomatic process, extending from the orbital margin superiorly to the maxillary teeth inferiorly. Its inferior border is characterized by a number of undulations formed by the roots of the maxillary dentition (Fig. 1.20).

- *Canine eminence*—prominent bulge formed by the root of the maxillary canine.
- *Incisive fossa*—lies medial to the canine eminence. Provides attachment for depressor septi, orbicularis oris, and nasalis.
- *Canine fossa*—lies lateral to the canine eminence. Provides attachment for levator anguli oris.
- *Infraorbital foramen*—extends posterosuperiorly as the infraorbital canal, grooving the orbital surface of the maxilla *en route* to the inferior orbital fissure. Transmits the infraorbital neurovascular bundle. Superior to levator anguli oris.
- *Nasal notch*—at the medial border of the maxilla. Forms the piriform aperture with its contralateral fellow and gives attachment to dilator nares.
- *Anterior nasal spine*—prominent midline process formed by the inferior ends of the nasal notches.

Posterior (infratemporal) surface

Smooth convex surface separated from the anterior surface by a bony ridge between the first molar tooth and the root of the zygomatic process, except for its continuity with the alveolar process. Forms the anterior wall of the pterygopalatine fossa medially and infratemporal fossa laterally.

- *Alveolar canals*—one or more canals transmitting the posterior superior alveolar neurovascular bundles.
- *Maxillary tuberosity*—the rounded most inferior border of the posterior surface, palpable with a finger hooked behind the last maxillary molar. It articulates with the pyramidal process of the palatine bone, forming the inferior aspect of the pterygomaxillary fissure.

Superior (orbital) surface

The orbital surface of the maxilla is smooth, almost flat, and forms the majority of the orbital floor. It articulates with the zygomatic bone laterally and with the lacrimal bone, orbital plate of the ethmoid bone, and orbital process of the palatine bone medially.

- *Lacrimal notch*—scalloped edge on the anteromedial border which articulates with the lacrimal bone, thereby completing the notch. The inferior oblique muscle originates in close proximity.
- *Lacrimal groove*—begins on the medial (orbital) surface of the frontal process and descends vertically on the nasal surface.

- *Posterior border*—free edge that helps to form the inferior orbital fissure; notched in the centre for the infraorbital groove.
- *Anterior border*—forms part of the orbital rim. Slopes superomedially, becoming the frontal process of the maxilla.

Medial (nasal) surface

Forms the lateral wall of the nasal cavity and dominated by a large opening into the maxillary antrum. This aperture is encroached upon and reduced in size in the articulated skull by the perpendicular plate of the palatine bone posteriorly; the inferior nasal concha inferiorly; and the uncinate process of the ethmoid and the lacrimal bone superiorly (Fig. 1.21 and Fig. 1.22). Anterior and inferior to the opening of the maxillary sinus, the nasal surface is smooth and forms the wall of the inferior meatus. Two grooves on the nasal surface contribute to the formation of the nasolacrimal and greater palatine canals:

- *Lacrimal groove*—anterior to the hiatus. Converted into the nasolacrimal canal by the lacrimal bone superiorly and the inferior nasal concha inferiorly. Opens into the inferior meatus.
- *Greater palatine canal*—formed by a groove on the rough surface posterior to the maxillary hiatus and a corresponding groove on the articulating perpendicular plate of the palatine bone. Transmits the greater and lesser palatine neurovascular bundles.
- *Conchal crest*—a curved ridge anterior to the lacrimal groove that articulates with the inferior concha.

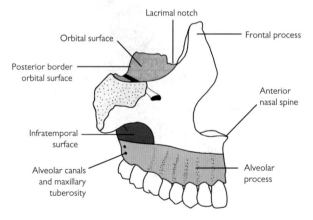

Fig. 1.19 Right maxilla surfaces and features, oblique view.
Reproduced courtesy of Daniel R. van Gijn.

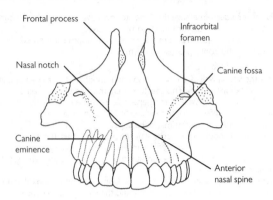

Fig. 1.20 The paired maxillae, anterior view.
Reproduced courtesy of Daniel R. van Gijn.

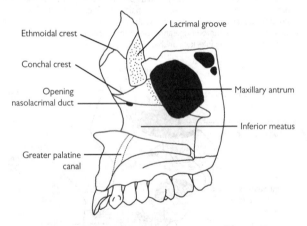

Fig. 1.21 The right maxilla, medial surface.
Reproduced courtesy of Daniel R. van Gijn.

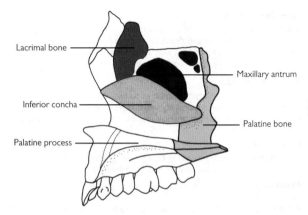

Fig. 1.22 The right maxilla and lacrimal, inferior concha, and palatine bones, medial view.

Reproduced courtesy of Daniel R. van Gijn.

Zygomatic process

The convergence point of the anterior, infratemporal, and orbital surfaces of the body. It has a rough, inverted triangular process that articulates with the zygomatic bone, indirectly connecting the maxilla to the temporal and frontal bones. Anteriorly it forms part of the anterior surface, posteriorly its concavity forms the anterior wall of the infratemporal fossa.

Frontal process

The prominent, strong upwards projection of the maxilla articulates with the lacrimal bone laterally, the nasal bone medially, and the nasal part of the frontal bone superiorly.

Medial wall

Forms part of the lateral wall of the nasal cavity between a rough area superiorly (articulating with the ethmoid bone) and the conchal crest inferiorly.

- *Ethmoidal crest*—oblique ridge articulating with the middle nasal concha at its posterior limit.

Lateral wall

Divided into an anterior and a posterior surface by the anterior lacrimal crest. Orbicularis oculi and levator labii superioris alaeque nasi are attached to the anterior surface.

- *Anterior lacrimal crest*—attachment for medial palpebral ligament and lacrimal fascia.
- *Lacrimal fossa*—formed by the lacrimal groove posterior to the anterior lacrimal crest and a corresponding groove on the lacrimal bone.

Alveolar process

The thick alveolar process of each maxilla contains up to eight alveoli or 'troughs' of variable size and depth for the maxillary teeth. Wider posteriorly, forming an arcade with the alveolar process of the contralateral maxilla. Buccinator overlies the alveolar process of the molar teeth.

Palatine process

A thick horizontal shelf that contributes to two-thirds of the hard palate. Forms the floor of the nasal cavity when articulated with its contralateral fellow. Consists of superior, medial, and inferior surfaces and medial and posterior borders.

Superior surface

Smooth and concave transversely. Forms most of the nasal floor.
• *Incisive canal*—lies anteriorly, near its median margin.

Medial border

Thicker anteriorly.
• *Nasal crest*—raised ridge, articulates with its contralateral fellow to form a groove for the vomer.

Inferior surface

Markedly concave, extensively pitted by the overlying mucoperiosteum and perforated by the foramina of nutrient vessels. Grooved on its posterolateral aspect by the nasopalatine neurovascular bundle *en route* to the incisive fossa (Fig. 1.23).
• *Incisive fossa*—conical midline opening between the two maxillae, posterior to the central incisors.
• *Incisive canals*—four canals found open in the incisive fossa (Fig. 1.24)
  • Two lateral (foramina of Stenson). Transmit the descending palatine artery and nasopalatine nerve.
  • Two midline (foramina of Scarpa). When present, they transmit the nasopalatine nerves.
• *Premaxilla*—the part of the hard palate anterior to a line running between the lateral incisor/canine space through the incisive fossa. Contains the incisor teeth and includes the anterior nasal spine.

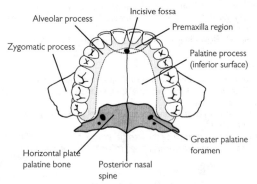

Fig. 1.23 The paired maxillae and paired palatine bones (yellow), inferior view.
Reproduced courtesy of Daniel R. van Gijn.

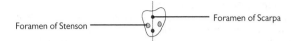

Fig. 1.24 Close-up view of the incisive fossa demonstrating the incisive canals.
Reproduced courtesy of Daniel R. van Gijn.

Maxillary fractures and a brief history of Rene Le Fort (1869–1951)

Introduction

The French surgeon Rene Le Fort is perhaps best known for his treatise 'Etude expérimentale sur les fractures de la mâchoire supérieure '(1901), which records the results of the delivery of (blunt) forces of varying magnitudes and direction to cadaveric heads in an attempt to identify predictable patterns of midface fractures (Fig. 1.25). Experiments included:

- 'Old person, almost edentulous. The cadaver was supine, with the head protruding over the table and hanging back. The mouth was wide open. A moderate blow with a wooden club fell level on the upper dental arch.'
- 'After decapitation, the head was hurled violently against the rounded edge of a marble table. The first blow did not seem to produce a fracture. After a second blow, one noted a fissure between the nasal orifice and canine fossa.'

There are three levels of maxillary fractures classically described by Le Fort. They may occur bilaterally and rarely occur in isolation. All by definition involve fracture of the pterygoid plates of the sphenoid bone and may be associated with other facial fractures and neurovascular injury. It is important to note that the Le Fort classification referred to blunt trauma, whereas modern, high-velocity injuries to the midface may cause more complicated, comminuted, less predictable patterns.

Le Fort I

Extends from the pterygoid plates through the lateral wall of the maxillary antrum towards the piriform aperture. Also known as a Guerin fracture. Separates the maxillary teeth from the upper face.

Le Fort II

A pyramidal fracture that extends from the pterygoid plates upwards towards the inferior orbital rim and medial orbital floor, then crosses the region of the nasofrontal suture.

Le fort III

Complete craniofacial dysjunction, in which the entire midface is separated from the skull base. The transverse fracture line runs from the pterygoid plates and involves the nasofrontal suture, medial orbital wall, orbital floor, zygomaticofrontal suture and zygomatic arch.

Alphonse Guerin (1816–1895)

'When a violent blow is struck backward on the face, as if one wanted to push in the part of the upper jaw lying below the nostrils, a transverse fracture is produced which passes about one centimetre below the malar bone and extends through the pterygoid processes; the latter processes are always fractured at the level of the lower end of the pterygomaxillary fissure i.e. where they have the least resistance.'

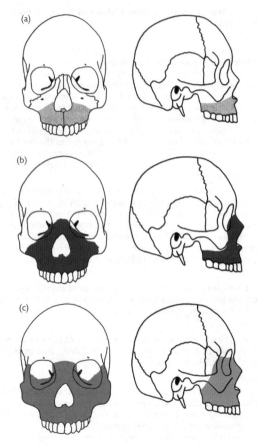

Fig. 1.25 (a) Le Fort I pattern (Guerin type). (b) Le Fort II pattern. (c) Le Fort III pattern (craniofacial dysjunction).

Reproduced courtesy of Daniel R. van Gijn.

Sphenoid bone

The sphenoid bone is a remarkable bone wedged, as its name suggests, between and within the temporal, zygomatic, frontal, parietal, occipital, and ethmoid bones. It forms the greater part of the central cranial base and middle cranial fossae. Wasp-like in appearance, it consists of a body, paired greater and lesser wings, and medial and lateral pterygoid plates, which resemble paired legs.

Body

The body of the sphenoid is approximately cuboidal, six-sided, and pneumatized by the paired sphenoid sinuses (which are interrupted by a septum in the median plane). It articulates anteriorly with the ethmoid and posteriorly with the basilar part of the occiput at the spheno-occipital synchondrosis (Fig. 1.26).

Superior (cerebral) surface (anterior to posterior)
- *Ethmoid spine*—triangular spine between the lesser wings; articulates with the cribriform plate of the ethmoid.
- *Jugum sphenoidale*—smooth, flattened area posterior to the ethmoidal spine on which the olfactory tracts lie.
- *Sulcus chiasmaticus*—transverse groove immediately posterior to the jugum and connecting the optic canals. Houses the optic chiasma.
- *Tuberculum sellae*—posterior extent of the sulcus chiasmaticus. Anterior attachment of the diaphragma sellae.
- *Middle clinoid processes*—at the lateral aspect of the tuberculum sellae. Connected to anterior clinoid process by the carotid clinoid ligaments. The space beneath transmits the cavernous part of ICA.
- *Sella turcica*—deeply concave area between the middle clinoid processes anteriorly and the dorsum sellae posteriorly. Contains the pituitary gland *in vivo*.
- *Dorsum sellae*—square plate of bone forming the posterior wall of the sella turcica. Deepened by the posterior clinoid processes. Provides posterior attachment for the diaphragma sellae. Its posterior sloping surface is continuous with the basiocciput, with which it forms the clivus.
- *Posterior clinoid process*—lateral tubercular projections of the dorsum sellae.
- *Petrosal process*—small process at the lateral margin of the dorsum sellae. Articulates with the apex of the petrous part of the temporal bone.

Lateral surface
Continuous with the greater wings and the medial pterygoid plates, interrupted only by the carotid sulcus.
- *Carotid sulcus*—F-shaped groove housing the internal carotid *en route* through the cavernous sinus.
- *Lingula*—thin lateral margin which helps to deepen the posterior carotid sulcus.

Etymology

- *Sphenoid*—described by Galen and from the Greek meaning 'wedge-like'. There are some who (rather romantically and perhaps optimistically) suggest that the intended and mis-translated origin was from '*sphecoid*' from the Greek *sphex* meaning wasp.

Anterior surface

- *Sphenoidal crest*—midline vertical crest that articulates with the perpendicular plate of the ethmoid and thus contributes to the bony nasal septum.
- *Sphenoidal conchae*—thin, curved plates on either side of the crest, which form part of the roof of the nasal cavity. (Often lost in the disarticulated skull). Their margins articulate with bones of the medial orbit as follows:
  - Inferiorly: a rough triangular lateral surface that articulates with the orbital process of the palatine bone.
  - Superiorly: articulates with the orbital plate of the frontal bone.
  - Laterally: articulates with the lamina papyracea of the ethmoid.
- *Sphenoidal foramen*—an aperture of variable size on the smooth medial aspect of the sphenoidal concha through which the sphenoidal sinus communicates with the sphenoethmoidal recess and upper nasal cavity.

Inferior surface

- *Sphenoidal rostrum*—a triangular spine that is a continuation of the sphenoidal crest. Received by the central groove of the vomer bone.
- *Vaginal process*—inferomedial protrusion from the base of the medial pterygoid plate. Supports the ala of the vomer on its upper surface. This arrangement forms a vomerovaginal canal of no known significance (may contain a branch of the sphenopalatine artery). The palatovaginal canal is a short tunnel between the vaginal process of the sphenoid and the sphenoid process of the palatine bone. It transmits the pharyngeal branches of the maxillary nerve and artery. Connects the nasopharynx and the pterygopalatine fossa.

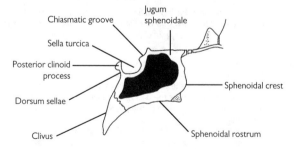

Fig. 1.26 Body of the sphenoid bone, sagittal view.
Reproduced courtesy of Daniel R. van Gijn.

Greater wing

The greater wing of the sphenoid projects laterally and superiorly from the sphenoid body and contributes to both the floor and wall of the middle cranial fossa. Has cerebral, temporal and lateral (temporal) surfaces. Its posterior and squamosal borders converge as a triangular apex between the petrous and squamosal parts of the temporal bone. Inferiorly from this apex the rough downward projecting sphenoid spine (spina angularis) arises (Fig. 1.27 and Fig. 1.28).

Cerebral surface

Concave and forms part of the middle cranial fossa housing the temporal lobes. Its medial border forms the inferior limit of the superior orbital fissure. It is punctuated by the following foramina from anterior to posterior in a laterally concave arc:

- *Foramen rotundum*—connects the middle cranial and pterygopalatine fossae. Transmits V_2.
- *Foramen ovale*—connects the middle cranial and infratemporal fossae. Transmits V_3, the accessory meningeal artery, and the lesser petrosal nerve.
- *Foramen spinosum*—transmits the middle meningeal vessels.
- *Emissary ethmoidal foramen (foramen Vesalii)*—inconsistent, small foramen medial to the foramen ovale. Transmits a vein between the cavernous sinus and the pterygoid venous plexus.

Lateral surface

Externally is divided into a vertical upper temporal and (almost) horizontal lower infratemporal area by the infratemporal crest (Fig. 1.29).

- *Infratemporal crest*—transverse ridge over the lateral surface of the greater wing dividing it into superior or temporal and inferior or infratemporal components.
- *Superior/temporal part*—forms part of temporal fossa; provides attachment for temporalis.
- *Inferior/infratemporal part*—includes the crest and forms the sloping roof of the infratemporal fossa. Continuous with the lateral pterygoid plate. The upper head of the lateral pterygoid muscle is attached to a small triangular process. Perforated from anterior to posterior by the foramen ovale and foramen spinosum along a virtual line connecting the free edge of the lateral pterygoid plate and the spina angularis.

Borders

- *Posterior border*:
  - Forms the anterior boundary of the foramen lacerum medially.
  - Situated at the base of the pterygoid plates, between the foramina ovale and lacerum. Houses the pterygoid canal (transmits the vidian neurovascular bundle *en route* to the pterygopalatine fossa) at its anterior edge.
  - Continues posterolaterally forming a *sulcus tubae* between it and the petrous temporal bone that houses the cartilaginous pharyngotympanic (Eustachian) tube.
- *Squamosal border*:
  - Projects superolaterally from the base of the spina angularis.
  - Articulates with the squamous border of the temporal bone.

- *Superior border:*
  - The squamous border changes direction acutely and runs anteroinferiorly at the sphenoid angle of the parietal bone. It articulates with the frontal bone at the frontosphenoid suture.
- *Anterior border (or lateral border of orbital surface):*
  - Heads inferiorly articulating with the posteromedial border of the zygomatic bone.

Orbital surface

An almost flat, quadrilateral surface, medially inclined so that the two sides partly face one another; the orbital surfaces form the posterior part of the lateral orbital wall. Has four borders (two articular and two free margins), contributes to two fissures, and one tubercle (Fig. 1.30).

- *Superior border*—articulates with the orbital plate of the frontal bone.
- *Lateral border*—articulates with the posteromedial border of the zygomatic bone.
- *Medial border*—forms the inferolateral boundary of the superior orbital fissure; a small tubercle at the junction of the superior two-thirds and inferior one-third provides one point of attachment for the common tendinous ring (anulus of Zinn).
- *Inferior border*—well defined. Forms the posterolateral border of the inferior orbital fissure.

Spina angularis

Found at the apex of the posterior and squamosal borders and arises immediately posterior to the foramen spinosum (Fig. 1.31).

Two nerves, two ligaments, and two other structures

- *Chorda tympani*—grooves the medial aspect after exiting the petrotympanic fissure.
- *Cartilaginous part pharyngotympanic tube*—passes on its medial aspect.
- *Auriculotemporal nerve*—passes on its lateral aspect.
- *Tensor tympani*—*en route* to the handle of the malleus.
- *Tensor veli palatini*—*en route* to the soft palate via the pterygoid hamulus.
- *Sphenomandibular ligament*—between the spine and lingula of the mandibular foramen, limiting mandibular opening.
- *Pterygospinous ligament*—extending from the superior aspect of the posterior border of the lateral pterygoid plate to the spina angularis. This may become ossified, forming a true foramen (of Civinini).

Lesser wing

Slender, triangular, and tapering lateral projection from the body of the sphenoid. Arises from a thin anterior root and thicker posterior root that, together with the body, form the optic foramen (Fig. 1.32).

Superior (upper) surface

Forms part of the floor of the anterior cranial fossa.
- *Anterior border*—articulates with the frontal bone.
- *Posterior border*—sharply defined. Forms the boundary between the anterior and middle cranial fossae and provides cover for the sphenoparietal sinus (*en route* to the cavernous sinus).

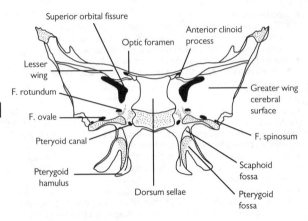

Fig. 1.27 The sphenoid bone, posterior view.
Reproduced courtesy of Daniel R. van Gijn.

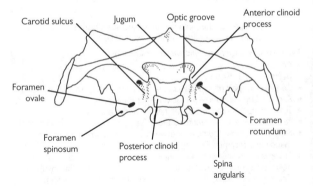

Fig. 1.28 The sphenoid bone, superior view.
Reproduced courtesy of Daniel R. van Gijn.

- *Anterior clinoid process*—medial end of the lesser wing. Provides attachment for the:
  - *Tentorium cerebelli*.
  - *Interclinoid ligament* (between anterior and posterior clinoid).
  - *Carotidoclinoid ligament* (between anterior and middle clinoid).

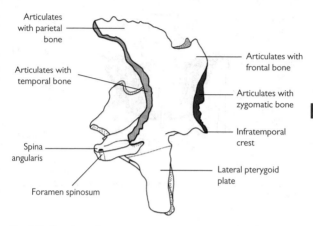

Fig. 1.29 The sphenoid bone, right lateral view.
Reproduced courtesy of Daniel R. van Gijn.

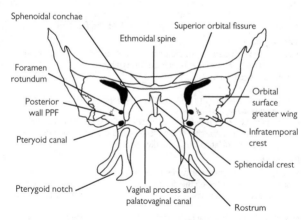

Fig. 1.30 The sphenoid bone, anterior view. PPF, pterygopalatine fossa.
Reproduced courtesy of Daniel R. van Gijn.

Inferior (lower) surface

Overhangs the orbit anteriorly (thus forming its posterior roof) and the middle cranial fossa posteriorly.

- Forms the upper border of the superior orbital fissure.
- Contributes to the attachment of the:
  - *Common tendinous ring*.
  - *Levator palpebrae superioris*.
  - *Superior oblique muscle* on medial aspect.

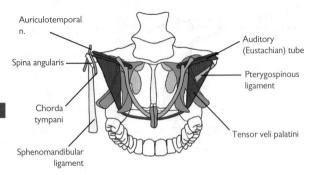

Fig. 1.31 The sphenoid and maxilla—demonstrating spina angularis and relations, posterior view.

Reproduced courtesy of Daniel R. van Gijn.

Pterygoid processes

The pterygoid processes arise from the interval between the body and greater wing of the sphenoid. Consist of a medial and lateral plate, with upper parts which are fused at their apex anteriorly: they diverge as they descend to form their constituent parts (Fig. 1.33 and Fig. 1.34).

Anterior features
- *Root*—broad-based, forms the posterior wall of the pterygopalatine fossa. From lateral to medial, it is perforated by:
  - *Foramen rotundum*.
  - *Pterygoid canal*.
  - *Palatovaginal notch* (forms a canal with the sphenoidal process of the palatine bone).
- *Pterygoid fissure*—the cleft formed between the splayed medial and lateral plates; the margins of the fissure articulate with the pyramidal process of the palatine bone and diverge behind.

Posterior features
- *Pterygoid fossa*—superior to the apex of the pterygoid fissure. A 'V'-shaped hollow between the divergent medial and lateral pterygoid plates. Provides attachment for tensor veli palatini and medial pterygoid muscles.
- *Scaphoid fossa*—an oval hollow formed by the concavity of the medial pterygoid plate superior to the pterygoid fossa. Provides attachment for part of tensor veli palatini.

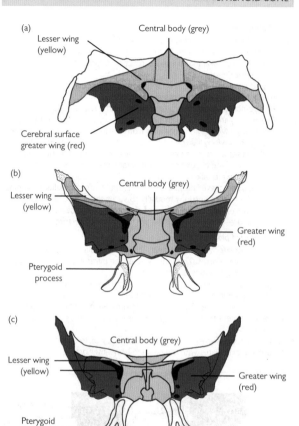

Fig. 1.32 Parts of the sphenoid bone: (a) superior view; (b) posterior view; (c) anterior view.

Reproduced courtesy of Daniel R. van Gijn.

Medial pterygoid plate

Thinner and longer than the lateral pterygoid plate, its inferior end terminates in the hook-like pterygoid hamulus. The pharyngobasilar fascia is attached to its posterior margin and the superior pharyngeal constrictor is attached inferiorly.

- *Pterygoid hamulus*—inferior continuation of the medial pterygoid plate, with the following attachments and features:
  - *Pterygomandibular raphe*—a tendinous band between buccinator (anteriorly) and the superior pharyngeal constrictor (posteriorly), Passes downwards and outwards from the hamulus to the posterior end of the mylohyoid line. When the mouth is opened wide, this raphe raises a fold of mucosa that indicates the internal, posterior boundary of the cheek. It is an important landmark for an inferior alveolar nerve block
  - *Tendon of tensor veli palatini*—travels lateral to the hamulus, wrapping around it to turn abruptly medially towards the soft palate.
- *Lateral surface*—medial boundary of the pterygoid fossa.
- *Medial surface*—lateral wall of the posterior nasal aperture.

Lateral pterygoid plate

Thin and quadrilateral. Diverges away from the medial pterygoid plates.
- *Lateral surface*—forms the medial wall of the infratemporal fossa. The lateral pterygoid muscle is attached to it.
- *Medial surface*—lateral wall of the pterygoid fossa. The deep head of medial pterygoid muscles is attached to it.
- *Posterior border*—free. A tubercle approximately midway along its length gives attachment to a pterygospinous ligament that runs to the spine of the sphenoid.
- *Anterior border*—forms the posterior boundary of the pterygomaxillary fissure and articulates with the palatine bone inferiorly.

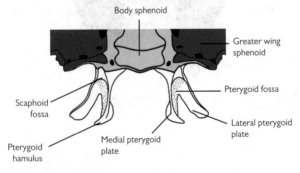

Fig. 1.33 The pterygoid processes, posterior view.
Reproduced courtesy of Daniel R. van Gijn.

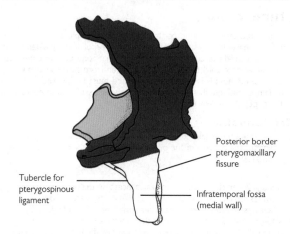

Posterior border
pterygomaxillary
fissure

Tubercle for
pterygospinous
ligament

Infratemporal fossa
(medial wall)

Fig. 1.34 The sphenoid bone, right lateral view.
Reproduced courtesy of Daniel R. van Gijn.

Ethmoid bone

The unpaired ethmoid bone occupies a central 'crumple zone' in the anterior skull base. It consists of four parts, the cribriform and perpendicular plates, and paired lateral masses or labyrinths that contribute to contribute to the anterior cranial fossa, nasal septum, and orbits, respectively (Fig. 1.35). The ethmoid is impressively fragile and must be handled with caution; a finger and thumb in the orbits of a cadaveric skull guarantee fracture of the paper-thin lamina papyracea (Fig. 1.36).

Cribriform plate

Occupies the ethmoidal notch of the frontal bone. Perforated sagittally by foramina for the passage of the olfactory nerves and their associated meninges and CSF.

Features
- *Crista galli*—thick, midline, triangular process on the upper surface; provides attachment for the falx cerebri from its posterior border and articulates with the frontal bone anteriorly (Fig. 1.36 and Fig. 1.37).
- *Alae*—two small projections from the shorter anterior border of the crista galli that form the posterior boundary of the foramen caecum.
- *Foramen caecum*—a frequently impervious foramen of variable size between the frontal bone and alae of the crista galli. May transmit a vein from the nasal cavity to the superior sagittal sinus.
- *Upper surface*—either side of the crista galli. Supports, and is gently grooved by, the frontal lobes and the olfactory bulbs.
- *Foramina*—numerous foramina on the upper surface, principally for the passage of the olfactory nerves, their associated meninges and CSF. A foramen in the groove between the cribriform plate and the orbital plates of the frontal bone transmits the anterior ethmoidal nerve and artery: on either side, the anterior ethmoidal neurovascular bundle enters the cranial cavity here from the orbit and proceeds to the nasal cavity via a slit just lateral to the crista galli.
- *Posterior border*—articulates with the spine of the sphenoid bone.

Perpendicular plate

Much like the fixed rudder of a sailing boat, the median sagittal, quadrilateral perpendicular plate of the ethmoid bone forms the superior part of the nasal septum.
- *Anterior border*—articulates with the crest of the united nasal bones and the nasal spine of the frontal bone.
- *Posterior border*—articulates with the sphenoidal crest superiorly and the vomer inferiorly.
- *Inferior border*—grooved to accept the septal cartilage.

Ethmoidal labyrinths

The labyrinths are suspended bilaterally beneath the cribriform plate and bounded laterally by vertical plates forming part of the medial orbital walls. They represent the anterior, middle, and posterior air cells of the ethmoid bone, invariably exposed in the disarticulated state (Fig. 1.37).

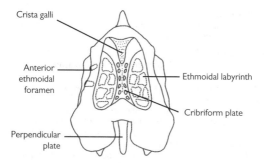

Fig. 1.35 The ethmoid bone, superior view.
Reproduced courtesy of Daniel R. van Gijn.

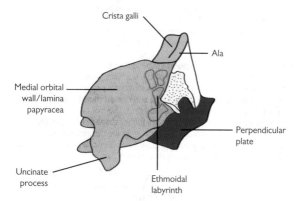

Fig. 1.36 The ethmoid bone, right lateral view.
Reproduced courtesy of Daniel R. van Gijn.

Superior surface
- Exposed air cells completed by the corresponding surface of the ethmoidal notch of the frontal bone.
- Interrupted by grooves for the anterior and posterior ethmoidal nerves and vessels.

Lateral surface (orbital plate)
The lamina papyracea forms most of the medial orbital wall and provides cover for the middle and posterior cells (the remaining anterior cells are covered by the lacrimal bone and frontal process of the maxilla). Articulates with the following five bones:
- Superiorly—orbital plate of frontal bone.
- Inferiorly—rests upon the maxilla and the orbital process of the palatine bone.
- Anteriorly—lacrimal bone (covers the remaining air cells).
- Posteriorly—sphenoid bone.

Posterior surface

Irregular exposed cells are closed by the sphenoidal conchae and orbital process of the palatine bone.

Medial surface (nasal plate)

Part of the lateral nasal wall; more complex and undulating than the smooth orbital plate. Features from superior to inferior:

- *Superior nasal concha*—thin and convex on its medial surface; covers the superior meatus into which the posterior ethmoid cells drain (Fig. 1.38).
- *Middle nasal concha*—long, curved plate that represents the most inferior extension of the nasal plate. Its lower free border articulates anteriorly with the frontal process of the maxilla and posteriorly with the perpendicular plate of the palatine bone.
- *Middle meatus*—between the middle concha and lateral nasal wall. It has numerous, occasionally inconsistent, features.
- *Uncinate process*—boomerang- or hook-shaped process with a variable superior attachment (anterior to lamina papyracea). Inferiorly is attached to the ethmoidal process of the inferior concha.
- *Bulla ethmoidalis*—a swelling on the lateral wall of the middle meatus caused by protruding anterior ethmoidal air cells, which open into the middle meatus either on or above the bulla, forming a rudimentary concha.
- *Hiatus semilunaris*—half-moon-shaped groove on the middle meatus; bound anteriorly by the crook of the uncinate, superiorly by the bulla ethmoidalis, and posteriorly by the ethmoidal process of the inferior concha. Drains the maxillary sinus, anterior ethmoidal cells, and, by way of the infundibulum and frontonasal duct, the frontal sinus.
- *Infundibulum*—a three-dimensional, funnel-shaped cleft between the uncinate and lateral wall of the nose, draining the anterior ethmoidal cells. Its tip occasionally continues further superiorly to drain the frontal sinus as a frontonasal recess (rather than a duct).

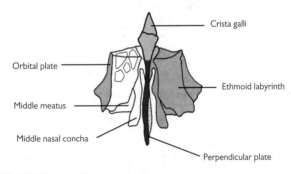

Fig. 1.37 The ethmoid bone, anterior view.
Reproduced courtesy of Daniel R. van Gijn.

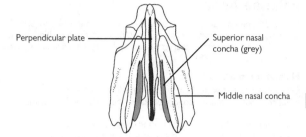

Fig. 1.38 The ethmoid bone, inferior view.
Reproduced courtesy of Daniel R. van Gijn.

Palatine bone

L-shaped bone consisting of horizontal and vertical surfaces and orbital, sphenoidal, and pyramidal processes. Contributes to three cavities (orbit, oral, and nasal), two fossae (pterygopalatine and pterygoid), and one fissure (inferior orbital) (Fig. 1.39).

Horizontal part

Quadrilateral with two surfaces and four borders (Fig. 1.40).

- *Superior (nasal) surface*—concave, forming the posterior floor of the nasal cavity.
- *Inferior (palatine) surface*—concave and rough surfaced. Forms the posterior quarter of the palate with its contralateral fellow. A transverse ridge near the posterior border provides attachment for the aponeurosis of tensor veli palatini.
- *Anterior border*—articulates with the palatine process of the maxilla.
- *Posterior border*—free margin, provides attachment for the soft palate and the musculus uvulae (uvula).
- *Lateral border*—continuation of the vertical part of the palatine bone; grooved by the sulcus for the greater palatine nerve.
- *Medial border*—thickest of the borders. Forms the posterior nasal crest with its contralateral fellow; articulates with the posterior border of the vomer.

Vertical part

Thin and oblong, with nasal and maxillary surfaces and four borders. The superior border has orbital and sphenoidal processes, separated by the sphenopalatine notch (Fig. 1.40).

Nasal surface

Forms the lateral wall of the nasal cavity, situated anterior to the medial pterygoid process. From inferior upwards, it bears the following features:

- *Surface for inferior meatus*—broad depression.
- *Conchal crest*—prominent horizontal ridge for articulation with the inferior nasal concha.
- *Surface for middle meatus*—concavity between the conchal crest inferiorly and the ethmoidal crest superiorly.
- *Ethmoidal crest*—articulates with the middle nasal concha. A shallow groove lies above forming part of the superior meatus.

Maxillary surface

- *Inferior two-thirds*—overlap the nasal surface of the body of the maxilla, helping to close and complete the posterior aspect of the maxillary hiatus and the greater palatine groove, respectively.
- *Posterosuperior surface*—forms the medial wall of the pterygopalatine fossa.

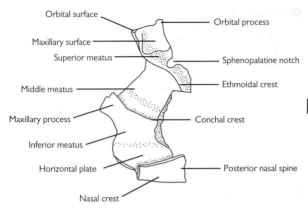

Fig. 1.39 The right palatine bone, medial view.
Reproduced courtesy of Daniel R. van Gijn.

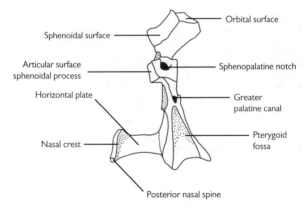

Fig. 1.40 The right palatine bone, posterior view.
Reproduced courtesy of Daniel R. van Gijn.

Pyramidal process

Projects backwards from the junction of the horizontal and vertical parts.
- *Posterior surface*—smooth area at the apex of the pyramidal process that completes the inferior aspect of the pterygoid fossa and offers some attachment for the medial pterygoid muscle.
- *Lateral surface*—articulates with the maxillary tuberosity where a triangular part can be seen between it and the lateral pterygoid plate, contributing to the floor of the pterygopalatine fossa.
- *Inferior surface*—transmits the lesser palatine neurovascular bundle through foramina of the same name.

Orbital process

A complex structure arising superolaterally from the perpendicular process with five surfaces, three articular and two non-articular (Fig. 1.41 and Fig. 1.42).

Articular surfaces
- *Ethmoid*—medial process. Articulates with the labyrinth and occasionally with the posterior ethmoidal and sphenoidal cells.
- *Sphenoid*—posterior process. Has an air sinus upon its surface. Articulates with the sphenoidal concha and communicates with the sphenoidal sinus.
- *Maxilla*—anterior process. Rough surface articulates with maxilla.

Non-articular surfaces
Triangular orbital surface makes a small contribution to the posterior floor of the orbit and the inferior orbital fissure.

Sphenoidal process

A thin plate posterior to and shorter than the orbital process. It presents three surfaces, three borders, and contributes to three fossae/foramina: the palatovaginal canal, pterygopalatine fossa, and sphenopalatine foramen (Fig. 1.42).

Surfaces
- *Superior*—articulates with sphenoidal concha. Overlapped by the vaginal process of the medial pterygoid plate to form the palatovaginal (or pharyngeal) canal.
- *Medial*—concave. Forms part of the roof and lateral wall of the nasal cavity.
- *Lateral*—has a rough component for articulation with the medial pterygoid plate and a smooth component which forms part of the medial wall of the pterygopalatine fossa.

Borders
- *Anterior*—forms the posterior boundary of the sphenopalatine notch.
- *Posterior*—articulates with the medial pterygoid plate.

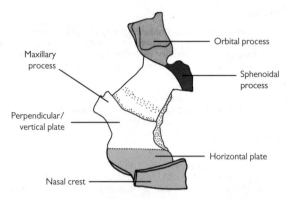

Fig. 1.41 The parts and processes of the right palatine bone, medial view.
Reproduced courtesy of Daniel R. van Gijn.

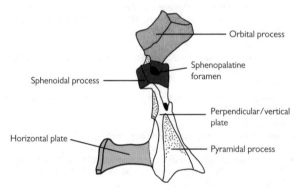

Fig. 1.42 The parts and processes of the right palatine bone, posterior view.
Reproduced courtesy of Daniel R. van Gijn.

Vomer

A thin, quadrilateral, midline structure forming the posteroinferior component of the nasal septum. Its anterior extremity articulates with the posterior margin of the maxillary incisor crest and descends between the incisive canals. It has two surfaces and four borders (Fig. 1.43).

Surfaces

Its surfaces have multiple markings for the vessels of the septum and a prominent groove for the nasopalatine neurovascular bundle, which travels across it obliquely in an anteroinferior direction.

Borders

Superior border

The thickest of the four borders (Fig. 1.44a).

- *Diverging alae*—articulate with the vaginal processes of the medial pterygoid plate, sphenoidal conchae, and the sphenoidal processes of the palatine bones.
- *Central groove*—receives the sphenoidal rostrum.
- *Vomerovaginal canal*—an inconsistent canal between the inferior surface of the alar and the vaginal process of the sphenoid. Medially related to the palatovaginal canal. Transmits the pharyngeal branch of the final (third) part of the maxillary artery.

Inferior border

Articulates with the nasal crest formed by the maxillae and horizontal processes of the palatine bones.

Posterior border

Free margin separating the posterior choanae. Thick and bifid superiorly and thin inferiorly.

Anterior border

Longest of the borders of the vomer, sloping obliquely in an anteroinferior direction and ending in an anterior angle (Fig. 1.44b).

- *Superior half*—articulates with the perpendicular plate of the ethmoid.
- *Inferior half*—presents a groove to receive the inferior margin of the nasal septal cartilage.

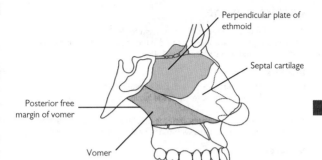

Fig. 1.43 The vomer (yellow) and its articulations, lateral view.
Reproduced courtesy of Daniel R. van Gijn.

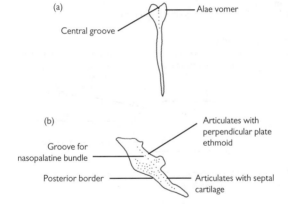

Fig. 1.44 (a) The vomer: (a) superior view; (b) lateral view.
Reproduced courtesy of Daniel R. van Gijn.

Lacrimal bone

A thin and fragile (paired) bone that has the dubious honour of being the smallest of the cranial bones. Located in the anteromedial orbit. Consists of four borders and two surfaces (Fig. 1.45).

Borders
- *Anterior border*—articulates with the frontal process of the maxilla.
- *Posterior border*—articulates with the lamina papyracea of the ethmoid bone.
- *Superior border*—articulates with the nasal notch of the frontal bone.
- *Inferior border*—articulates with the orbital surface of the maxilla.

Surfaces
Lateral (orbital) surface
- *Posterior lacrimal crest*—attachment to orbital septum.
- *Lacrimal hamulus*—hook-like end of the lacrimal crest.
- *Lacrimal sulcus*—lodges the lacrimal sac and the frontal process of the maxilla.
- *Descending process*—articulates with the lacrimal process of the inferior concha.

Medial (nasal) surface
- Lines by mucous membrane, forms part of the middle meatus, and abuts the anterior ethmoidal air cells.

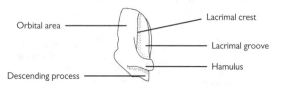

Orbital area

Descending process

Lacrimal crest

Lacrimal groove

Hamulus

Fig. 1.45 Right lacrimal bone, lateral aspect.
Reproduced courtesy of Daniel R. van Gijn.

Inferior nasal concha

A separate bone that consists of two borders, two surfaces, and four processes (Fig. 1.46 and Fig. 1.47). It 'closes off' the inferior portion of the maxillary hiatus by articulating with the following:
- The nasal surface of the maxilla anteriorly.
- The perpendicular plate of the palatine bone posteriorly.
- The inferior portion of the lacrimal bone anterosuperiorly via its lacrimal process.
- The posterior aspect of the uncinate process of the ethmoid bone via its ethmoidal process.

Borders

- *Superior border*—articulates anteriorly with the conchal crest of the maxilla and the conchal crest of the palatine bone posteriorly.
- *Inferior border*—free edge and thicker than the upper border.

Surfaces

- *Medial surface*—convex and furrowed by longitudinal grooves for vessels.
- *Lateral surface*—concave. Forms the superior and medial boundary of the inferior meatus.

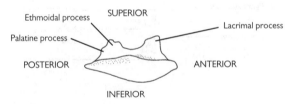

Fig. 1.46 Left inferior concha, medial ('nasal') surface.
Reproduced courtesy of Daniel R. van Gijn.

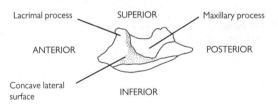

Fig. 1.47 Left inferior concha, lateral surface.
Reproduced courtesy of Daniel R. van Gijn.

Nasal bone

The nasal bones are small, quadrangular paired, central facial bones that bridge the gap between the frontal processes of the maxillae. They articulate at the internasal suture and bear four borders and two surfaces (Fig. 1.48).

Borders

- *Superior*—articulates with the frontal bone at the frontonasal suture.
- *Inferior*—articulates/overlaps with the upper lateral cartilage.
- *Lateral*—articulates with the frontal process of the ipsilateral maxilla at the nasomaxillary suture.
- *Medial*—articulates with its contralateral fellow at the internasal suture.

Surfaces

- *External surface*—convex, with attachments for procerus and nasalis muscles.
- *Internal surface*—concave and grooved by the anterior ethmoidal nerve before it continues as the external nasal nerve.

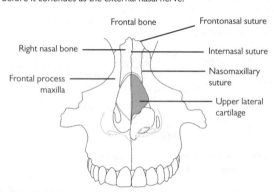

Fig. 1.48 Paired nasal bones, anterior view.
Reproduced courtesy of Daniel R. van Gijn.

Chapter 2

The mandible

Introduction

The mandible is the largest of the facial bones, occupying a prominent position upon and providing the foundation for the lower third of the face. Despite holding the honour of being the strongest bone in the face, its protrusive location makes it vulnerable to injury, particularly in relation to aggressively placed fists, steering wheels, and concrete.

Anatomically, the mandible consists of a symmetrical, horseshoe-shaped body continuous with paired broad rami posteriorly. The former houses the lower teeth within the alveolus while the latter provides attachment for the four principal muscles of mastication from its medial and lateral surfaces and coronoid and condylar processes. In addition to the aforementioned muscles of mastication, the mandible gives origin to the muscles of the tongue, the floor of the mouth, and some muscles of facial expression.

Surgically, the terminology becomes a little more confusing and includes the midline 'symphysis', where the two halves of the mandible are strongly joined, and 'parasymphysis', or the area bound between the distal aspect of the lower canine teeth.

In addition to mastication, the mandible and its intimately related structures are involved in airway maintenance and speech. Pathology and trauma affecting the mandible therefore may result in significant, and on occasion life-threatening, dysfunction and pain.

Body

The U-shaped body of the mandible consists of two halves that meet developmentally at the faint symphysis menti (🕘 Fig. 2.4, p. 70). Each half consists of an upper and lower border, with external and internal surfaces, and extends as far posteriorly as the third molar tooth, behind which, via the angle, the ramus begins (Fig. 2.1 and Fig. 2.2).

Key features

- *Mental protuberance*—the triangular-shaped inferior extent of the midline symphysis menti.
- *Mental tubercles*—raised lateral aspects of the mental protuberance. Flank a central depression.
- *Chin*—combination of the mental protuberance and tubercles.
- *Mental foramen*—lies in the interspace between the two premolar teeth approximately equidistant from the upper and lower borders. Accommodates the mental neurovascular bundle.
- *External oblique line*—extends posteriorly from the mental tubercles. It continues below the mental foramen becoming progressively more ridge-like as it becomes the anterior border of the ramus.
- *Digastric fossa*—occupies a space on the inner surface of the inferior border of the body of the mandible, near the midline bilaterally. It gives attachment to the anterior belly of digastric.
- *Alveolar process*—the tooth-bearing portion. Consists of buccal and lingual bony plates interrupted by interdental and interdental septa that define the 16 alveoli or sockets of the mandibular teeth.
- *Mylohyoid line*—an oblique line on the internal surface marking the attachment of the mylohyoid muscle. It extends from the posterior symphyseal area to a point roughly 1 cm below the upper border on the distal aspect of the third molar. The pterygomandibular raphe and its attached superior constrictor and buccinator muscles are found at its posterior end.
- *Mylohyoid groove*—groove on the inner surface of the mandible running obliquely forward and downward from the lingula. Houses the mylohyoid neurovascular bundle.
- *Submandibular fossa*—a concavity on the inner surface below the mylohyoid line. Associated with the submandibular gland.
- *Sublingual fossa*—shallow depression above the mylohyoid line lateral to the genial tubercles. Lodges the sublingual glands.
- *Genial tubercles*—small (occasionally fused) elevations in the posterior symphyseal area. Usually divided into upper and lower mental spines which give attachment to the genioglossus and geniohyoid respectively.
- *Genial (lingual) foramen*—an inconsistent foramen into a blind ending canal carrying a branch of the lingual artery.

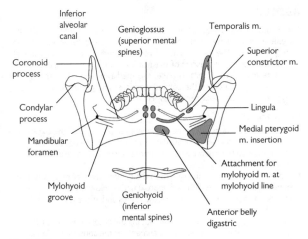

Fig. 2.1 Mandible, posterior view.
Reproduced courtesy of Daniel R. van Gijn.

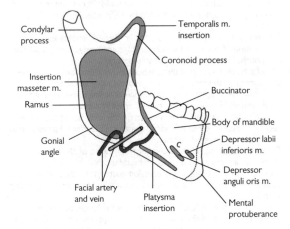

Fig. 2.2 Mandible, right lateral view.
Reproduced courtesy of Daniel R. van Gijn.

Ramus

The paired ascending, quadrilateral part of the mandible that includes the angle. It consists of two surfaces, four borders, and the coronoid and condylar processes. The ramus and aforementioned processes provide attachment for the four muscles of mastication, namely, the masseter to the otherwise featureless lateral surface, the medial pterygoid to the medial surface, the temporalis to the coronoid process and ramus, and the lateral pterygoid to the condylar processes (Fig. 2.3).

Key features

- *External oblique ridge*—a more prominent continuation of the external oblique line up the anterior border of the ramus. Provides inferior attachment to buccinator and has important surgical correlations (Champy's lines) (Fig. 2.4).
- *Mandibular foramen*—through which the inferior alveolar neurovascular bundle gains entrance. Situated approximately midway between the anterior and posterior borders of the ramus and at the level of the mandibular occlusal plane.
- *Lingula*—sharp triangular spur overlapping the anterior aspect of the mandibular foramen. Provides attachment for the sphenomandibular ligament.
- *Mandibular (sigmoid) notch*—the deep concavity at the upper border of the ramus—situated between the coronoid process anteriorly and the condyle posteriorly. It is crossed by the masseteric neurovascular bundle.
- *Coronoid process*—thin, triangular, and fin-shaped process and continuation of the external oblique ridge anteriorly and sigmoid notch posteriorly. Provides attachment to temporalis.
- *Condylar process*—roughly ovoid when viewed from above, with the long axes of both meeting at an angle of 145 degrees at the anterior border of the foramen magnum. Connects to the ramus via the thin condylar neck. Fibrocartilage-covered articular surface.
- *Pterygoid fovea*—a shallow depression on the anterior aspect of the neck of the condyle just inferior to the articular surface. For attachment of the lateral pterygoid muscle.
- *Temporal crest*—the ridge descending from the tip of the coronoid process to an area behind the third molar tooth.
- *Retromolar fossa*—triangular depression posterior to the third molar tooth. Bound by the temporal crest medially and external oblique ridge laterally.
- *Gonial angle*—the angle of the mandible at the lower, posterior, and lateral-most point of the ramus. Used as a cephalometric landmark and shows intersex variation. Presents rough oblique ridges for the masseter laterally, medial pterygoid medially, and stylomandibular ligament in between. Note difference between surgical and anatomical angle.
- *Mandibular canal*—carries the inferior alveolar neurovascular bundle and extends from the mandibular foramen, descending obliquely forward within the ramus and subsequently body, passing inferior to (and supplying the teeth within) the alveoli, eventually opening at the mental foramen as the mental nerve after looping back upon itself. Continues briefly anteriorly as the incisive canal carrying the incisive nerve to the anterior teeth.

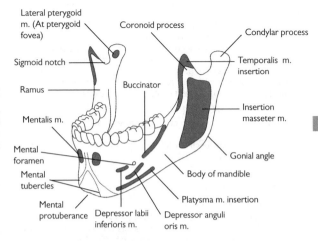

Fig. 2.3 Overview of the anatomy of the mandible seen in anterolateral view.
Reproduced courtesy of Daniel R. van Gijn.

Mandibular fractures

Foramina, teeth, and bony buttresses provide areas of strength and weakness, accounting for the condyle as the commonest site of fracture, followed by the body. Two fractures coexisting are common, and a second should be sought on assessment. Clinical assessment may identify blood in the floor of the mouth, malocclusion, a palpable step, trismus (lockjaw), mandible mobility, or mental nerve paraesthesia.

Fracture classification

- Open or closed.
- Fracture pattern (comminuted, simple, unicortical).
- Anatomical location.
- Fracture orientation—favourable or unfavourable, dependent on the forces of the musculature, which reduces (favourable) or distracts (unfavourable) the fracture.

Management of mandibular fractures

Determination of management is dependent on the patient's age and stage of dentition, coexisting injuries, fracture pattern, anatomical location, and deforming forces acting to distract the fracture. The aims of treatment are to restore occlusion, facilitate fracture healing, and permit physiotherapy and rehabilitation.

Management options
- *Conservative*—soft diet for 6 weeks and may be employed for stable or minimally displaced condylar fractures.
- *Intermaxillary fixation* (IMF)—utilizes screws, plates, wires, or arch bars for a non-rigid fixation. It may be used for condylar fractures, comminuted fractures or paediatric fractures.
- *Open reduction internal fixation* (ORIF)—provides a rigid or non-rigid/ functionally stable fixation and permits immediate mobilization.

Load sharing versus load bearing
- *Load sharing*—stability with friction of bone ends and plate across fracture site.
- *Load bearing*—bears functional forces at the fracture site; larger plates and bicortical screws.

Biomechanics of the mandible

Zones of tension and compression
Forces applied to the mandible cause varying zones of tension and compression. The superior border of the mandible is designated the *tension zone* and the inferior border the *compression zone* (Fig. 2.5).

Lines of ideal osteosynthesis
Maxime Champy (1976) described ideal lines of osteosynthesis within the mandible. These allow the use of small, easily bendable miniplates, allowing for a less invasive intraoral approach to the mandible with minimal periosteal stripping—while still providing optimal fixation and stability.

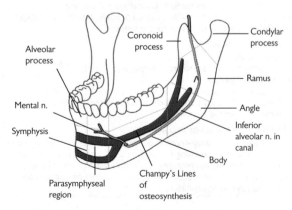

Fig. 2.4 Parts of the mandible and Champy's lines of osteosynthesis.
Reproduced courtesy of Daniel R. van Gijn.

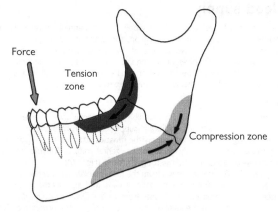

Fig. 2.5 Zones of tension (red) and compression (yellow) of the mandible—with an anteriorly placed force (grey arrow).

Reproduced courtesy of Daniel R. van Gijn.

Blood supply

A sound knowledge of the blood supply to the mandible is clinically important to the dental implant surgeon, the orthognathic surgeon in the planning and postoperative success of mandibular osteotomies, and the inquisitive emergency physician in the initial diagnosis and management of mandibular fractures. As with the bony anatomy of the mandible, it is convenient to consider the body and ramus separately.

Body

The main nutrient artery of the mandible is the inferior alveolar artery (first part of maxillary artery). Additional supply comes from branches of the facial and lingual arteries that supply the muscles attached to the posterior symphysial region, namely genioglossus, geniohyoid, mylohyoid, the anterior belly of digastric, and the tongue proper (Fig. 2.6):

- *Inferior alveolar artery*—arises from the first (mandibular) part of the maxillary artery. Enters the mandibular canal and supplies the bone, dentition, and adjacent soft tissues from within. Divides into incisive and mental branches at the level of the first premolar—the former supplies the anterior teeth and supporting tissues while the latter anastomoses with the inferior labial and submental arteries of the facial artery.
- *Sublingual artery*—branches from the lingual artery. Supplies the sublingual gland, mylohyoid, and neighbouring muscles and anastomoses with the submental branch of the facial artery.
- *Submental artery*—from the facial artery. Anastomoses with the sublingual and mylohyoid arteries and supplies the skin in the submental area. Along with the sublingual artery, it may perforate the lingual plate—with the potential for brisk bleeding into a confined space (e.g. sublingual space) in the event of iatrogenic damage or trauma to this region.
- *Mylohyoid artery*—a branch of the inferior alveolar artery, given off before it enters the mandibular canal. Runs within the mylohyoid groove with the nerve to mylohyoid (V_3) to supply the mylohyoid muscle.

Ramus

The ramus and the coronoid process, are supplied by the inferior alveolar artery and by the vessels that supply the masseter, medial pterygoid, and temporalis muscles (Fig. 2.7):

- *Masseteric branch* (maxillary artery).
- *Facial artery* (external carotid artery).
- *Transverse facial* (superficial temporal artery).
- *Pterygoid branches* (from second part of the maxillary artery).
- *Anterior deep, middle, and posterior deep temporal arteries* (from second part of the maxillary artery).

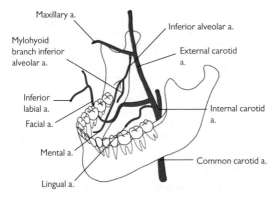

Fig. 2.6 The blood supply of the mandible, superolateral view.
Reproduced courtesy of Daniel R. van Gijn.

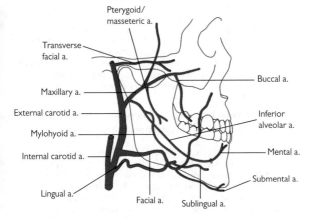

Fig. 2.7 Blood supply of the mandible, right lateral view.
Reproduced courtesy of Daniel R. van Gijn.

Mandibular nerve

The nerve supply of the mandible is from the third division of the trigeminal nerve, the mandibular nerve (V_3). It consists of a larger (anterior) sensory root, which provides general sensation to the skin of the lower face, temporal region, and the lips, floor of the oral cavity and anterior two-thirds of the tongue, and the gingivae and dentition of the mandible—and a smaller (posterior) motor root to the muscles of mastication. While separated intracranially, the motor and sensory roots unite extracranially shortly after exiting the foramen ovale. Before dividing into its anterior and posterior divisions, it gives off a meningeal branch and the nerve to medial pterygoid.

- *Meningeal branch*—loops back intracranially via the foramen spinosum with the middle meningeal artery. Supplies the dura of the middle and anterior cranial fossa.
- *Nerve to medial pterygoid*—supplies medial pterygoid, tensor tympani, and tensor veli palatini.

Anterior division (motor with one exception)

The smaller anterior division supplies the four muscles of mastication and a sensory branch to the cheek (Fig. 2.9).

- *Nerve to lateral pterygoid*.
- *Nerve to masseter*—passes through the mandibular notch posterior to the tendon of temporalis, enters the deep surface of masseter and contributes an articular branch to the temporomandibular joint (TMJ).
- *Deep temporal nerves*—anterior, middle, and posterior branches. Pass over lateral pterygoid to enter the deep surface of temporalis.
- *Long buccal nerve*—passes between the two heads of lateral pterygoid (supplying its motor aspect in the process), anterior to masseter. Supplies the skin covering the buccinators anteriorly and sensation to the buccal mucosa.

Posterior division (sensory with one exception)

The larger posterior division has three sensory branches and one motor branch (Fig. 2.9 and Fig. 2.11).

- *Auriculotemporal nerve*—characteristic two roots surrounding the middle meningeal artery. Passes posterior to the TMJ (supplying it in the process) and loosely follows the course of the superficial temporal artery. Supplies the superior auricle and adjacent skin, the external auditory canal and the tympanic membrane, the skin overlying the parotid sheath and the parotid gland proper. Caries postganglionic parasympathetic fibres to the parotid gland from the otic ganglion.
- *Lingual nerve*—passes on the surface of medial pterygoid and continues more superficially between it and the ramus of the mandible. At the junction of the ramus and the body of the mandible it is intimately related to the periosteum of the lingual surface of the mandible. It passes under the pterygomandibular raphe (and the attached superior pharyngeal constrictor) and lies deep to the inferior alveolar nerve. Supplies general sensation to the anterior two-thirds of the tongue, the floor of the mouth, and lingual mucosa.

- *Inferior alveolar nerve*—the largest branch of the posterior division, descending superficial to medial pterygoid with the lingual nerve. After passing between the sphenomandibular ligament and mandibular ramus, it enters the mandibular canal via the mandibular foramen together with the inferior alveolar artery. Before entering the foramen, it gives off the nerve to mylohyoid which runs within the mylohyoid groove and supplies mylohyoid and the anterior belly of digastric. The inferior alveolar nerve supplies the mandibular dentition and the mandible. It exits the mental foramen as the mental nerve, which supplies sensation to the anterior chin, lower lip and buccal gingivae of the lower anterior teeth.

Dental nerve blocks
Inferior alveolar nerve block (IANB)
The IANB is used extensively in dental practice for the anaesthesia of structures innervated by the mandibular nerve during dental/surgical procedures. It involves the deposition of a local anaesthetic solution into the pterygomandibular space via an intraoral route.

Technique
Several techniques are described (direct, indirect, Gow-Gates, Akinosi closed mouth) although the direct is probably the most common. This involves insertion of a needle into the pterygomandibular space by piercing mucosa and buccinators, so that the tip of the needle contacts bone just superior to the lingula, i.e. at the point just before the inferior alveolar nerve enters the mandibular foramen (Fig. 2.10).

Landmarks
- *Pterygomandibular depression*—site of injection. Between the mucosa overlying the pterygomandibular raphe medially and the mucosa overlying the anterior border of the ramus laterally (Fig. 2.8).
- *Coronoid notch*—point of maximum concavity on the anterior border of mandibular ramus. Serves to mark the level of injection.
- *Occlusal plane*—injection should be approximately parallel to and 10 mm above the lower occlusal plane.
- *Contralateral premolar teeth*—the syringe should extend over the premolars on the contralateral side to the injection.

Pterygomandibular space
The pterygomandibular space is a triangular space which contains the inferior alveolar neurovascular structures. It is bounded laterally by the medial surface of the mandibular ramus, medially by the medial pterygoid muscle, superiorly by the lateral pterygoid muscle, posteriorly by the parotid gland, and anteriorly by buccinator, the superior pharyngeal constrictor and the pterygomandibular raphe.

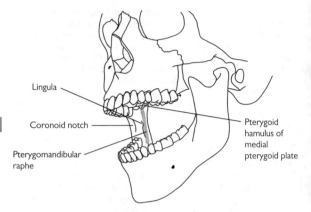

Fig. 2.8 The position of the pterygomandibular raphe and associated clinically relevant structures, open mouth view.

Reproduced courtesy of Daniel R. van Gijn.

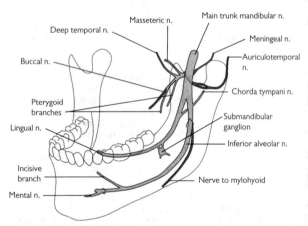

Fig. 2.9 The mandibular division of the trigeminal nerve. Yellow denotes the anterior (principally sensory) root and grey denotes the posterior (principally motor) root.

Reproduced courtesy of Daniel R. van Gijn.

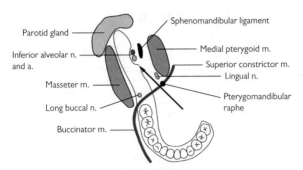

Fig. 2.10 The anatomy of the inferior alveolar nerve block and pterygomandibular space, transverse view. Arrow demonstrates route of needle.

Reproduced courtesy of Daniel R. van Gijn.

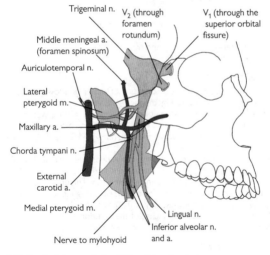

Fig. 2.11 Detail of the mandibular division of the trigeminal nerve.

Reproduced courtesy of Daniel R. van Gijn.

Muscles of mastication

The four muscles of mastication are the paired lateral and medial pterygoids, the temporalis muscles, and the powerful masseter (Fig. 2.13 and Fig. 2.14). They are derived embryologically from the first pharyngeal arch and, as such, receive their innervation from the mandibular division of the trigeminal nerve (V_3). All act individually on the mandible, with the common goal to masticate, ie. to chew, tear, and grind food. The muscles fill the otherwise potential void of the infratemporal fossa and define its boundaries, relying upon its neurovascular components.

Masseter

A thick, three-layered quadrilateral muscle covering the lateral aspect of the ramus. It lies deep to the parotid gland and is crossed by the parotid duct.

* *Origin*—zygomatic arch (superficial: anterior two-thirds of lower border; middle: deep surface and posterior one-third of lower border; deep: deep surface of the zygomatic arch and lateral surface of the coronoid process of the mandible).
* *Insertion*—ramus of mandible and coronoid process.
* *Action on mandible*—elevates and protrudes.
* *Nerve supply*—anterior division of V_3, masseteric branch.
* *Blood supply*—masseteric branch of the maxillary artery (external carotid artery), facial artery, and transverse facial artery (superficial temporal artery) (Fig. 2.15).

Lateral pterygoid

A short, thick, conical muscle consisting of upper and lower heads, lying deep to temporalis, covered by the pterygoid venous plexus (Fig. 2.14).

* *Origin*—upper head: infratemporal surface of the greater wing of sphenoid; lower head: lateral surface of the lateral pterygoid plate.
* *Insertion*—the heads converge onto the pterygoid fovea, TMJ capsule, and articular disc.
* *Action on mandible*—protrudes mandible, depresses chin. Individually: side-to-side grinding motion—movement to the opposite side. Assists geniohyoid and digastric in opening the mouth. The upper heads' continued action on the articular disc on clenching (i.e. closed jaw) is important in a possible aetiology of TMJ dysfunction.
* *Nerve supply*—muscular branches of the anterior division of V_3.
* *Blood supply*—muscular branches of the maxillary artery.

Medial pterygoid

The deepest of the muscles of mastication is a thick, quadrilateral muscle with deep and superficial heads. It mirrors the masseter, forming a pterygomasseteric sling acting to support the angle of the mandible (Fig. 2.16).

* *Origin*—deep head: medial surface of the lateral pterygoid plate. Superficial head: maxillary tuberosity and pyramidal process of the palatine bone.
* *Insertion*—fibres pass posterolaterally, inserting onto the medial aspect of the ramus and angle of the mandible up to the level of the mandibular foramen.

- *Action on mandible*—elevation of the mandible and protrusion with lateral pterygoids; side-to-side grinding.
- *Nerve supply*—medial pterygoid branch of V₃.
- *Blood supply*—pterygoid branches of the maxillary artery.

Temporalis

A large, fan-shaped muscle occupying the space of the temporal fossa. Its bulk and location are most pronounced in its absence, as exemplified by temporal hollowing resulting from disruption of the deep temporal arteries with resultant ischaemia and muscular atrophy, or fat wasting secondary to malnutrition or medication.

- *Origin*—floor of the temporal fossa (up to the inferior temporal line) and deep temporal fascia.
- *Insertion*—coronoid process and ramus of mandible.
- *Action on mandible*—elevation (anterior fibres) and retrusion (posterior fibres). Contributes to side-to-side grinding.
- *Nerve supply*—deep temporal nerves (branches of V₃).
- *Blood supply*—anterior, middle, and posterior deep temporal branches (second part of the maxillary artery), superficial temporal arteries.

> **Temporal fossa**
>
> The floor of the temporal fossa is formed by the articulation of four bones (greater wing of sphenoid, parietal, squamous temporal, and frontal) at the pterion. The fossa is superior to the zygomatic arch (thus distinguishing itself from the infratemporal fossa which lies inferior to the arch) and filled by the mass of the temporalis muscle and temporal fascia.

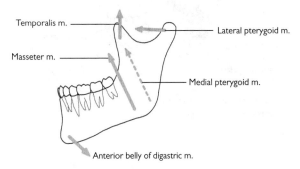

Fig. 2.12 Direction of pull of the muscles acting upon the mandible.
Reproduced courtesy of Daniel R. van Gijn.

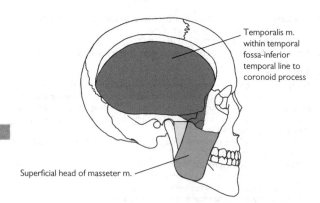

Fig. 2.13 Temporalis and masseter muscles, lateral view.
Reproduced courtesy of Daniel R. van Gijn.

Temporalis m.
within temporal
fossa-inferior
temporal line to
coronoid process

Superficial head of masseter m.

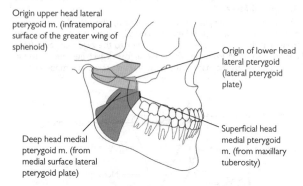

Origin upper head lateral
pterygoid m. (infratemporal
surface of the greater wing of
sphenoid)

Origin of lower head
lateral pterygoid
(lateral pterygoid
plate)

Deep head medial
pterygoid m. (from
medial surface lateral
pterygoid plate)

Superficial head
medial pterygoid
m. (from maxillary
tuberosity)

Fig. 2.14 Attachments of lateral and medial pterygoid muscles.
Reproduced courtesy of Daniel R. van Gijn.

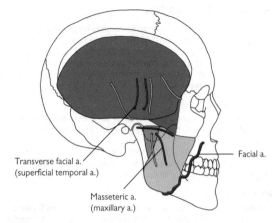

Fig. 2.15 Blood supply to the muscles of mastication.
Reproduced courtesy of Daniel R. van Gijn.

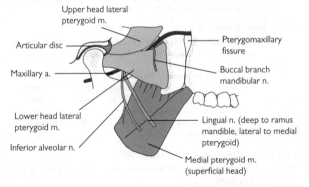

Fig. 2.16 The muscles of mastication and relationships.
Reproduced courtesy of Daniel R. van Gijn.

Age-related changes

The bones of the maxilla and mandible are unique in their ability to bear teeth. The presence of dentition, and the associated eruption and potential later loss, has significant consequences on the growth and senescence of the mandible (Fig. 2.17). This, in turn, has implications for how the mandible is affected by pathology and how this is subsequently managed by the maxillofacial or dental surgeon.

Developing mandible

• The mandibular canal and mental foramen lie close to the inferior border of the body—the latter angled forwards below the first molar tooth.
• The condyle is short, thick, and underdeveloped and lies below the level of the coronoid process (subsequent condylar growth is thought to be a response to changes in function and influenced by loading of the TMJ).

Adult mandible

• Elongation of the body to accommodate teeth and ongoing forward protrusion of the chin give the mental foramen its final, adult, anterior-facing position.
• Deposition of alveolar bone superiorly and bone inferiorly results in the adult position of the mental foramen—approximately midway between the upper and lower borders of the mandibular body.

Edentulous mandible

• Periodontal disease, loss of teeth, and the subsequent loss of bony alveolar support has dramatic effects on the height of the mandibular body.
• With ongoing alveolar resorption, the mental foramen, mandibular canal and its associated nerve all lie progressively closer to the superior border. In the event of bony dehiscence, the latter occasionally lies vulnerable, beneath the oral mucosa only.
• The edentulous mandible has significant implications for the maxillofacial and dental implant surgeon.

Problems of the edentulous mandible

The fractured edentulous mandible presents a challenge to the oral and maxillofacial surgeon:
• Alveolar bone resorption through loss of teeth weakens the mandible.
• Loss of cross-sectional area, and increased reliance on periosteal blood supply, diminish the potential for fracture healing and increase the chance of vascular compromise during intraoperative periosteal stripping.
• Medical comorbidities in the elderly also adversely affect fracture healing.
• Fractures tend to occur in the body region—with unfavourable muscle pull.
• Bilateral 'bucket handle' body fractures in the pencil-thin edentulous mandible are particularly difficult, given the pull of the suprahyoid muscles and generally require ORIF.

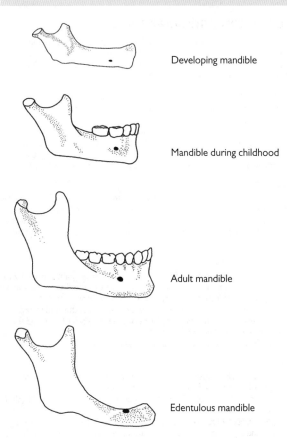

Developing mandible

Mandible during childhood

Adult mandible

Edentulous mandible

Fig. 2.17 Changes in the shape of the mandible related to eruption and loss of teeth. Note the evolving position of the mental foramen relative to the alveolar process of the mandible.

Reproduced courtesy of Daniel R. van Gijn.

Temporomandibular joint

The TMJ is a synovial, fibrocartilage-lined joint between the mandibular condyle inferiorly and the glenoid fossa of the temporal bone superiorly (Fig. 2.18). Together with its opposite number it forms a cranio-mandibular articulation, connected by the intervening mandible.

Glenoid fossa

Smooth and concave and formed by the squamous and petrous parts of the temporal bone.
- Bound by the articular eminence anteriorly and the postglenoid tubercle posteriorly (ridge dividing the fossa from the external acoustic meatus).
- *Glaser's squamotympanic fissure*—divides the fossa into an articular surface anterolaterally and a non-articular surface posteromedially.

Mandibular condyle

Covered with dense articular fibrocartilage, the convex mandibular condyle measures approximately 15–20 mm wide and 8–10 mm from front to back.
- *Pterygoid fovea*—prominent depression on the medial aspect below the articular surface. Provides site of attachment for the lateral pterygoid muscle.

Fibrous capsule

The fibrous capsule is divided into an upper and lower joint capsule by the articular disc—with fibres attached separately from the disc to the glenoid fossa (loose) and from the disc to the mandibular condyle (tight).
- *Upper part*—between the disc and temporal bone. Attached to the articular tubercle, the circumference of the mandibular fossa, and the squamotympanic fissure above.
- *Lower part*—attached to the neck of the mandible.

Ligaments

- *Sphenomandibular ligament*—a thin, flat ligament (separate from the capsule), extending from the spina angularis of the sphenoid to the lingula of the mandible. Thought to limit opening of the mandible (slack when in occlusion). A remnant of Meckel's cartilage.
- *Stylomandibular ligament*—condensation of deep cervical fascia. Extends from the styloid process to the posterior aspect of the angle of the mandible. Possibly limits excessive anterior translation of the TMJ.
- *Temporomandibular (lateral) ligament*—strongest ligament of the joint. Attached to the root of the zygomatic arch above and to the lateral surface and posterior border of the neck of the condyle below. Consists of superficial band ligament and medial band ligament. Prevents posterior displacement.
- *Superficial band ligament*—from the lateral surface of the articular eminence to the posterior aspect of the mandibular neck.
- *Medial band ligament*—runs horizontally from the crest of the articular tubercle to the lateral surface of the condyle and disc.

Relations of TMJ

- *Superiorly*—middle cranial fossa. Separated by thin plate of temporal bone.
- *Medially*—middle meningeal artery and proximal branches of the maxillary artery.
- *Laterally*—upper aspect of the parotid capsule and associated upper divisions of the facial nerve.
- *Anteriorly*—lateral pterygoid muscle within the infratemporal space.
- *Posterior*—tegmen tympani of the temporal bone and middle ear cavity.
- *Inferiorly*—maxillary artery.

Blood supply

- The predominant blood supply to the TMJ is via the superficial temporal artery laterally and the maxillary artery medially.
- The principal venous drainage is by way of the lateral pterygoid venous plexus.

Nerve supply

The disc proper is not innervated. The capsular ligament and posterior bilaminar extension of the disc are innervated by:

- *Auriculotemporal nerve.*
- *Masseteric nerve.*
- *Postganglionic sympathetic nerves.*

Articular disc

An oval-shaped disc between the mandibular condyle inferiorly and glenoid fossa superiorly. It is concave and shallow centrally with a thicker anulus peripherally. Its position is essentially a balance between the attachments of the lateral pterygoid anteriorly and the elastic bilaminar (retrodiscal) zone posteriorly. It acts to stabilize the condyle within the TMJ and reduce wear on the joint.

Attachments

- The periphery of the disc fuses with the capsular ligament surrounding the lower joint compartment.
- Anteriorly, the disc is continuous (via its capsular attachment) with the tendon of lateral pterygoid.
- The disc has thickened bands anteriorly and posteriorly and a thinner intermediate zone.
- *Bilaminar region*—a region of loose tissue attached posteriorly to the disc which splits into two laminae: the upper lamina (elastic) is attached to the squamotympanic fissure and the lower lamina (non-elastic) is attached to the condyle.

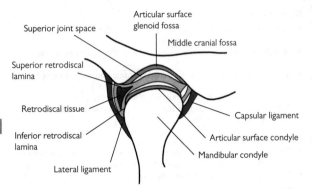

Fig. 2.18 The right temporomandibular joint, lateral view.
Reproduced courtesy of Daniel R. van Gijn.

Temporomandibular joint dysfunction (TMJD)

Problems of the TMJ are common—with a lifetime incidence of approximately 50%, affecting women more than men. Signs and symptoms include pain, clicking, trismus, crepitus, and locking episodes in the open or closed position. Causes include trauma and parafunctional habits including bruxism and finger nail biting.

- *Internal derangement*—refers to the abnormal positioning and movement of the articular disc characterized by locking and clicking.
- *Myofascial pain*—refers to pain and tightness in the muscles of mastication in the presence of an otherwise normal TMJ.
- *TMJ arthropathy*—osteoarthritis, rheumatoid arthritis, traumatic arthritis, and infective arthritis may all affect the TMJ.

Management
- *Conservative*—address parafunctional habits/precipitants. Straight-line jaw exercises, bite-raising appliances, analgesics, tricyclic antidepressants.
- *Surgical*—arthroscopy and arthrocentesis/manipulation. Open procedures that address the disc (meniscopexy—fixing the disc to zygomatic periosteum; meniscectomy—disc removal), eminectomy (removing articular eminence of zygomatic arch), and joint replacement.

Dentition and occlusion

Unlike 'polyphyodonts' whose teeth are replaced throughout life, humans have just two generations of teeth—a deciduous or primary set (from 6 months) and a permanent or adult set (from 6 years). There are 20 deciduous teeth and the normal adult has 32 permanent teeth—eight in each quadrant and evenly divided between the maxillary (16) and mandibular (16) arches (Fig. 2.19).

Structure

The principal forms of teeth are the incisors, canines, premolars, and molar teeth (Fig. 2.20).

- *Incisors* (Latin 'to cut')—cutting teeth with thin crowns (incisal edge).
- *Canines* (Latin 'of the dog')—for tearing. Short, cone-shaped crown tapering to a point.
- *Premolars*—bicuspid (two cusps) and similar in their labial appearance to the canine; not present in the deciduous dentition.
- *Molars* (Latin 'to grind'/millstone)—for grinding; multiple cusps.

Parts

Each tooth consists of an enamel-coated dentine crown and a cementum-covered root. Periodontal ligaments anchor the root within the surrounding alveolar bone, providing proprioceptive information and the target structure in the practice of exodontia. Internally lies the pulp chamber coronally and pulp (root) canals apically, collectively the pulp cavity houses the neurovascular supply to the tooth and is ultimately responsible for the pain of pulpitis (Fig. 2.21).

Innervation

- *Maxillary arch*—anterior, middle, and posterior superior alveolar nerves (V_2): the anterior and middle superior alveolar nerves arise from the infraorbital nerve and the posterior superior alveolar nerve arises directly within the pterygopalatine fossa from the maxillary nerve).
- *Mandibular arch*—inferior alveolar nerve (V_3).

Blood supply

- *Posterior superior alveolar artery*—from the third part of the maxillary artery (within pterygopalatine fossa). Supplies the maxillary molar and premolar teeth, adjacent gingivae, and maxillary sinus.
- *Anterior superior alveolar artery*—from the infraorbital artery. Passes through the canalis sinuosus to supply the maxillary incisor and canine teeth.
- *Middle superior alveolar arteries*—from the infraorbital artery.
- *Inferior alveolar artery*—branch of the maxillary artery. Traverses the mandibular canal and supplies mandibular molars and premolars and the incisors via its mental and incisive branches. Supplies the mandible proper.

Terminology

- *Mesial*—closer to midline. Anterior-most.
- *Distal*—further away from midline. Posterior-most.
- *Labial/buccal*—aspect of tooth adjacent to lips/cheeks.
- *Lingual*—aspect of tooth facing the tongue (mandibular arch).
- *Palatal*—aspect of tooth facing hard palate (maxillary arch).
- *Occlusal*—biting surface of premolar/molar teeth.
- *Incisal*—biting surface of incisor/canine teeth.

> **Eye teeth**
>
> Colloquial term for canines due to their position in line with the eye and relative proximity of their long roots to the orbit.
>
> *'To give one's eye teeth'*—to give something one considers very precious (usually in exchange for an object/situation one desires); 'Your real sea dog will give his eye-teeth for a glass of grog'. Eye teeth were considered valuable because once they appeared it meant that a child had grown a full set of teeth (and possibly then had acquired some knowledge of the world).

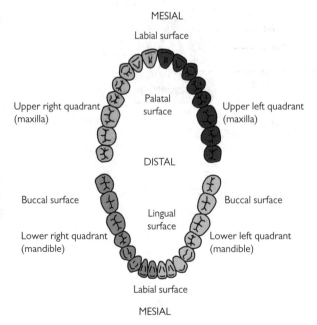

Fig. 2.19 Dental quadrants and terminology.
Reproduced courtesy of Daniel R. van Gijn.

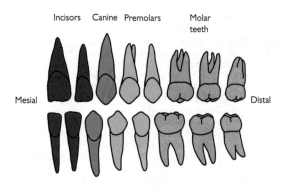

Fig. 2.20 Adult maxillary and mandibular dental arches.
Reproduced courtesy of Daniel R. van Gijn.

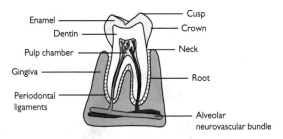

Fig. 2.21 Anatomy of a tooth.
Reproduced courtesy of Daniel R. van Gijn.

Occlusion

Overview

Dental occlusion refers to the way the teeth contact. It forms the mainstay of objective outcome in trauma surgery, orthognathic surgery, orthodontics, and reconstructive surgery. The *intercuspal position* (ICP) is the occlusal position in which cusps of the maxillary and mandibular teeth are fully interdigitated or in maximum intercuspation.

- *Trauma*—the maxillary and mandibular arches may be wired together in the ideal occlusion during repair of fractures of the mandible and maxilla. This is called intermaxillary fixation (IMF).
- *Orthognathic surgery*—literally meaning 'straight jaw' and where oral and maxillofacial surgery and orthodontics unite; the subspecialty involved with correcting growth abnormalities in the facial skeleton resulting in severe malocclusions.

Malocclusion

An appreciable deviation—both aesthetically and functional from the ideal. Edward Angle's (1855–1930) molar classification is probably the most recognized and used internationally (Fig 2.22). The mesiobuccal cusp of the upper first molar should occlude with the sulcus/groove between the mesial and distal cusps of the lower first permanent molar.

Normal occlusion: The mesiobuccal cusp of the upper first molar occludes with the buccal groove of the lower first permanent molar.

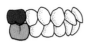

Class I malocclusion: As per normal occlusion with the presence of crowding and rotations

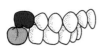

Class II malocclusion: The mesiobuccal cusp of the upper first molar occludes *anterior* to the buccal groove of the lower first molar. May be subclassified according to the incisor relationship as *Division 1* (overjet) or *Division 2* (overbite)

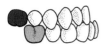

Class III malocclusion: The mesiobuccal cusp of the upper first molar occludes *posterior* to the buccal groove of the lower first molar

Fig. 2.22 Angle's classification of occlusion—based on the mesiobuccal cusp of the maxillary first molar (red) and buccal groove of the mandibular first molar (yellow).
Reproduced courtesy of Daniel R. van Gijn.

Chapter 3

The skull base

Introduction

The skull base is a complex amalgamation of bones and their respective fossae, foramina, and fissures and of multiple surgical specialties, blurring the boundaries between ear, nose, and throat (ENT) surgeons, plastic surgeons, neurosurgeons, radiologists, and oral and maxillofacial surgeons. This rough terrain is an area much loved by examiners and anatomists, and conversely (and universally) feared by students. The skull base divides the neurocranium from the viscerocranium and can be considered as having a superior/intracranial surface and an inferior/extracranial surface, the cranial base.

Intracranial surface

The intracranial region can be divided into the terraced anterior, middle, and posterior cranial fossae: the anterior fossa is the most superior.

Cranial base

The pertinent features of the cranial base are dealt with in their respective chapters, reflecting its contribution to the pharynx, auditory system, TMJ, and hard palate. It can be functionally divided into an anterior, middle and posterior regions (Fig. 3.1).

Anterior cranial base
- Extends from the upper incisors to the posterior border of the hard palate.
- Includes the orbits and paranasal sinuses.

Middle cranial base
From the posterolateral wall of the maxillary sinuses to a line drawn through the anterior margin of the foramen magnum/petro-occipital suture.
- *Pharyngeal area*—forms the roof of the nasopharynx and the origin for the pharyngobasilar fascia (to the pharyngeal tubercle).
- *Tubal area*—the cartilaginous pharyngotympanic (Eustachian) tube sits in the narrow groove between the petrous bone and the greater wing of the sphenoid.
- *Neurovascular area*—contains the carotid and jugular foramina and their respective transmitted structures, separated by the caroticojugular spine.
- *Styloid area*—the styloid process and the styloid apparatus, namely those structures derived from the second branchial arch: stylopharyngeus muscle, stylohyoid muscle and ligament, styloglossus muscle, and stylomandibular ligament.
- *Auditory area*—a small area anterolateral to the neurovascular area which contains the petrotympanic fissure (transmits the chorda tympani).
- *Articular area*—anterior to the auditory area. Contains the mandibular fossa and is bound by the capsule of the TMJ.
- *Infratemporal fossa*.

Posterior cranial base
- *Occipital (muscular) area*.

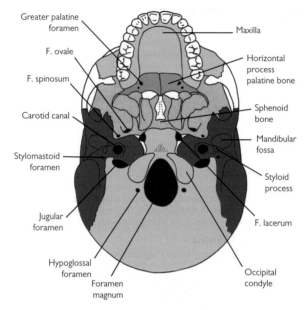

Fig. 3.1 Cranial base. Sphenoid bone yellow, temporal bones red.
Reproduced courtesy of Daniel R. van Gijn.

Anterior cranial fossa

The anterior cranial fossa (ACF) is the most superior and the shallowest of the three intracranial fossae. It lies above the nasal and orbital cavities and houses the frontal lobes, olfactory nerves, bulbs, and tracts and associated meninges (Fig. 3.2).

Boundaries

- *Anteriorly*—bound by the frontal crest and intracranial surface of the frontal bone/frontal sinus.
- *Posterolaterally*—sharply demarcated by the paired concave crests of the free edges of the lesser wings of the sphenoid (sphenoid ridge).
- *Posteromedially*—the jugum sphenoidale, which represents the anterior margin of the chiasmatic groove and connects the anterior clinoid processes.
- *Laterally*—frontal bone.
- *Floor*—the convex orbital plates of the frontal bone bilaterally, the depressed cribriform plates of the ethmoid bone centrally, and the lesser wings of the sphenoid posteriorly. The frontoethmoid suture line marks the inferior extent and is an important orbital surgical landmark.

Features and foramina

- *Frontal crest*—continuous with the sagittal sulcus which houses the superior sagittal sinus. The falx cerebri is attached to its margins.
- *Crista galli*—the cockerel's comb/crest. A true median landmark radiologically that separates the olfactory bulbs and provides attachment for the falx cerebri (Fig. 3.3 and Fig. 3.4).
- *Foramen caecum*—the primitive/previous tract connecting the ACF and dermal surface of the nose. The dural diverticulum that exists embryologically invariably involutes and the foramen caecum ossifies. It is associated with a variety of midline nasal pathologies including dermoid cysts and encephaloceles.
- *Anterior and posterior ethmoidal foramina*—transmit arteries of the same name.
- *Cribriform plate*—Latin, 'sieve-like'. Transmits fibres of the olfactory nerve and their associated meninges and is the floor of the olfactory fossa. The thickness/depth of the olfactory fossa is classified by the Keros classification (1962) and identifies anatomy at risk of erosion/prone to defect and subsequent CSF leak.
- *Fovea ethmoidalis*—roof of the ethmoid bone, lateral to and raised above, the cribriform plate. Separates the ethmoid air cells from the ACF.

Anterior cranial fossa skull base fracture

Fractures involving the posterior wall of the frontal sinus/cribriform plates assume the risk of dural breach—and the subsequent risk of CSF leak and ascending intracranial infection and abscess. Anosmia (complete loss of smell) may arise due to sheering of the olfactory nerve fibres as they traverse the cribriform plate.

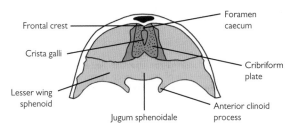

Fig. 3.2 Anterior cranial fossa, superior view.
Reproduced courtesy of Daniel R. van Gijn.

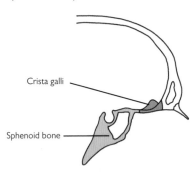

Fig. 3.3 Anterior cranial fossa, sagittal view.
Reproduced courtesy of Daniel R. van Gijn.

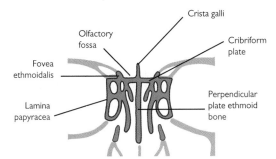

Fig. 3.4 Ethmoid bone, coronal view.
Reproduced courtesy of Daniel R. van Gijn.

Middle cranial fossa

The middle cranial fossa (MCF) houses the temporal lobes and sits deeper than the ACF. It can be subdivided into a deep lateral part and a narrower and shallower medial/central component. Its principal foramina (superior orbital fissure (SOF), foramina rotundum, ovale, and spinosum) form a crescent; with the exception of the foramen spinosum, each transmits a division of the trigeminal nerve (Fig. 3.5).

Boundaries

See Fig. 3.6.
- *Anteriorly*—crescentic margin formed by the free edge of the lesser wings of the sphenoid, the anterior part of the optic groove, and the anterior clinoid processes.
- *Posteriorly*—anterior surface of the petrous temporal bones.
- *Laterally*—squamous temporal bones, sphenoidal angle of parietal bone, and greater wing of sphenoid.

Medial part

Elevated above the lateral components of the MCF and is formed by the body of the sphenoid bone. It is bound anteriorly by the anterior margin of the optic groove and posteriorly by the dorsum sellae (Fig. 3.7). Its features from anterior to posterior are the:
- Chiasmatic groove.
- Tuberculum sellae—forms the anterior wall of the sella turcica.
- Anterior and middle clinoid processes.
- Sella turcica—the dural-lined central fossa housing the pituitary gland and flanked by the paired cavernous sinuses.
- Dorsum sellae—forms the posterior wall of the sella turcica.

Lateral part

See Figs. 3.8–3.10. Deep to support the temporal lobes of the brain. Its lateral walls are grooved by impressions formed by the middle meningeal vessels (Fig. 3.9).

Features
- *SOF*—communicates between the cavernous sinus and the orbit. Transmits cranial nerves III, IV, V$_1$, and VI, the superior ophthalmic vein, and a branch of the inferior ophthalmic vein (Fig. 3.10).
- *Foramen rotundum*—connects the MCF and pterygopalatine fossa and transmits the maxillary division of the trigeminal nerve. Inferomedial to the SOF at the base of the greater wing of the sphenoid.
- *Foramen ovale*—connects the MCF with infratemporal fossa. Its contents can easily be remembered by the mnemonic *OVALE*—Otic ganglion, V$_3$, Accessory meningeal artery, Lesser petrosal nerve (cranial nerve IX), and Emissary veins.
- *Foramen lacerum*—situated at the most anterior end of the apex of the petrous temporal bone; forms the roof of the fossa of Rosenmüller (posterolateral pharyngeal recess). Bound medially by the basilar part of the occipital bone. Structures transmitted include emissary veins connecting the pterygoid venous plexus and cavernous sinus and meningeal branches of the ascending pharyngeal artery. The

ICA passes along its superior surface. The greater petrosal nerve enters posterolaterally and exits anteriorly as part of the nerve of the pterygoid canal (Vidian nerve).

- *Foramen spinosum*—in the greater wing of the sphenoid. Transmits the middle meningeal artery and vein and owes its name to its proximity to the spine of the sphenoid on its inferior aspect.
- *Hiatuses for the greater and lesser petrosal nerves.*
- *Carotid canal*— within petrous temporal bone. Transmits the ICA which enters the MCF above the foramen lacerum. The entrance to the carotid canal is found externally (termed the carotid foramen), anterior to the jugular fossa (Fig. 3.8).
- *Fossa for trigeminal ganglion.*
- *Arcuate eminence*—bony projection of the superior semicircular canal.
- *Tegmen tympani*—thin plate of bone covering the tympanic cavity, antrum, and Eustachian tube. Separates the middle ear from the dura mater of the temporal lobe of the cerebral hemisphere.
- *Foramen Vesalii*—variable small foramen between the scaphoid fossa and foramen ovale. When present, it transmits the sphenoidal emissary vein and connects the pterygoid venous plexus within the infratemporal fossa with the cavernous sinus (thus represents a pathway for spread of infection from extracranial to intracranial/cavernous sinus).

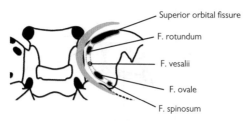

Superior orbital fissure
F. rotundum
F. vesalii
F. ovale
F. spinosum

Fig. 3.5 Crescentic arrangement of middle cranial fossa foramina.
Reproduced courtesy of Daniel R. van Gijn.

Etymology

- *Spinosum*—from Latin *spina* meaning 'thorn'. Refers to its location next to the spine of sphenoid.
- *Lacerum*—Latin for 'mangled' or 'torn', referring to its irregular appearance.
- *Tegmen*—Latin for 'cover' or 'roof'.
- *Andreas Vesalius*—considered the founding father of human anatomy. Sixteenth-century Flemish anatomist and author of *De humani corporis fabrica* ('On the fabric of the human body').

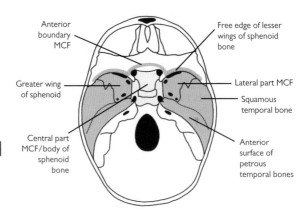

Fig. 3.6 Middle cranial fossa (MCF), central and lateral parts.
Reproduced courtesy of Daniel R. van Gijn.

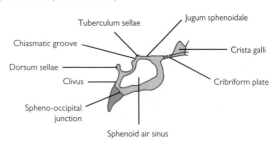

Fig. 3.7 Middle cranial fossa, central part.
Reproduced courtesy of Daniel R. van Gijn.

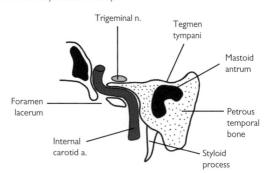

Fig. 3.8 Right carotid canal, coronal view.
Reproduced courtesy of Daniel R. van Gijn.

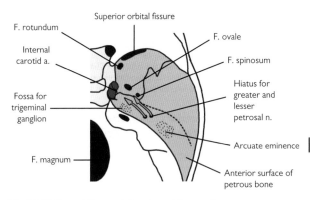

Fig. 3.9 Middle cranial fossa, right lateral aspect (grey area).
Reproduced courtesy of Daniel R. van Gijn.

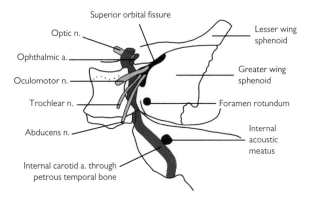

Fig. 3.10 Relationship of structures in the middle cranial fossa.
Reproduced courtesy of Daniel R. van Gijn.

Posterior cranial fossa

The posterior cranial fossa (PCF) is the deepest, most posterior component of the cranial cavity and houses the brainstem and cerebellum. At its lowest part it is monopolized by the central foramen magnum. The PCF is formed by the occipital bone and the posterior surfaces of the petrous temporal bones (Fig. 3.11). The triangular circumference of the latter is bounded by the superior and inferior petrosal sinuses and the sigmoid sinus (Fig. 3.12).

Boundaries of the posterior cranial fossa

- *Anteriorly*—posterior surface of the petrous part of the temporal bone.
- *Posterior*—occipital bone.
- *Lateral*—squamous and mastoid parts of the temporal bone.

Features

See Fig. 3.13.

- *Internal acoustic meatus*—transmits neurovascular structures (facial and vestibulocochlear nerves and labyrinthine artery and vein) from the PCF to the inner and middle ears.
- *Foramen magnum*—Latin, meaning large opening. Oval and broader posteriorly. Contains the medulla oblongata (with meninges), CSF, right and left vertebral arteries and veins with the vertebral plexuses of sympathetic nerves, and the spinal accessory nerves. The anterior (midline) margin is the basion and the posterior (midline) margin is the opisthion.
- *Groove for superior petrosal sinus*—drains the cavernous sinus into the transverse sinus. Receives the labyrinthine, inferior cerebral, and cerebellar veins.
- *Jugular foramen*—the large, irregularly shaped conduit between the jugular fossa of the petrous temporal bone and the jugular process of the occipital bone. Traditionally subdivided by the jugular spine into an anteromedial pars nervosa and posterolateral pars vascularis. The former transmits the inferior petrosal sinus and glossopharyngeal nerve (and Jacobsen's tympanic branch) while the latter transmits the vagus (and Arnold's auricular branch/the Alderman's nerve), and the accessory nerve and jugular bulb (Fig. 3.14).
- *Hypoglossal canal*—traverses the occipital condyles from posteromedial to anterolateral and transmits the hypoglossal nerve.
- *Vestibular aqueduct*—situated on the posterior surface of the petrous temporal bone. Transmits the endolymphatic duct and sac from the inner ear to the posterior cranial fossa.

Acoustic neuroma

Acoustic neuroma is a benign tumour of the Schwann cells of the vestibulo-cochlear nerve, and is the most common lesion of the cerebellopontine angle. Initial presentation is unilateral hearing loss when confined to the bony internal auditory meatus that may be falsely attributed to ageing. Other otological symptoms include tinnitus and dizziness. With tumour enlargement, adjacent cranial nerves may be compressed, with the following sequelae:

- *Facial nerve*—ipsilateral facial weakness.
- *Trigeminal nerve*—ipsilateral facial sensory loss.
- *Abducens nerve*—ipsilateral paralysis of lateral rectus (conjugate gaze palsy).

Etymology

- *Magnum*—Latin meaning 'great'. Consider use of the term 'magnum' in bottle of wine (1.5 L) and firearm (0.44 Magnum revolver).
- *Ludwig Levin Jacobson (1783–1843)*—lends his name to the tympanic branch of the glossopharyngeal nerve. Referred otalgia may originate from pathology arising within the sensory net of cranial nerves V, VII, IX, and X.
- *Philipp Friedrich Arnold (1803–1890)*—professor of anatomy and physiology at Heidelberg. Described the reflex of coughing/syncope on stimulation of the external acoustic meatus and lends his name to the auricular branch of the vagus nerve.
- *Alderman's nerve*—an alternative name for the auricular branch of the vagus nerve. Stimulating the external acoustic meatus is thought to provoke gastric emptying: apparently aldermen would stick their fingers in their ears to induce gastric emptying following a gluttonous meal.

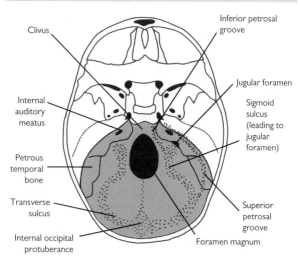

Fig. 3.11 Posterior cranial fossa (grey area).
Reproduced courtesy of Daniel R. van Gijn.

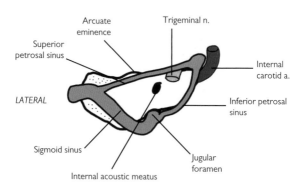

Fig. 3.12 Petrosal venous sinuses (posterior surface, left petrous temporal bone).
Reproduced courtesy of Daniel R. van Gijn.

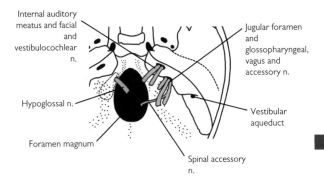

Fig. 3.13 Features of the posterior cranial fossa.
Reproduced courtesy of Daniel R. van Gijn.

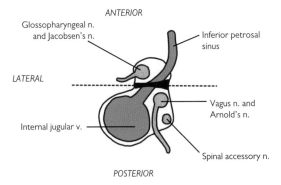

Fig. 3.14 Pars nervosa (above dotted line) and pars vascularis (below dotted line)
(extracranial view of right jugular fossa).
Reproduced courtesy of Daniel R. van Gijn.

Pituitary fossa

The pituitary fossa is a dural-lined hollow within the central part of the sphenoid bone and MCF. It resembles a Turkish saddle, hence its alternative, elegant, name of sella turcica (Fig. 3.15).

Boundaries
- *Lateral*—dural slings between anterior and posterior clinoid processes.
- *Anterior*—middle clinoid process (laterally).
- *Posterior*—dorsum sellae, a vertical strut of bone.
- *Floor*—roof of the sphenoid air sinuses.
- *Roof*—the diaphragm sella, a fold of dura attached to the anterior and posterior clinoid processes.

Contents
- Pituitary gland.
- Pituitary vessels.
- Anterior and posterior intercavernous sinuses connecting the right and left cavernous sinuses.
- CSF.

Relations
- *Laterally*—cavernous sinus. The ICA lies in a shallow groove in the lateral wall of the body of the sphenoid as it ascends from the carotid canal through the cavernous sinus (Fig. 3.16).
- *Anteriorly*—sphenoid sinus. The optic canals proceed laterally from the sulcus chiasmatis, which is posterior to the jugum sphenoidale forming the upper anterior boundary of fossa.
- *Posteriorly*—basilar artery and pons.
- *Inferiorly*—sphenoid sinus.
- *Superiorly*—optic chiasm lies posterosuperior to the sulcus chiasmatis.

Etymology
- *Pituitary*—from Latin *pituitarius* meaning 'mucous'; *pituita* meaning 'phlegm' or 'clammy moisture'. Name assigned to gland because it was thought to be responsible for secreting mucus through the nose.
- *Sella turcica*—meaning 'Turkish seat'. The saddle-shaped depression in the body of the sphenoid bone.
- *Clivus (of Blumenbach)*—meaning 'slope'. The gentle slope formed from the sphenoid body and basiocciput. Johann Friedrich Blumenbach (1752–1840).

Empty sella syndrome
Damage to the pituitary gland may be congenital, neoplastic, or iatrogenic; it becoming flattened and shrinks. CSF occupies the space of the pituitary fossa and gives the appearance of an 'empty sella' on magnetic resonance imaging.

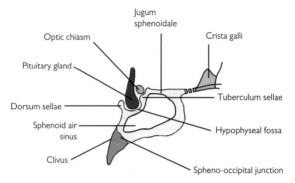

Fig. 3.15 Floor of the middle cranial fossa and pituitary fossa.
Reproduced courtesy of Daniel R. van Gijn.

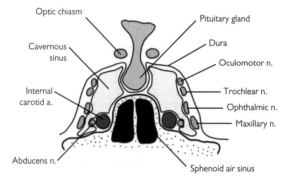

Fig. 3.16 Relations of the pituitary gland.
Reproduced courtesy of Daniel R. van Gijn.

Cavernous sinus

Dural venous sinuses lying on either side of the pituitary fossa, connected via the anterior and posterior intercavernous sinuses. Each extends from the orbital apex to the apex of the petrous temporal bone and invests the cavernous segment of the ICA. Tributaries include the superior and inferior ophthalmic veins, superficial middle cerebral vein, inferior cerebral veins, and sphenoparietal sinus. The multiple cavities (or caverns) within the cavernous sinuses are separated by fibrous septa.

Boundaries

- *Medial*—sphenoid air cells and pituitary gland.
- *Lateral*—uncus of the temporal lobe.
- *Anterior*—medial end of the SOF.
- *Posterior*—apex of the petrous temporal bone.
- *Roof*—dura attached to the anterior and middle clinoid processes.
- *Floor*—greater wing of the sphenoid.

Drainage

- To the transverse sinus via the superior petrosal sinus.
- To the IJV via the inferior petrosal sinus.
- To the pterygoid plexus via veins travelling through the foramen ovale and foramen lacerum.
- To the facial vein via the superior ophthalmic vein.

Contents

See Fig. 3.17.
- The cavernous segment of the ICA.
- Sympathetic plexus travel through the sinus on the ICA.
- Abducens nerve (lateral to internal carotid siphon).
- Oculomotor and trochlear nerves laterally.
- V_1 and V_2 course in the lateral wall.

Pathway for intracranial infection and cavernous sinus thrombosis

Pathology
- Narrow sinus drainage channels become blocked with inspissated mucus.
- Mucous stasis results in subsequent infection.
- Frontal and sphenoidal sinuses are in close proximity to the dura and cavernous sinus.
- Extension of infection to frontal lobe and abscess development may occur.
- May cause development of cavernous sinus thrombosis.
- Midface infection (commonly furuncle) may be a frequent cause.

Features of cavernous sinus thrombosis
Symptoms relate primarily to venous obstruction and/or impingement of adjacent cranial nerves:
- *General*—headache, fever, proptosis, periorbital oedema, chemosis.
- *Cranial nerve signs*—ophthalmoplegia (lateral gaze often initially due to location of VI), forehead paraesthesia (V_1), and ptosis and mydriasis (III).

(a)

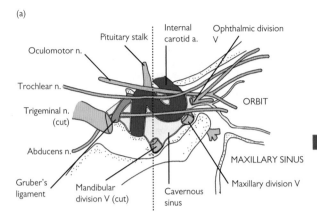

(b)

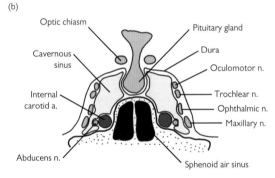

Fig. 3.17 (a) Relations of the cavernous sinus, sagittal section (optic nerve/chiasm not shown). (b) Coronal section through dotted line in Fig. 3.17a.

Reproduced courtesy of Daniel R. van Gijn.

Etymology

- *Cavernous*—meaning 'full of cavities/caverns' or 'porous'.
- *Clinoid*—from 'cline' meaning 'bed'. *Clinical* teaching refers to bedside teaching and shares a common stem.

Circle of Willis

A complex arterial anastomosis, the circle of Willis, unites the internal carotid and vertebrobasilar systems on the base of the brain: there is considerable individual variation in the pattern and calibre of vessels that make up the circle. It lies in the subarachnoid space and allows cross-circulation of the brain. (Fig. 3.18). The ICA contributes up to 90% to the circle.

Anterior circulation

After traversing the neck without branching, the ICA enters the skull via the carotid canal of the petrous temporal bone, taking a series of right-angled turns before passing anteriorly through the cavernous sinus as the carotid siphon. It leaves the cavernous sinus by piercing the dura medial to the anterior clinoid processes, before bifurcating into its terminal branches, the anterior and middle cerebral arteries.

Branches within carotid canal
- *Caroticotympanic artery to middle ear.*
- *Vidian artery.*

Branches within cavernous sinus
- *Dural and meningeal branches.*
- *Inferior hypophysial branches.*

Intracranial branches of the internal carotid artery
- *Anterior cerebral*—passes superior to the optic nerve. Is joined by the anterior communicating artery which divides it into pre-communicating (A1) and post-communicating (A2) segments.
- *Middle cerebral*—continuation of the ICA. Supplies the frontal, parietal, and superior temporal lobes.
- *Ophthalmic*—runs in the optic canal with the optic nerve. Surrounded by dural sheath.
- *Posterior communicating*—communicates with the posterior cerebral arteries from the posterior circulation.
- *Anterior choroidal*—supplies the choroid plexus of the third and lateral ventricles. May arise from the middle cerebral artery.

Posterior circulation

Constituted by the paired vertebral arteries (from the first part of the subclavian arteries), which ascend cranially through the vertebral foramina of the upper six cervical vertebrae. After exiting the foramina in the lateral masses of the atlas, they pass posteromedially on the posterior arch of the atlas, piercing the spinal dura and atlanto-occipital membrane to enter the cranial cavity via the foramen magnum. They lie on the anterior surface of the medulla oblongata and unite at the inferior border of the pons to form the basilar artery, which supplies the superior spinal cord, brainstem, cerebellum, and posteroinferior cerebral cortex and contributes to the circle of Willis.

Branches of the vertebral artery
- *Anterior and posterior spinal arteries.*
- *Posterior inferior cerebellar artery (PICA)*—supplies inferior surface cerebellum and part of the medulla. Displays anatomical variation.

Branches of the basilar artery
- *Anterior inferior cerebellar artery (AICA)*—closely related to the facial and vestibulocochlear nerves. May branch from the vertebral arteries.
- *Internal auditory*—travels with the facial and vestibulocochlear nerves through the internal auditory meatus.
- *Lateral pontine.*
- *Superior cerebellar*—supplies the superior surface of the cerebellum.
- *Posterior cerebral*—linked to the ipsilateral ICA and anterior circulation via the posterior communicating artery. Supplies the majority of the temporal and occipital lobes.

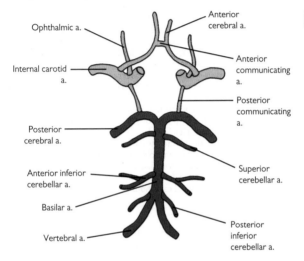

Fig. 3.18 Circle of Willis.
Reproduced courtesy of Daniel R. van Gijn.

- *Thomas Willis (1621–1675)*—English physician and author of *Cerebri anatome* (illustrated by Sir Christopher Wren) in which the term 'neurology' was first coined. Contains a description of the eponymous circulatory anastomosis. Willis is also credited with first using the term *mellitus* (meaning honeyed or sweet) to describe the sweet taste of glycosuria (*Willis's disease* was the old name for diabetes mellitus) and the accessory nerve, sometimes known as the nerve of Willis.

Venous drainage

A system of both paired and unpaired, valveless, deep, and superficial veins empty into the dural venous sinuses, which lie between the endosteal and meningeal layers of the dura mater. The sinuses drain mainly into the right and left IJV.

Paired sinuses

See Fig. 3.19.

- *Transverse sinus*—drains the occipital, superior sagittal, and straight sinuses, emptying into the sigmoid sinus.
- *Sigmoid sinus*—lies in a deep groove on the petrous part of the temporal bone. A continuation of the transverse sinus at the termination of the tentorium cerebelli, receiving the superior petrosal sinus. As its name suggest, it is S-shaped. Travels posteromedial to the mastoid air cells, terminating at the jugular bulb, where it is continuous with the IJV in the jugular foramen.
- *Superior petrosal sinus*—connects the cavernous sinus anteriorly with the transverse sinus posteriorly. Drains the cerebellar, inferior cerebral, and labyrinthine veins.
- *Inferior petrosal sinus*—connects the cavernous sinus anteriorly with the superior bulb of the IJV posteriorly. Located between the petrous temporal and basilar occipital bones.
- *Sphenoparietal sinus*—drains into the cavernous sinus and is located along the lesser wing of the sphenoid, receiving the middle meningeal, superficial middle cerebral (Sylvian), and anterior temporal diploic veins.
- *Basilar venous plexus*—a plexiform network connecting the inferior and superior petrosal sinuses and cavernous and intercavernous sinuses.

Unpaired sinuses

See Fig. 3.20.

- *Superior sagittal sinus*—largest sinus extending from the anterior falx cerebri to the occipital protuberance and confluence of the sinuses. Receives the diploic, cerebral, and meningeal veins. Deviates towards the right and is continuous with the right transverse sinus.
- *Inferior sagittal sinus*—courses along the inferior aspect of the falx cerebri, terminating in the straight sinus.
- *Straight sinus*—receives drainage from the great cerebral vein and inferior sagittal sinus, and drains into the confluence of the sinuses.
- *Occipital sinus*—lies on the occipital bone and is the smallest venous sinus, receiving venous drainage from the margin of the foramen magnum (internal vertebral plexus of veins), drains into the confluence of the sinuses.
- *Anterior and posterior intercavernous sinuses*—lie on the anterior and posterior margins of the diaphragm sellae, respectively and connect the right and left cavernous sinuses and the basilar plexus.
- *Confluence of the sinuses*—common venous space at the internal occipital protuberance. Receives the superior sagittal sinus, straight sinus, and occipital sinus and leads into the transverse sinuses.

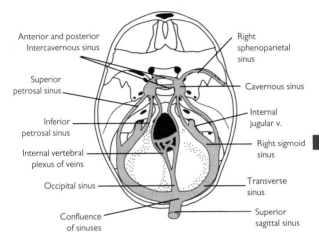

Fig. 3.19 Intracranial venous sinuses, superior view.
Reproduced courtesy of Daniel R. van Gijn.

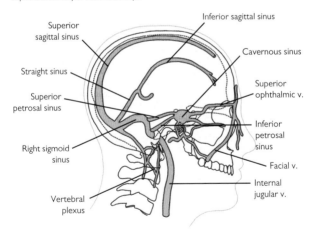

Fig. 3.20 Intracranial venous sinuses, lateral view.
Reproduced courtesy of Daniel R. van Gijn.

Infratemporal fossa

The infratemporal fossa is an irregular-shaped cavity with no anatomical floor found deep to the mandibular ramus and zygomatic arch and posterior to the maxilla. It serves as a thoroughfare for neurovascular structures entering or leaving the cranial cavity: in some descriptions, it encompasses the masticator and parapharyngeal spaces. Its principal occupants are the muscles of mastication, the first and second parts of the maxillary artery, the pterygoid venous plexus, the mandibular division of the trigeminal nerve (V₃) and the otic ganglion.

Boundaries

There is a lack of consensus in the surgical literature concerning the boundaries and contents of the infratemporal fossa. Despite its name, it lies predominantly below the infratemporal crest of the greater wing of the sphenoid (Fig. 3.21).

- *Medial*—lateral pterygoid plate, pterygomaxillary fissure, superior pharyngeal constrictor, tensor veli palatini and levator veli palatini.
- *Lateral*—mandibular ramus.
- *Anterior*—posterior surface of the maxilla and inferior orbital fissure (perpendicular to pterygopalatine fissure).
- *Posterior*—carotid sheath, prevertebral fascia.
- *Roof*—greater wing of sphenoid bone and squamous temporal bone.

Contents

See Fig. 3.22.

- *Muscles*—insertions of temporalis, medial, and lateral pterygoid muscles. The lateral pterygoid acts as a key landmark (medial pterygoid and V₃ lie deep, the maxillary artery lies superficially, the lingual and inferior alveolar nerves are inferior, the pterygoid venous plexus lies within, and the deep temporal neurovascular bundle is superior).
- *Artery*—the first and second parts of the maxillary artery and its branches. The artery passes between the two heads of the lateral pterygoid and into the pterygopalatine fossa.
- *Fat*—part of the buccal fat pad.
- *Vein*—pterygoid venous plexus.
- *Nerve*—V₃ and branches. Chorda tympani, posterior superior alveolar nerve and otic ganglion.
- *Ligament*—sphenomandibular ligament.

Foramina and fissures

See Fig. 3.23.

- *Foramen ovale*—transmits V₃.
- *Sphenoidal emissary foramen (of Vesalius)*—lies medial to foramen ovale (when present). Transmits an emissary vein.
- *Foramen spinosum*—meningeal branch of V₃. Transmits the middle meningeal artery and vein.
- *Mandibular foramen*—inferior alveolar neurovascular bundle.
- *Pterygomaxillary fissure*—transmits the maxillary artery and tributaries of the pterygoid venous plexus.
- *Petrotympanic fissure*—transmits the chorda tympani (from medial aspect), the anterior tympanic artery and vein, and the anterior ligament of the malleus.

- *Foramen lacerum.*
- *Alveolar foramina and maxillary tuberosity*—transmit the posterior superior alveolar neurovascular bundle.

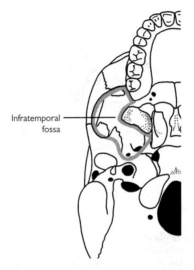

Fig. 3.21 Boundaries of the right infratemporal fossa, base of skull.
Reproduced courtesy of Daniel R. van Gijn.

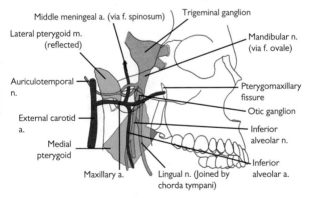

Fig. 3.22 Structures within the infratemporal fossa.
Reproduced courtesy of Daniel R. van Gijn.

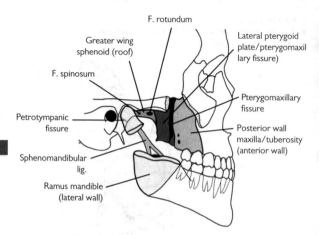

Fig. 3.23 Boundaries and foramina of the right infratemporal fossa.
Reproduced courtesy of Daniel R. van Gijn.

Stylohamular plane

A surgical plane extending from the pterygoid hamulus to the styloid process. The jugular foramen and carotid canal lie medial to this plane and therefore lateral skull base dissections in this region are limited by this plane.

Pterygopalatine fossa

A small, inverted pyramidal space immediately inferolateral to the apex of the orbit; an area that unnecessarily strikes concern into the heart of students. It is effectively a medial continuation of the infratemporal fossa, beyond the bottleneck of the pterygomaxillary fissure laterally and restrained by the nasopharynx medially. It communicates with the nasal cavity, nasopharynx, MCF and cavernous sinus, the orbital cavity and the infratemporal fossa, and so it is a true keystone to understanding the anatomy of this region.

Boundaries

See Fig. 3.24.

- *Medial*—perpendicular plate of the palatine bone.
- *Lateral*—pterygomaxillary fissure.
- *Anterior*—superomedial surface of the infratemporal maxilla.
- *Superior*—the greater wing of the sphenoid and the IOF.
- *Posterior*—root of the pterygoid process and anterior surface of the greater wing of the sphenoid.

Contents

See Fig. 3.25.

Maxillary nerve

Passes through the foramen rotundum to the posterior wall of the pterygopalatine fossa. All its extracranial branches arise from within the fossa: branches arise either directly from the nerve or from the pterygopalatine ganglion. Its terminal branch, the infraorbital nerve, runs laterally to enter the orbit via the inferior orbital fissure where it acts as a landmark to delineate the infratemporal fossa laterally and the pterygopalatine fossa medially.

Main trunk

- *Zygomatic nerve*—enters the orbit via the inferior orbital fissure. Divides into the zygomaticofacial and zygomaticofacial nerves.
- *Infraorbital nerve*—the terminal branch of the maxillary nerve.
- *Posterior superior alveolar nerve*.

Ganglionic branches

- Meningeal, ganglionic, zygomatic, posterior, middle and anterior superior alveolar nerves, and infraorbital nerves.

Pterygopalatine ganglion

The largest of the peripheral parasympathetic ganglia, situated deep in the pterygopalatine fossa adjacent to the sphenopalatine foramen. Many of the branches are sensory and are not connected with the ganglion functionally, but simply pass through to the maxillary nerve.

- Anterior to the pterygoid canal and foramen rotundum.
- Inferior to the maxillary nerve as it traverses the pterygopalatine fossa.
- Preganglionic parasympathetic fibres to pterygopalatine ganglion travel initially in the greater petrosal branch of the facial nerve, subsequently as part of the nerve of the pterygoid canal.
- The nerve of the pterygoid canal enters the ganglion posteriorly.

- *Postganglionic parasympathetic fibres*—join the maxillary nerve. Some may travel in the zygomatic and zygomaticotemporal branches of V_3 to the lacrimal gland, but most are now believed to travel directly to the gland via orbital branches.
- *Postganglionic sympathetic fibres*—pass through the ganglion without synapsing and supply vessels and orbitalis (having arisen in the superior cervical ganglion). Travel via the internal carotid plexus.
- Sensory branches of the maxillary nerve travel through the pterygopalatine ganglion without synapsing (orbital, nasopalatine, posterior superior nasal, greater palatine, lesser palatine, and pharyngeal nerves).

Blood supply
- The maxillary artery passes via the pterygomaxillary fissure from the infratemporal fossa to the pterygopalatine fossa, where it terminates as the third part of the artery. Its branches accompany similarly named nerves.
- *Branches*—posterior superior alveolar, infraorbital, artery of pterygoid canal, pharyngeal, greater palatine and sphenopalatine arteries.
- Veins are small and variable. The sphenopalatine vein is the most consistent, draining the posterior nasal cavity and passing into the pterygopalatine fossa via the sphenopalatine foramen. Ultimately it enters the pterygoid venous plexus via the pterygomaxillary fissure.
- The inferior ophthalmic vein drains into the pterygoid venous plexus via the inferior orbital fissure.

Communications and foramina
- *Medial*—nasal cavity via the sphenopalatine foramen (transmits sphenopalatine artery, nasopalatine nerve, and posterior superior nasal nerves).
- *Anterior*—orbit via medial end of the inferior orbital fissure.
- *Lateral*—infratemporal fossa via the pterygomaxillary fissure.
- *Posterior*—MCF/Meckel's cave via the foramen rotundum (transmits V_3). The pterygoid canal in the posterior wall transmits the nerve of the pterygoid (Vidian) canal. The palatovaginal (pharyngeal) canal transmits the pharyngeal branch of the maxillary artery and the pharyngeal nerve (V_2).

Pterygopalatine ganglion
Largest of the peripheral parasympathetic ganglia. Principally secretomotor to the lacrimal gland and the mucosae of the nasal cavity and paranasal sinuses, and hence known as the 'ganglion of hayfever'.

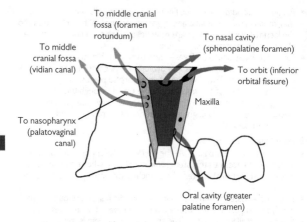

Fig. 3.24 Foramina, boundaries, and communications of the right pterygopalatine fossa. Middle, red: perpendicular plate of the palatine bone. Left, yellow: root of the pterygoid process and anterior surface of the greater wing of the sphenoid bone. Right, grey: the greater wing of the sphenoid bone. Viewed through the pterygomaxillary fissure.

Reproduced courtesy of Daniel R. van Gijn.

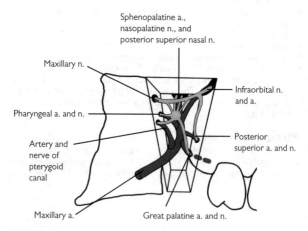

Fig. 3.25 Structures in the right pterygopalatine fossa.

Reproduced courtesy of Daniel R. van Gijn.

Summary tables

See Tables 3.1–3.3.

Table 3.1 Summary table of cranial foramina and their respective contents

Opening	Contents (cranial nerve)
Cribriform plate	Olfactory nerve (I)
Optic canal	Optic nerve (II)
	Ophthalmic artery
Superior orbital fissure	Oculomotor nerve (III)
	Trochlear nerve (IV)
	Ophthalmic division of trigeminal nerve (V$_1$)
	Abducens nerve (VI)
	Superior ophthalmic vein
Foramen rotundum	Maxillary division of trigeminal nerve (V$_2$)
Foramen ovale	Mandibular division of trigeminal nerve (V$_3$)
	Accessory meningeal artery
Foramen spinosum	Middle meningeal artery
Internal auditory canal	Facial nerve (VII)
	Vestibulocochlear nerve (VIII)
Jugular foramen	Glossopharyngeal nerve (IX)
	Vagus nerve (X)
	Spinal accessory nerve (XI)
	Internal jugular vein
Hypoglossal canal	Hypoglossal nerve (XII)
Foramen magnum	Lower end of medulla oblongata and meninges
	CSF
	Vertebral arteries and veins and associated sympathetic plexuses
	Spinal arteries
	Hypoglossal nerves (XII)
	Spinal accessory nerve (XI)
	Apical ligament of the dens and the tectorial membrane pass through it to attach to the internal basiocciput

Table 3.2 Skull base cranial nerve syndromes

Syndrome and causes	Structures affected (cranial nerve)	Symptoms
Superior orbital fissure syndrome (Rochon-Duvigneaud syndrome) (Tolosa Hunt syndrome is an inflammatory cause of superior orbital fissure syndrome) Trauma, tumours, inflammatory conditions (granulomatosis with polyangiitis (formerly Wegener's granulomatosis), sarcoid, polyarteritis nodosa)	Oculomotor nerve (III) Trochlear nerve (IV) Ophthalmic division of trigeminal nerve (V_1) Abducens nerve (VI)	Ophthalmoplegia/ diplopia Forehead paraesthesia Ptosis Exophthalmos
Orbital apex syndrome Trauma, tumours, inflammatory conditions (granulomatosis with polyangiitis, sarcoid, polyarteritis nodosa)	Optic nerve (II) Oculomotor nerve (III) Trochlear nerve (IV) Ophthalmic division of trigeminal nerve (V_1) Abducens nerve (VI)	As for superior orbital fissure syndrome—with blindness on the affected side because the optic nerve is involved
Cavernous sinus syndrome Vascular (thrombosis, aneurysms), tumours, and inflammatory conditions	Oculomotor nerve (III) Trochlear nerve (IV) Ophthalmic and maxillary divisions of trigeminal nerve (V_1 and V_2) Abducens nerve (VI)	Ophthalmoplegia Orbital congestion Paraesthesia in V_1 and V_2 distribution Horner's syndrome (involvement of sympathetic fibres associated with internal carotid artery /abducens nerve)
Petrous apex syndrome (Gradenigo's syndrome) Suppurative otitis media with subsequent inflammation at petrous apex	Ophthalmic division of trigeminal nerve (V_1) Abducens nerve (VI)	Retro-orbital pain Reduced corneal sensitivity Lateral rectus palsy/ diplopia Otitis media May spread to jugular foramen and involve cranial nerves IX, X, and XI

Table 3.3 Summary of syndromes associated with compression of cranial nerves

Syndrome	Structures affected (cranial nerve)	Symptoms
Jugular foramen syndrome (Vernet's syndrome) Primary tumours (glomus jugulare tumours, meningioma, vestibular schwannoma), trauma, jugular venous thrombosis	Glossopharyngeal nerve (IX) Vagus nerve (X) Spinal accessory nerve (XI)	Difficulty swallowing Hoarse voice/dysphonia Ipsilateral soft palate paralysis Uvular deviation towards normal side Numbness posterior 1/3 tongue Loss of gag reflex Paresis of ipsilateral SCM and trapezius muscles
Retropharyngeal space syndrome (Villaret's syndrome) Tumour/trauma involving retroparotid/retropharyngeal space ICA pathology	Glossopharyngeal nerve (IX) Vagus nerve (X) Spinal accessory nerve (XI) Hypoglossal nerve (XII) Sympathetic trunk	As per Vernet's syndrome plus: Deviation of tongue to the affected side Horner's syndrome (enophthalmos, miosis, partial ptosis, anhidrosis, enophthalmos)
Condylar jugular syndrome (Collet–Sicard syndrome) Metastatic disease	Glossopharyngeal nerve (IX) Vagus nerve (X) Spinal accessory nerve (XI) Hypoglossal nerve (XII)	As per Vernet's syndrome plus: Deviation of tongue to affected side
Carotid canal syndrome	ICA Venous plexus Sympathetic plexus	Horner's syndrome

Chapter 4

The cranial nerves

Introduction

There are 12 pairs of cranial nerves that are individually named and numbered using Roman numerals in a rostrocaudal sequence. Unlike spinal nerves, only some cranial nerves are mixed in function, i.e. they carry both sensory and motor fibres; others are purely sensory or motor and some may also carry pre- or postganglionic parasympathetic fibres.

- The olfactory nerve (I) is concerned with olfaction (the sense of smell).
- The optic nerve (II) contains the axons of retinal ganglion cells.
- The oculomotor nerve (III) innervates levator palpebrae superioris and four of the extraocular muscles (superior, inferior, and medial rectus and inferior oblique). It also contains preganglionic parasympathetic axons that synapse in the ciliary ganglion.
- The trochlear nerve (IV) innervates superior oblique.
- The trigeminal nerve (V) has extensive sensory, motor, and autonomic components. It has three main divisions, ophthalmic (V_1), maxillary (V_2), and mandibular (V_3). The ophthalmic division has three main branches, the lacrimal, frontal, and nasociliary nerves, which collectively innervate the upper part of the face (conjunctiva, skin over the forehead, upper eyelid, and much of the external surface of the nose). The maxillary division contains sensory fibres destined for the nose, lower eyelid, cheek, palate, maxillary teeth, and gingivae and mucosa of the nasopharynx behind the pharyngotympanic tube. Sensory branches of the mandibular division supply the mandibular teeth and gingivae, the fibrous capsule of the TMJ, the skin in the temporal region, part of the auricle and the lower lip, the lower part of the face, and the mucosa of the anterior two-thirds (presulcal part) of the tongue and the floor of the oral cavity. Motor branches of the mandibular division innervate the muscles of mastication, tensor veli palatini, tensor tympani, anterior belly of digastric, and mylohyoid. The auriculotemporal nerve carries postganglionic secretomotor parasympathetic fibres to the parotid gland.
- The abducens nerve (VI) innervates the ipsilateral lateral rectus.
- The facial nerve (VII) contains motor axons that supply muscles derived from the second branchial arch, namely the mimetic facial muscles, buccinator, stapedius, platysma, the posterior belly of digastric, and stylohyoid. It also contains sensory axons that carry taste from the anterior two-thirds of the tongue via the chorda tympani, and cutaneous sensation, including pain, from the posterior aspect of the external acoustic meatus (NB: the innervation of this region is complex). Preganglionic parasympathetic neurons in the superior salivatory nucleus pass via either the chorda tympani to the submandibular ganglion or the greater petrosal nerve and the nerve of the pterygoid canal to the pterygopalatine ganglion.
- The vestibulocochlear nerve (VIII) consists of the vestibular nerve, concerned with balance, and the cochlear nerve, concerned with hearing.

- The glossopharyngeal nerve (IX) contains motor fibres to stylopharyngeus; parasympathetic secretomotor fibres to the parotid gland (derived from the inferior salivatory nucleus); sensory fibres to the tympanic cavity, pharyngotympanic tube, fauces, tonsils, nasopharynx, uvula, and posterior (postsulcal) third of the tongue; and gustatory fibres from the circumvallate papillae.
- The vagus nerve (X) is a large mixed nerve, containing branchiomotor nerve fibres, general visceral afferents, and preganglionic parasympathetic fibres. It has a more extensive course and distribution than any other cranial nerve, running through the neck, thorax, and abdomen.
- The accessory nerve (XI) is conventionally described as having a cranial root composed of a variable number of small rootlets that emerge from the postolivary groove of the dorsolateral medulla, caudal to the rootlets of the vagus, and join the pharyngeal plexus, and a spinal root that supplies trapezius and sternocleidomastoid.
- The hypoglossal nerve (XII) is motor to all the muscles of the tongue except palatoglossus.

Olfactory nerve

The first, shortest, and most rostral of the cranial nerves. It represents an extension of the central nervous system (CNS) and conveys the sense of smell (Fig. 4.1).

- Olfactory epithelium covers the superior medial vertical lamellae of the superior turbinates, a similar small portion of the middle turbinates, and the corresponding nasal septum.
- Olfactory receptor neurons are bipolar. Their cell bodies lie in the olfactory epithelium; a single unbranched apical dendrite bearing sensory receptors extends to the epithelial surface, and a basally directed unmyelinated axon passes in the opposite direction, joining other axons to form bundles that coalesce and ultimately pass through the cribriform plate (ethmoid bone) to enter the olfactory bulb, where they synapse in glomeruli on mitral and other cells.
- Olfactory supporting cells ensheath these bundles of axons and have elicited considerable interest as a possible source of transplantable cells capable of supporting CNS axonal regeneration.
- Olfactory axons are wrapped in meningeal sheaths (the anatomical basis of CSF rhinorrhoea occurring usually after trauma or surgery involving the anterior skull base).

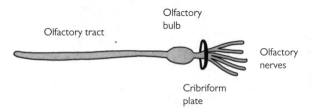

Fig. 4.1 The olfactory nerve, schematic.
Reproduced courtesy of Daniel R. van Gijn.

Anosmia

- Anosmia is the absence of the function of smell (distinct from *ageusia* which is the absence of taste function).
- Causes may be traumatic, infective, or congenital.
- Head trauma may cause anosmia/hyposmia *indirectly* due to mechanical obstruction secondary to injuries to the nose/sinuses or *directly* via shearing of the primary olfactory axons as they pass through the cribriform plate.
- *Kallmann syndrome*—congenital hypogonadotropic hypogonadism characterized by delayed onset of puberty and cleft lip/palate associated with anosmia/hyposmia.

Optic nerve

The second cranial nerve carrying special sensory information for sight
(Fig. 4.2). Like the olfactory nerve it is essentially an outposting of the CNS
with ocular, orbital, canalicular, and intracranial components. It is largely
supplied by the ophthalmic and central retinal arteries.
- Carries axons of retinal ganglion cells which converge at the optic disc
  to form the optic nerve.
- Pierces the sclera just medial to the posterior pole of the eyeball and
  takes a slightly tortuous course in the orbit that enables it to adapt to
  movements of the eyeball.
- Surrounded by the long and short ciliary nerves and vessels close to the
  back of the eyeball.
- Leaves the orbit through the optic canal (sphenoid bone) where it
  is accompanied by the ophthalmic artery (ICA) and surrounded by
  extensions of the three layers of the meninges and CSF.
- Intracranial portions of the optic nerves join at the optic chiasm. Gyrus
  recti of frontal lobes lie above the nerve. The optic tract is separated
  from the nerve by the anterior cerebral and anterior communicating
  arteries.
- The central artery of the retina enters the optic nerve about halfway
  along its length and provides the sole arterial supply for the eyeball.

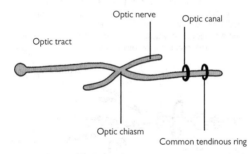

Fig. 4.2 The optic nerve, schematic.
Reproduced courtesy of Daniel R. van Gijn.

Visual defects
- Pre-chiasmatic optic nerve lesions (traumatic, neoplastic,
  inflammatory, or vascular) result in ipsilateral loss of vision.
- Bitemporal hemianopia is the hallmark presentation of chiasmatic
  lesions. Lesions include pituitary macroadenomas, gliomas, and
  craniopharyngiomas.
- The post-chiasmatic (or retro-chiasmatic) region includes the optic
  tracts, lateral geniculate nucleus, and optic radiations. Lesions are
  predominantly central (optic cortex) from infarcts, trauma, or vascular
  malformations and result in contralateral homonymous hemianopia.

Oculomotor nerve

The third cranial nerve, with three main functions: motor to levator palpebrae superioris (involved in elevation of the eyelid), supplies four of the extraocular muscles (ipsilateral inferior and medial rectus and inferior oblique and contralateral superior rectus), and innervates the pupil and lens (Fig. 4.3).

- Motor nucleus near the midline, in the ventral part of the periaqueductal grey of the rostral midbrain; level of the superior colliculus, ventral to the cerebral aqueduct, dorsal to the medial longitudinal fasciculus (which links the motor nuclei of III, IV, and VI).
- Runs along lateral dural wall of the cavernous sinus.
- Branches into superior and inferior divisions that enter the orbit via the superior orbital fissure inside the common tendinous ring, separated by the nasociliary nerve (branch of V_1).
- Carries preganglionic parasympathetic fibres (cell bodies in Edinger–Westphal nucleus in midbrain) to the ciliary ganglion where they synapse: postganglionic fibres run in short ciliary nerves to supply sphincter pupillae and the ciliary muscle.
- Ciliary ganglion lies in loose areolar tissue near the orbital apex, posterolateral to the globe, between the optic nerve and lateral rectus; it can be injured, e.g. during surgical repair of orbital fractures.
- Parasympathetic axons are located near the periphery of the oculomotor nerve, which means that visceromotor signs and symptoms, e.g. subtle ptosis or mildly diminished pupillary reactivity, may appear prior to the onset of, or without any extraocular muscle dysfunction, as a result of external compression of the nerve.

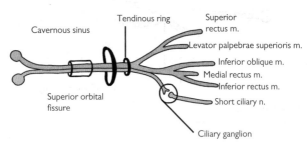

Fig. 4.3 The oculomotor nerve, schematic.
Reproduced courtesy of Daniel R. van Gijn.

Oculomotor nerve palsy

The third cranial nerve supplies all extraocular muscles except lateral rectus and superior oblique. Paralysis of the nerve causes a downward and abducted gaze, upper lid ptosis, and pupillary dilatation.

Causes

Intracranial

- Herniation of the uncus—compresses oculomotor nerve against the petroclinoid ligament.
- Trauma or raised intracranial pressure forces brainstem inferiorly, compressing the nerve against the petroclinoid ligament.
- Posterior cerebral artery aneurysms.

Extracranial

- Superior orbital fissure syndrome—most commonly due to trauma, causing palsy of all nerves passing through the fissure (oculomotor, trochlear, branches of V_1 and abducens) and the superior and inferior branches of the ophthalmic vein.

Trochlear nerve

The fourth cranial nerve and the longest intracranial course. It supplies a single muscle, the superior oblique (Fig. 4.4).

- The only cranial nerve to emerge from the dorsal surface of the brainstem.
- Runs along the lateral dural wall of the cavernous sinus.
- Crosses the oculomotor nerve and enters the orbit through the superior orbital fissure, outside the common tendinous ring, above levator palpebrae superioris and medial to the frontal and lacrimal nerves.
- Enters the superior surface of superior oblique.

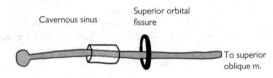

Cavernous sinus

Superior orbital fissure

To superior oblique m.

Fig. 4.4 The trochlear nerve, schematic.
Reproduced courtesy of Daniel R. van Gijn.

Trigeminal nerve

Trigeminal literally means three twins (*tri-* + *geminus* (twin), Latin). The trigeminal nerve is the fifth cranial nerve and has three main divisions, ophthalmic, maxillary, and mandibular, that are conventionally abbreviated to V_1, V_2, and V_3, respectively. Each division is associated with a developing facial process that gives rise to a specific area of the adult face: the ophthalmic nerve is associated with the frontonasal process, the maxillary nerve with the maxillary process, and the mandibular nerve with the mandibular process. The trigeminal nerve has an extensive sensory distribution that includes the skin, conjunctivae, oral and (para)nasal mucosae, the upper and lower teeth, gingivae, periodontal ligaments, and the TMJ. Its branches carry the motor supply to the muscles of mastication and the nerve is functionally connected to all four pairs of parasympathetic ganglia in the head. Almost all the sensory fibres have their cell bodies in the trigeminal (Gasserian) ganglion in the middle cranial fossa; uniquely, proprioceptive fibres have their cell bodies in the mesencephalic nucleus in the midbrain. Motor fibres have their cell bodies in the motor nucleus of the trigeminal nerve.

Ophthalmic division V_1

See Fig. 4.5.
- The ophthalmic nerve passes forwards along the lateral dural wall of the cavernous sinus, giving off the *lacrimal*, *frontal*, and *nasociliary* nerves before it reaches the superior orbital fissure. These branches travel through the orbit and supply the conjunctiva, skin over the forehead, upper eyelid, and much of the external surface of the nose.

Maxillary division V_2

See Fig. 4.6.
- The maxillary nerve leaves the skull via the foramen rotundum and enters the upper part of the pterygopalatine fossa where many of its extracranial branches are given off. It crosses the pterygopalatine fossa, giving off two large branches containing fibres destined for the nose, palate, and pharynx that pass through the pterygopalatine ganglion without synapsing. The maxillary nerve then inclines sharply laterally on the posterior surface of the orbital process of the palatine bone and on the upper part of the posterior surface of the maxilla in the inferior orbital fissure (which is continuous posteriorly with the pterygopalatine fossa).
- It travels outside the orbital periosteum and gives off zygomatic and posterior superior alveolar branches. About halfway between the orbital apex and the orbital rim, the maxillary nerve turns medially to enter the infraorbital canal, becoming the infraorbital nerve.
- Named branches from the main trunk are meningeal, ganglionic, zygomatic, posterior, middle, and anterior superior alveolar, and infraorbital nerves.
- Named branches from the pterygopalatine ganglion are orbital, nasopalatine, posterior superior nasal, greater and lesser palatine, and pharyngeal.

Mandibular division V₃

See Fig. 4.7.
- The largest division of the trigeminal nerve and unlike the other two divisions it is a *mixed* nerve.
- Its *sensory* branches supply the teeth and gums of the mandible, the skin in the temporal region, part of the auricle (including the external meatus and tympanic membrane) and the lower lip, the lower part of the face, and the mucosa of the anterior two-thirds (presulcal part) of the tongue and the floor of the oral cavity.
- The *motor* branches innervate the muscles of mastication, tensor veli palatini, tensor tympani, anterior belly of digastric, and mylohyoid (i.e. the muscles derived from the first branchial arch).
- The large sensory root and small motor root both leave the skull via the foramen ovale and unite just outside the skull.
- The combined nerve passes between tensor veli palatini and lateral pterygoid, gives off a meningeal branch and the nerve to medial pterygoid, and divides into a *small anterior* and *large posterior* trunk.
- The anterior trunk gives off branches to the four main muscles of mastication (masseter, temporalis, medial pterygoid, and lateral pterygoid muscles) and a (long) buccal branch which is sensory to the cheek (do not confuse this with the buccal branch of the facial nerve, which is a motor nerve).
- The posterior trunk gives off the auriculotemporal, lingual, and inferior alveolar nerves, and motor fibres that supply mylohyoid and the anterior belly of digastric.

Trigeminal neuralgia

Introduction
Trigeminal neuralgia (or *tic douloureux*) is a clinical manifestation of intense paroxysms of sharp pain resulting from disorders of the trigeminal nerve, seen most commonly in women between 50 and 70 years of age. It is almost always unilateral and can affect any branch of the trigeminal nerve in response to certain 'trigger points', although is most commonly experienced in the maxillary and mandibular divisions.

Cause
Most commonly vascular compression of the trigeminal nerve (e.g. by the superior cerebellar artery) in the middle cranial fossa or venous pressure at the cerebellopontine angle. It is important to consider/exclude demyelination (multiple sclerosis), and posterior fossa tumours including vestibular schwannomas and meningiomas.

Management
Following exclusion of space-occupying lesions, treatment is initially medical with anticonvulsant medication such as carbamazepine and/or gabapentin. Surgical options include *peripheral destructive* procedures (including cryotherapy of infraorbital nerve), *central* neurosurgical procedures (including microvascular decompression) and central destructive (thermal, chemical, or mechanical) procedures involving the trigeminal ganglion.

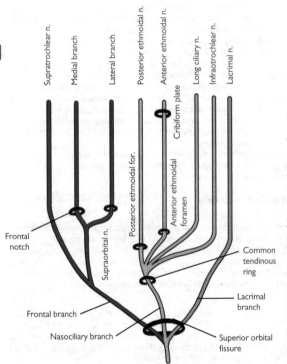

Supratrochlear n.

Medial branch

Lateral branch

Posterior ethmoidal n.

Anterior ethmoidal n.

Cribiform plate

Long ciliary n.

Infraotrochlear n.

Lacrimal n.

Posterior ethmoidal for.

Anterior ethmoidal foramen

Frontal notch

Supraorbital n.

Frontal branch

Nasociliary branch

Common tendinous ring

Lacrimal branch

Superior orbital fissure

Fig. 4.5 The ophthalmic division (V₁) of the trigeminal nerve, schematic.
Reproduced courtesy of Daniel R. van Gijn.

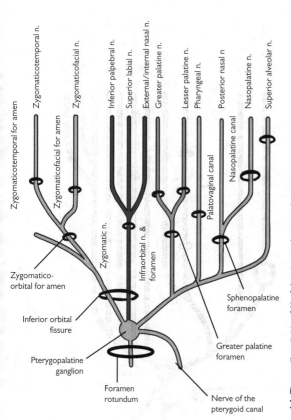

Fig. 4.6 The maxillary division (V₂) of the trigeminal nerve, schematic.
Reproduced courtesy of Daniel R. van Gijn.

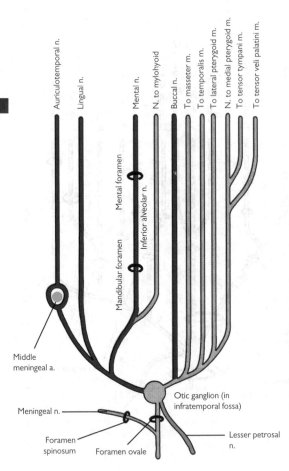

Fig. 4.7 The mandibular division (V_3) of the trigeminal nerve, schematic.
Reproduced courtesy of Daniel R. van Gijn.

Abducens nerve

The sixth cranial nerve and motor innervation to lateral rectus muscle. It has nucleus, cisternal, cavernous, and orbital parts (Fig. 4.8).

- Axons of VII loop around the abducens nucleus, producing the facial colliculus in the floor of the fourth ventricle.
- Long intracranial course, which may make localization of pathology difficult.
- Exits the brainstem at the border of the pons and medullary pyramids.
- Usually runs through Dorello's canal (Fig. 4.9).
- At the apex of the petrous temporal bone the nerve makes a sharp turn anteriorly to enter the cavernous sinus.
- Lies lateral to the ICA in the cavernous sinus (whereas III, IV, and V_2 run along the lateral dural wall of the sinus).
- Enters the orbit through the superior orbital fissure within the common tendinous ring, at first below, and then between, the two divisions of the oculomotor nerve and lateral to the nasociliary nerve.
- Enters the medial (deep) surface of lateral rectus.

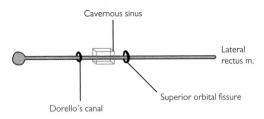

Cavernous sinus

Lateral rectus m.

Superior orbital fissure

Dorello's canal

Fig. 4.8 The abducens nerve, schematic.
Reproduced courtesy of Daniel R. van Gijn.

Dorello's canal—Primo Dorello (1872–1963), Italian anatomist

Dorello's canal is a bow-shaped canal between the medial-most aspect of the petrous ridge (petrous apex) and the superolateral part of the clivus—bound superiorly by the petrosphenoidal ligament (of Gruber). It is a fibro-osseous conduit (rather than a true canal) through which the abducens nerve courses from the pontine cistern to the cavernous sinus.

Grüber's ligament—Wenzel Grüber (1814–1890), Russian anatomist

The eponymous name for the petrosphenoidal ligament that forms the superior boundary of Dorello's canal.

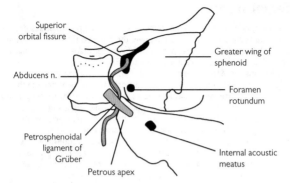

Fig. 4.9 The petrosphenoidal ligament and path of abducens nerve through Dorello's canal, schematic.

Reproduced courtesy of Daniel R. van Gijn.

Facial nerve

The facial nerve is the seventh cranial nerve and supplies muscles derived from the second branchial arch, namely the mimetic facial muscles (often called the muscles of facial expression), buccinator, stapedius, platysma, the posterior belly of digastric, and stylohyoid (Fig. 4.10).

- Neurons in the face area of the motor cortex (supranuclear neurons) project bilaterally to facial motor neurons that control muscles in the upper face (frontalis, orbicularis oculi) but contralaterally to facial motor neurons that innervate the muscles of the middle and lower face. (It should be remembered that sparing of the forehead in facial paralysis is not necessarily pathognomonic of a central lesion.)
- After it leaves the brainstem, the facial nerve is conventionally divided into *intracranial* (cisternal), *intratemporal*, and *extratemporal* portions. The intratemporal portion is subdivided into meatal, labyrinthine, tympanic (horizontal), and mastoid (vertical) segments.

Intratemporal

- The mastoid segment of the facial nerve gives off the nerve to the stapedius, the chorda tympani, and a sensory auricular branch. The nerve to stapedius is a small twig given off behind the pyramidal eminence that passes forwards through a small canal to reach stapedius. Damage to this branch, with consequent paralysis of stapedius, leads to hypersensitivity to loud noises (hyperacusis).
- The chorda tympani runs in a bony canal to enter the tympanic cavity, where it curves anteriorly across the pars flaccida of the tympanic membrane between its mucous and fibrous layers, medial to the upper part of the handle or neck of the malleus and above the insertion of tensor tympani, to reach the anterior wall of the tympanic cavity, where it enters another bony canal (of Huguier).
- The chorda tympani exits the skull at the petrotympanic fissure and enters the infratemporal fossa where it joins the lingual nerve.
- The chorda tympani carries axons mediating the special sense of taste from the anterior two-thirds or presulcal part of the tongue (but not from the taste buds studding the walls of the circumvallate papillae) and preganglionic parasympathetic axons that will synapse on postganglionic neurons in the submandibular ganglion.

Extratemporal

- The main trunk of the facial nerve exits the skull via the stylomastoid foramen. It lies below the tympanic plate, lateral to the bases of the styloid process and the carotid sheath and posterior to the parotid gland.
- The nerve gives off the posterior auricular nerve (to supply the occipital belly of occipitofrontalis, auricularis superior, and the intrinsic auricular muscles) and a muscular branch that supplies the posterior belly of digastric and stylohyoid.
- It next enters the parotid gland high up on its posteromedial surface and divides within the gland, usually just behind and superficial to the retromandibular vein and ECA, into upper temporofacial and lower cervicofacial trunks.

- The trunks branch further to form a parotid plexus (pes anserinus) from which five main terminal branches, temporal, zygomatic, buccal, marginal mandibular, and cervical, ultimately emerge. These branches diverge within the substance of the parotid and leave the gland via its anteromedial surface, medial to its anterior margin. Numerous microdissection studies have demonstrated considerable individual variations in branching patterns and anastomoses between branches, both within the parotid and on the face.
- The facial nerve has both intra- and extracranial connections with the cutaneous branches of all three divisions of the trigeminal nerve (including branches of the auriculotemporal, buccal, mental, lingual, infraorbital, zygomatic, and ophthalmic nerves); with branches of the vestibulocochlear, glossopharyngeal, and vagus nerves; and with branches of the cervical plexus (including the great auricular, greater and lesser occipital, and transverse cervical nerves). These cutaneous connections may facilitate the perineural spread of tumours that arise either within the parotid or on the face.

Bell's palsy

Complete unilateral facial weakness and a diagnosis of exclusion—responsible for approximately 75% of facial nerve palsies. In addition to facial weakness (involving the forehead), it may present with numbness or pain around the ear, loss of taste, and hyperacusis due to paralysis of the stapedius muscle. The proposed cause is viro-vascular trauma to the nerve resulting in oedema and compression of the nerve within its canal.

Investigations

Investigations include magnetic resonance imaging to exclude space-occupying and demyelinating lesions, serology to exclude Lyme disease (*Borrelia*) and Ramsay Hunt syndrome (varicella zoster virus), and (occasionally) nerve conduction studies.

Treatment

Treatment includes systemic steroids (within 72 hours), antiviral medication (minimal evidence), and protection of the eye if incomplete eye closure. Approximately 80% will make a complete recovery. Botox and surgery have a role in helping to balance facial symmetry and improve synkinesis (involuntary movement of part of the face when intentionally trying to move another).

Sir Charles Bell (1774–1842)

Scottish surgeon, anatomist, physiologist, and neurologist, among other notable talents. His description of facial nerve palsy remains appropriate today:

'The face is twisted to the right side. The left nostril does not move in respiration. The eye-lids of the left side are not closed when he winks, although, when he attempts it, the eye-ball is turned up, the cheek is relaxed, and the forehead on the left side unruffled.'

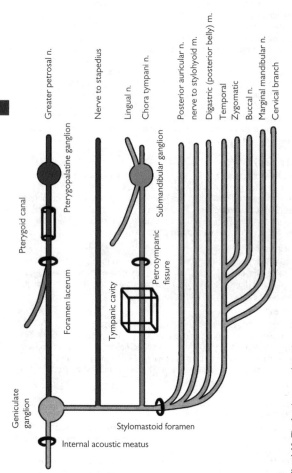

Fig. 4.10 The facial nerve, schematic.
Reproduced courtesy of Daniel R. van Gijn.

Vestibulocochlear nerve

The eighth cranial nerve. It contains mainly sensory fibres concerned with balance (vestibular component) and hearing (cochlear component), and efferent fibres that terminate on cochlear and vestibular sensory cells (Fig. 4.11).

- Exits the brainstem at the cerebellopontine angle.
- Runs through the posterior cranial fossa together with VII, the nervus intermedius, and labyrinthine vessels.
- Enters the petrous temporal bone via the porus acusticus (internal auditory canal/internal acoustic meatus), and divides into an anterior trunk, the cochlear nerve, and a posterior trunk, the vestibular nerve.

Vestibulocochlear nerve schwannoma

Overview

Vestibular schwannoma or acoustic neuroma (a misnomer as they are neither acoustic nor neuromas) is a benign intracranial tumour of the myelinating Schwann cells. The cause is essentially unknown but may be due to chromosomal defects. The majority of cases are sporadic although some may be related to *neurofibromatosis type 2* (MISME syndrome— multiple inherited schwannomas meningiomas and ependymomas).

Presentation

Triad of ipsilateral sensorineural hearing loss, tinnitus, and vestibular/vertigo symptoms. Larger tumours may result in facial nerve weakness and facial paraesthesia.

Treatment

Treatment strategies include observation, microsurgical removal/debulking of the tumour, and radiotherapy.

Glossopharyngeal neuralgia

Overview

A rare condition predominantly affecting men, resulting in paroxysms of intense, stabbing type in the distribution of the glossopharyngeal nerve, including the tonsillar region, base of the tongue, and the ipsilateral ear.

Causes

Causes include compression from aberrant vessels, cerebellopontine angle tumours, an elongated styloid process (Eagle syndrome), peritonsillar abscess, demyelinating disorders, or a carotid aneurysm.

Management

Diagnosis is normally made following clinical examination and magnetic resonance imaging—the former to distinguish from trigeminal neuralgia owing to the location of the pain and the latter to exclude tonsillar, pharyngeal, and cerebellopontine angle lesions. Treatment includes prescription of antiseizure/antidepressant medication, local anaesthetic injections, and microsurgical decompression

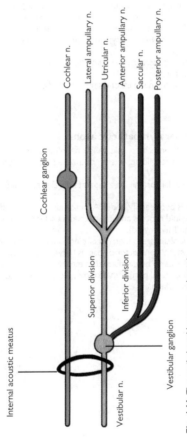

Fig. 4.11 The vestibulocochlear nerve, schematic.
Reproduced courtesy of Daniel R. van Gijn.

Glossopharyngeal nerve

The ninth cranial nerve and nerve of the third pharyngeal arch. It is a mixed nerve with sensory, motor, and parasympathetic components (Fig. 4.12).

Sensory

- General sensation from the skin of the auricle, tympanic cavity including tympanic membrane, pharyngotympanic tube, fauces, tonsils, nasopharynx, uvula, and postsulcal tongue. Neuronal cell bodies in superior or inferior glossopharyngeal ganglia in the jugular foramen.
- Sensory innervation of oropharynx is responsible for initiating gag reflex.
- Special sensation of taste from circumvallate papillae (presulcal), and from postsulcal tongue.
- Visceral sensation from the carotid sinus and body.

Motor

- To stylopharyngeus.

Preganglionic parasympathetic axons

Via lesser petrosal branch to otic ganglion (infratemporal fossa) where they synapse. Postganglionic axons distributed to parotid gland via auriculotemporal nerve (V_3).

- Exits skull via jugular foramen in a separate dural sheath, anterior to X and XI.
- Passes forwards between IJV and ICA; descends anterior to the ICA and deep to the styloid process and its attached muscles (stylopharyngeus, styloglossus, and stylohyoid).
- Innervates stylopharyngeus then either pierces the lower fibres of the superior pharyngeal constrictor or passes between the superior and middle constrictors to be distributed to the tonsil, the mucosae of the pharynx and postsulcal part of the tongue, the circumvallate papillae, and oral mucous glands.

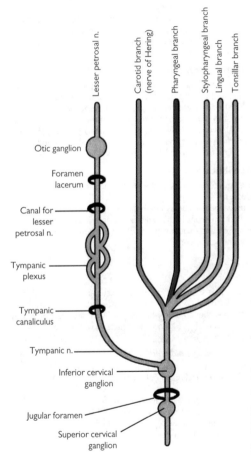

Fig. 4.12 The glossopharyngeal nerve, schematic.
Reproduced courtesy of Daniel R. van Gijn.

Vagus nerve

The tenth cranial nerve with a very extensive distribution, from brainstem to the splenic flexure of the colon. It is a mixed nerve with sensory, motor, and parasympathetic components (Fig. 4.13).

- Exits skull via jugular foramen with XI. Has two sensory ganglia, superior (jugular) and inferior (nodose).
- Descends vertically in the neck in the carotid sheath, posterior to and between the IJV and ICA until it reaches the upper border of the thyroid cartilage. Then passes between the IJV and common carotid artery (CCA) to the root of the neck.

Sensory distribution

- Axons carry visceral sensory information from the larynx, oesophagus, trachea, and abdominal and thoracic viscera and from chemoreceptors in the aortic bodies and stretch receptors in the aortic arch.
- Somatic sensory information from the skin of the back of the auricle (Arnold's/Alderman's nerve) and external auditory canal, parts of the external surface of the tympanic membrane, and the pharynx.
- Taste sensation from the epiglottis (possibly).

Motor distribution

- Innervates striated muscles of the pharynx and the larynx, and palatoglossus.
- Carries preganglionic parasympathetic axons that synapse on postganglionic neurons in the walls of the viscera and innervate smooth muscle and exocrine glands of the pharynx, larynx, and thoracoabdominal viscera.

Vagus nerve

Overview

Pathology affecting the vagus nerve can occur anywhere along its substantial course. The majority of lesions may be subtle due to its predominantly parasympathetic nature. Features include deviation of the uvula away from the side of the lesion and ipsilateral vocal cord paralysis and loss of the pharyngeal reflex.

Classification of lesions according to level

- *Supranuclear*—may also involve cranial nerves IX, XI, and XII.
- *Brainstem*—lesions include neoplasms, vascular lesions, and demyelination.
- *Jugular foramen*—skull base trauma, neoplasms (glomus jugulare, meningioma), or Vernet syndrome (palsies of IX, X, and XI).
- *Extracranial*—may be cause by neoplasms (infiltration or schwannomas) or trauma (including iatrogenic).

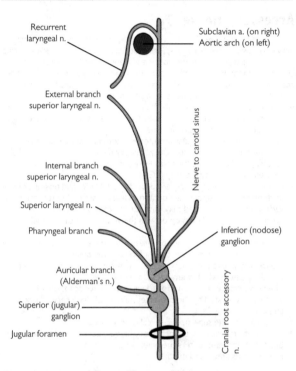

Fig. 4.13 The vagus nerve, schematic.
Reproduced courtesy of Daniel R. van Gijn.

Etymology

- *Vagus*—from the Latin meaning 'wandering' or 'straying'. It was historically known as the pneumogastric nerve owing to its parasympathetic supply to the heart, lungs, and gastrointestinal tract. The words vagabond and vagrant share a common stem.
- *Nodose*—from the Latin *nodosus* meaning 'knot' or 'swollen'.

Accessory nerve

The 11th cranial nerve. The conventional description is that the accessory nerve has two roots, a large spinal root (spinal accessory nerve) arising from cervical segments of the spinal cord, and a smaller cranial root with cell bodies in the nucleus ambiguus of the brainstem that is regarded as accessory to the vagus (Fig. 4.14). Some more recent descriptions regard the cranial root as part of X rather than a part of the accessory nerve.

- 'Spinal root' enters the skull via the foramen magnum, behind the vertebral artery, and passes laterally to join the 'cranial root' either before or within the jugular foramen.
- Exits the skull via the jugular foramen in a common dural sheath with X.
- Outside the jugular foramen, the accessory nerve passes either medial or lateral to IJV, crosses the transverse process of the atlas and is crossed by the occipital artery (ECA).
- It descends medial to the styloid process, stylohyoid, and posterior belly of digastric to the upper part of sternocleidomastoid. It enters the deep surface of the muscle and may form an anastomosis with fibres from C2 or C3 (ansa of Maubrac); or with the ventral root of C1 (McKenzie branch).
- The accessory nerve may not progress beyond sternocleidomastoid, but usually it emerges above the midpoint of the posterior border of the muscle (above the emergence of the great auricular nerve): note that the point at which it emerges is very variable.
- The nerve crosses the posterior triangle on levator scapulae, from which it is separated by the prevertebral layer of deep cervical fascia and adipose tissue.
- It is related to the superficial cervical lymph nodes.
- Superior to the clavicle, the accessory nerve passes behind the anterior border of trapezius, enters the deep surface of the muscle, and innervates its upper and middle fibres.

Accessory nerve

Injury to the accessory nerve is predominantly iatrogenic in nature secondary to neck dissection (more specifically during the dissection of level 2b during the skeletonization/identification of the nerve). Injury results in weakness of the ipsilateral sternocleidomastoid (affecting head rotation away from the side of the lesion) and trapezius muscles. Shoulder stiffness and pain may be a feature.

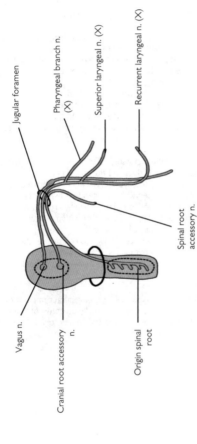

Fig. 4.14 The accessory nerve, schematic.
Reproduced courtesy of Daniel R. van Gijn.

Hypoglossal nerve

The 12th cranial nerve. It innervates all the intrinsic (transverse, superior and inferior longitudinal, vertical) and three of the extrinsic muscles of the tongue (styloglossus, hyoglossus, and genioglossus) (Fig. 4.15).

* Emerges from the brainstem as a series of rootlets.
* Within the posterior cranial fossa, these rootlets run laterally behind the vertebral artery, usually in two bundles that perforate the dura mater opposite the hypoglossal canal (occipital bone) and unite after passing through the canal.
* Outside the skull, the hypoglossal nerve initially lies in a plane medial to the IJV, ICA, and IX, X, and XI (these three nerves exit the skull via the jugular foramen). It then passes inferolaterally behind the ICA and IX and X to lie between the ICA and IJV: all of these structures are deep to the posterior belly of digastric.
* Descends almost vertically between the ICA and IJV, anterior to X.
* The nerve usually crosses the upward loop of the lingual artery close to the tip of the greater cornu of the hyoid and then runs upwards and forwards on hyoglossus (which separates it from the lingual artery), deep to stylohyoid, the tendon of digastric, and the posterior border of mylohyoid.
* Between mylohyoid and hyoglossus, it lies below the deep part of the submandibular gland and its duct and the lingual nerve.
* Fibres from C1 travel with the hypoglossal nerve before leaving it in the superior root of the ansa cervicalis (descendens hypoglossi), usually as the hypoglossal nerve curves round the occipital artery. As their name implies, these fibres descend, anterior to or within the carotid sheath, and supply the superior belly of omohyoid.
* The superior root of the ansa cervicalis is joined by the inferior root (C2, C3) to form the ansa hypoglossi, from which branches supply the sternohyoid, sternothyroid, and inferior belly of omohyoid.

Hypoglossal nerve

Hypoglossal nerve injury occurs mainly during surgery or trauma to the neck and results in weakness (and eventually atrophy) of the ipsilateral muscles. This results in a deviation of the tongue towards the side of the lesion.

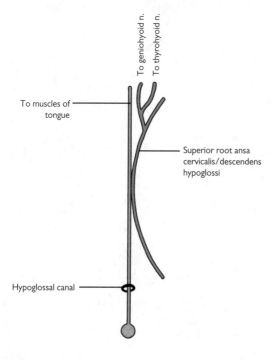

To geniohyoid n.

To thyrohyoid n.

To muscles of tongue

Superior root ansa cervicalis/descendens hypoglossi

Hypoglossal canal

Fig. 4.15 The hypoglossal nerve, schematic.
Reproduced courtesy of Daniel R. van Gijn.

Chapter 5

The neck

Introduction

Surgical exploration of the neck is often described as being akin to a 'safari in tiger country', owing to its elegant yet intimately arranged group of vital structures tightly packed between bilateral, large neurovascular bundles that await a wrong move at every turn. The neck occupies the space between the clavicles and thoracic inlet inferiorly (or *outlet* depending on which way one is approaching), to the base of the skull and inferior border of the mandible superiorly. At its core lies the cervical part of the vertebral column, providing the all-important support for the skull above and strength and movement to the neck proper.

The anterior neck (anterior to the flexor musculature) provides a vulnerable passage for the major neurovascular supply *to* and drainage *from* the head, neck, and intracranial region, while simultaneously transmitting the upper aerodigestive tract and housing the thyroid and parathyroid endocrine glands. In the posterior neck, a large mass of extensor musculature is situated posterior to the cervical vertebrae—the most prominent being the aptly named large trapezius muscles.

Cranial nerves IX–XII descend into the neck: IX (glossopharyngeal) and XII (hypoglossal) meander towards the oropharynx and tongue, respectively; XI (accessory) deflects backwards to supply the large SCM and trapezius muscles; while X (*vagus*) wanders inferiorly within the carotid sheath between and posterior to the CCA and IJV, before disappearing into the thoracic and abdominal cavities beyond.

Skin of the neck and platysma

The skin of the neck is flexible, thin, and intimately related to the subcutaneous tissue and embedded platysma muscle. It is ordinarily under some tension and its encircling lines of relaxed skin tension provide a convenient means of disguising surgical scars.

Cutaneous blood supply

The blood supply to the skin of the neck is derived from a rich network within platysma and a subdermal plexus, arising primarily from the facial, occipital, posterior auricular, and subclavian arteries.

- *Anterior cervical skin*—superior thyroid artery (from the ECA); transverse cervical artery (from the subclavian artery).
- *Posterior cervical skin*—occipital artery (ECA), deep cervical and transverse cervical arteries (subclavian artery).
- *Superior cervical skin*—SCM branch of the occipital artery, submandibular and submental branches of the facial artery.

Cutaneous nerve supply

Sensation to the skin of the neck is supplied by the cutaneous branches of the cervical plexus: the anterior rami of C2–C4 supply the skin of the posterior neck and scalp, the lateral and anterior aspects of the neck, and angle of the mandible. They converge and become superficial (piercing the deep cervical fascia) at the *punctum nervosum* (erroneously called Erb's point), a point along the posterior border of the SCM at the junction of its superior one-third and inferior two-thirds (Fig. 5.1). The first three branches *ascend* while the three supraclavicular branches *descend*:

- *Lesser occipital (C2)*—appears from the posterior border of SCM and ascends on its posterior border to supply the auricle and inferior occipital scalp.
- *Greater auricular (C2, C3)*—largest ascending branch, divides into anterior and posterior branches at the inferior pole of the parotid gland; anterior branch supplies skin of face over parotid and posterior branch supplies skin over mastoid process and posterior surface of auricle.
- *Transverse cervical (C2, C3)*—runs obliquely forward from the posterior border of SCM deep to platysma and divides into superior branches (to submandibular region/forms plexus with cervical branch of VII) and inferior branches (supplying anterior and lateral aspects of the neck).
- *Supraclavicular (C3, C4)*—divides into medial, intermediate, and lateral branches. Medial supplies midline from sternoclavicular joint to skin over second rib; intermediate supplies skin over pectoralis major and deltoid; lateral supplies skin over posterosuperior shoulder.

Platysma

The platysma muscle is a highly variable, wide, flat sheet of muscle extending from the mandible to the clavicles and lies enclosed within the superficial fascia of the neck together with cutaneous nerves and lymphatics. A common variant is in the level of its midline interdigitation: the majority of cases interdigitate approximately 1–2 cm below the mandibular symphysis, with a midline dehiscence inferiorly (Fig. 5.2).

- *Origin*—subcutaneous tissues of supra/infraclavicular regions.
- *Insertion*—inferior border of mandible (*pars mandibularis*), skin of lower lip (*pars labialis*), cheek, angle of mouth (*pars modiolaris*), and orbicularis oris.
- *Action*—draws corner of mouth inferiorly and apart (wider). Wrinkles and tightens the skin of the neck.
- *Innervation*—cervical branch of the facial nerve.
- *Blood supply*—submental branch of facial artery, superior thyroid artery, and superficial cervical artery.

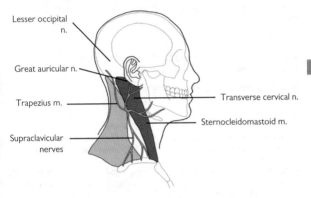

Fig. 5.1 Cutaneous innervation of the neck.
Reproduced courtesy of Daniel R. van Gijn.

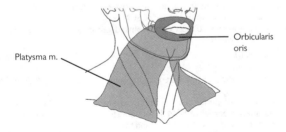

Fig. 5.2 Platysma muscle.
Reproduced courtesy of Daniel R. van Gijn.

Triangles of the neck

The triangles of the neck describe a topographically and (occasionally) surgically convenient focused division of the neck. The principal reference point is the SCM muscle which divides the neck into anterior and posterior triangles on each side. Both can be arbitrarily subdivided into smaller triangles (Fig. 5.3).

Anterior triangle

An inverted triangle anterior to the SCM with its base superior and apex inferior. It can be subdivided into the *digastric*, *muscular*, *carotid*, and *submental* triangles.

Boundaries
- *Anterior*—midline neck.
- *Posterior*—anterior border of SCM/manubrium sterni.
- *Base*—inferior border of mandible.

Subdivisions of anterior triangle

Digastric triangle
See Fig. 5.4.
- *Boundaries*—lower border of the mandible and the anterior and posterior bellies of the digastric muscle. Its floor consists of mylohyoid and hyoglossus and it is covered by deep cervical fascia, platysma, superficial fascia, and skin.
- *Contents*—submandibular gland and lymph nodes, facial artery and vein, tail of parotid gland (posteriorly), and submental and mylohyoid arteries and nerves (running on mylohyoid).

Muscular triangle
See Fig. 5.3.
- *Boundaries*—midline (hyoid bone to sternum), superior belly of omohyoid, and anterior border of SCM.
- *Contents*—infrahyoid muscles (thyrohyoid, omohyoid, sternothyroid, and sternohyoid).

Carotid triangle
See Fig. 5.5 and Fig. 5.6.
Owes its name to the fact that it contains parts of the ICA, ECA, and CCA.
- *Boundaries*—superior belly of omohyoid, posterior belly of digastric, and anterior border of SCM. Floor consists of middle and inferior constrictor muscles, thyrohyoid, and hyoglossus.
- *Contents*—IJV, ICA, ECA (ascending pharyngeal, occipital, facial, lingual, superior thyroid branches of ECA), descendens hypoglossi, CCA.

Submental triangle
See Fig. 5.7.
- *Boundaries*—unpaired midline triangle bound by both anterior bellies of the digastric muscles and the body of the hyoid bone; floor formed by mylohyoid muscles.
- *Contents*—submental lymph nodes, anterior jugular veins.

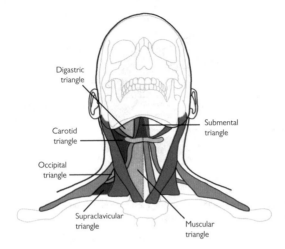

Fig. 5.3 Triangles of the neck, overview.
Reproduced courtesy of Daniel R. van Gijn.

Etymology
- *Platysma*—Greek meaning 'flat plate'; consider the broad and flat webbed feet of the (duck billed) platypus.
- *Carotid*—from the Greek *karoticus* meaning 'to stupefy'. External pressure over the carotid(s) was recognized to put one to sleep; the word *garrotte* meaning to cause death by strangulation has a similar stem.

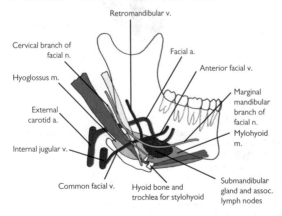

Fig. 5.4 The digastric triangle and its contents.
Reproduced courtesy of Daniel R. van Gijn.

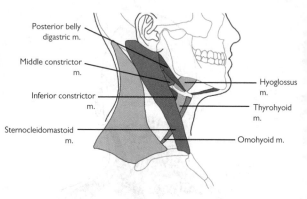

Fig. 5.5 The floor of the carotid triangle and adjacent structures.
Reproduced courtesy of Daniel R. van Gijn.

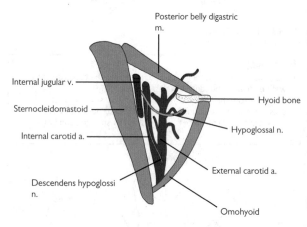

Fig. 5.6 The carotid triangle and its contents.
Reproduced courtesy of Daniel R. van Gijn.

Posterior triangle

The posterior triangle is separated from the anterior triangle by the SCM and forms the posterior compartment of the neck. The inferior belly of omohyoid divides it into a superior *occipital triangle* and an inferior *supraclavicular triangle* (Fig. 5.8).

Boundaries
- *Anterior*—posterior border of SCM.
- *Posterior*—anterior border of trapezius.
- *Inferior*—middle border of clavicle.

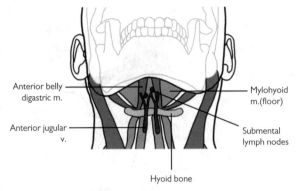

Fig. 5.7 The submental triangle and its contents.
Reproduced courtesy of Daniel R. van Gijn.

- *Roof*—skin, superficial fascia (containing platysma), and the investing layer of deep cervical fascia which is pierced inferiorly by supraclavicular nerves and external jugular vein (EJV).
- *Floor*—prevertebral fascia overlying splenius capitis, levator scapulae, and scaleni anterior and medius.

Contents
- *Vessels*—the third part of the subclavian, transverse cervical, and suprascapular arteries. Lower part of EJV and its tributaries (receives transverse cervical and suprascapular veins).
- *Nerves*—spinal accessory nerve, cutaneous branches of cervical plexus, trunks of brachial plexus (upper, middle, lower).
- *Lymph nodes*—level V along the posterior border SCM.
- *Fat*.

Subdivisions of posterior triangle

Occipital triangle
See Fig. 5.9.
- *Boundaries*—posterior border of the SCM anteriorly, the anterior border of trapezius posteriorly, and inferior belly of omohyoid inferiorly.
- *Contents*—include the spinal accessory nerve, upper branches of the brachial plexus, supraclavicular nerve, transverse cervical vessels, and branches of the cervical plexus.

Supraclavicular triangle
- Bound by the posterior border of the SCM anteriorly, the anterior border of trapezius posteriorly, and inferior belly of omohyoid superiorly. The floor is formed by the first rib, scalenus medius, and serratus anterior and the roof is formed by skin, superficial fascia, platysma, and the investing layer of deep cervical fascia.
- Contents include the third part of the subclavian artery, trunks of the brachial plexus, the nerve to subclavius, and lymph nodes.

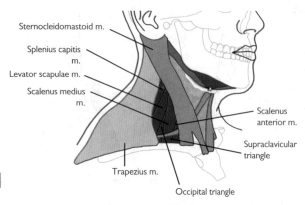

Fig. 5.8 The posterior triangle and its subdivisions.
Reproduced courtesy of Daniel R. van Gijn.

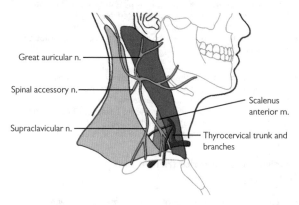

Fig. 5.9 The occipital triangle and its contents, lateral view.
Reproduced courtesy of Daniel R. van Gijn.

Muscles of the posterior neck

The posterior cervical musculature can be divided into four layers (Figs. 5.10–5.12). From superficial to deep these are the trapezius (*layer one*), splenius capitis and splenius cervicis (*layer two*), semispinalis capitis and longissimus capitis and cervicis (*layer three*), and the four muscles that form the boundaries of the suboccipital triangle (*layer four*). The *ligamentum nuchae* (Fig. 5.13) is a large posterior midline fibrous structure extending from the external occipital protuberance to the spinous process of C7 and forming an intermuscular septum between the muscles of the posterior neck. Collectively, these muscles function as extensors (bilateral contraction) and lateral flexors (unilateral contraction) of the neck.

Layer one

See Fig. 5.10.

- *Trapezius*—covers the entire cervical spine and is attached to the superior nuchal line, external occipital protuberance, and ligamentum nuchae. Supplied by the spinal accessory and C3/4 spinal nerves.

Layer two

See Fig. 5.10.

- *Splenius capitis*—a flat muscle attached to the ligamentum nuchae and the spinous processes of C7–T3 vertebrae, inserting laterally onto the occipital bone and deep to SCM on the mastoid process. Supplied by C3/4 cervical nerves.
- *Splenius cervicis*—inferior and fused to splenius capitis and deep to levator scapulae. Originates from the transverse processes of T3–T6 vertebrae and inserts into the transverse processes of C1–C3 vertebrae. Supplied by C3/4 cervical nerves.

Layer three

See Fig. 5.11.

- *Semispinalis capitis*—originates from the T1–T5 vertebrae and inserts into the spinous processes of C1–C5 vertebrae. Supplied by greater occipital nerve.
- *Longissimus capitis*—part of the erector spinae muscle group. Lies between semispinalis capitis and longissimus cervicis. Originates from the T1–T4 vertebrae and lower three/four cervical vertebrae to insert onto the posterior aspect of the mastoid process.
- *Longissimus cervicis*—originates from long tendons arising from the transverse processes of the T1–T5 vertebrae and inserts into the transverse processes of C2–C6 vertebrae.

Layer four (suboccipital triangle)

The suboccipital region is the deepest point of the posterior neck and contains a group of four small muscles. It lies inferior to the external occipital protuberance of the occipital bone and immediately posterior to the atlas and axis vertebrae. The *suboccipital triangles* are paired muscular triangles formed by three of the aforementioned four muscles (Fig. 5.12).

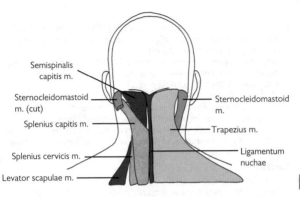

Fig. 5.10 Posterior neck muscles—demonstrating layer one (light grey) and layer two muscles (yellow).

Reproduced courtesy of Daniel R. van Gijn.

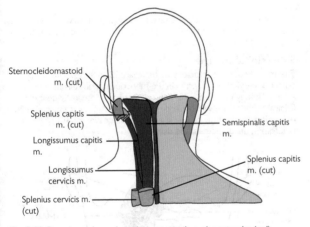

Fig. 5.11 Posterior neck muscles—demonstrating layer three muscles (red).

Reproduced courtesy of Daniel R. van Gijn.

Muscles
- *Rectus capitis posterior major*—originates from the spinous process of the axis and inserts into the inferior nuchal line of the occipital bone. Innervated by the suboccipital nerve.
- *Rectus capitis posterior minor*—originates from the posterior tubercle of the atlas and inserts into the inferior nuchal line of the occipital bone. Innervated by the suboccipital nerve.
- *Obliquus capitis superior*—originates from the transverse process of the atlas and inserts into the occipital bone between the superior and inferior nuchal lines. Innervated by the suboccipital nerve.
- *Obliquus capitis inferior*—originates from the spinous process of the axis and inserts into the transverse process of the atlas. Innervated by the suboccipital nerve.

Boundaries
- *Superolateral*—obliquus capitis superior.
- *Superomedial*—rectus capitis posterior major.
- *Inferolateral*—obliquus capitis inferior.
- *Roof*—semispinalis capitis.
- *Floor*—atlanto-occipital membrane and posterior arch of C1 vertebra.

Contents
The third part of the vertebral artery, the suboccipital nerve (dorsal ramus of C1), and the suboccipital venous plexus. The greater occipital nerve and occipital artery are within the roof.

Suboccipital triangle

The most important structure to be aware of in surgery involving the posterior cervical spine region in the suboccipital triangle is the vertebral artery. Although injury is rare, consequences are potentially devastating. Clinical sequelae are variable and reflect variations in anatomy and circulation dominance, but include lateral medullary syndrome (Wallenberg syndrome), quadraparesis, and death.

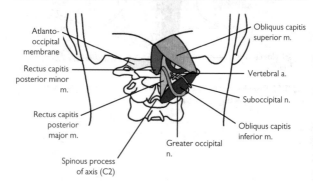

Fig. 5.12 The muscles, greater occipital nerve, and vertebral artery within the occipital triangle.

Reproduced courtesy of Daniel R. van Gijn.

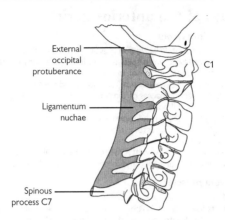

Fig. 5.13 Ligamentum nuchae and attachments, lateral view.
Reproduced courtesy of Daniel R. van Gijn.

Muscles of the anterior neck

Sternocleidomastoid

Largest and most superficial cervical muscle, covered by the investing layer of deep cervical fascia which splits around it. SCM divides the neck into anatomical anterior and posterior triangles (Fig. 5.14).

- *Origin and insertion*—manubrium (tendinous) and medial clavicle (muscular), mastoid process of temporal bone, and lateral superior nuchal line (occipital bone).
- *Arterial supply*—occipital and superior thyroid arteries.
- *Nerve supply*—spinal accessory (motor) and cervical plexus (sensory, proprioception).
- *Actions*—contralateral cervical rotation and ipsilateral cervical flexion (unilaterally), cervical flexion and forced inhalation (bilaterally).

Suprahyoid muscles

Stylohyoid

Divides at its lower end to allow passage for the intermediate tendon of digastric. Acts to elevate and draw the hyoid posteriorly during swallowing.

- *Origin and insertion*—styloid process (temporal bone) and greater cornu of the hyoid bone.
- *Nerve supply*—facial nerve.

Digastric

Consists of two bellies (anterior and posterior) joined by an intermediate tendon. It forms the inferior border of the digastric/submandibular triangle.

- *Origin*—digastric fossa of the mandible (anterior belly) and mastoid notch of temporal bone (posterior belly).
- *Insertion*—intermediate tendon (hyoid bone).
- *Arterial supply*—submental branch of facial artery (anterior belly) and occipital artery (posterior belly).
- *Nerve supply*—the two bellies have different embryological derivations, which explains their different innervations. The anterior belly is innervated by the mylohyoid nerve (posterior division of V_3), the posterior belly is innervated by the facial nerve.
- *Action*—opens the mouth by depressing the mandible.

Mylohyoid

Muscular diaphragm forming the floor of the mouth and separating the oral cavity from the submandibular space. The two halves of the mylohyoid unite in a midline raphe.

- *Origin*—mylohyoid line of the mandible.
- *Insertion*—body of the hyoid bone.
- *Blood supply*—mylohyoid branch of the inferior alveolar artery (first part of maxillary artery).
- *Nerve supply*—mylohyoid nerve (from inferior alveolar nerve from V_3).
- *Action*—elevates the floor of the oral cavity, hyoid bone, and tongue. Depresses mandible.

Geniohyoid

Superficial to mylohyoid muscle.

- *Origin*—inferior mental spine (mandible).
- *Insertion*—anterior surface of the body of the hyoid bone.
- *Blood supply*—branches of the lingual artery.
- *Nerve supply*—C1 via hypoglossal nerve (from ansa cervicalis).
- *Action*—draws the hyoid up and forward during swallowing. Depresses the mandible when the hyoid is fixed.

Infrahyoid muscles ('TOSS')

A group of four paired muscles in the anterior neck, all originating from or inserting onto the hyoid bone. All are innervated by the ansa cervicalis of the cervical plexus *except* for the thyrohyoid, which is supplied by the first cervical spinal nerve via the hypoglossal nerve. They act collectively to depress the hyoid bone and larynx during speech and swallowing.

Thyrohyoid

- *Origin*—oblique line of the thyroid cartilage.
- *Insertion*—body and greater cornu of the hyoid bone.

Omohyoid

- *Origin*—superior border of scapula and superior transverse ligament of scapular notch (inferior belly). Intermediate tendon.
- *Insertion*—intermediate tendon (inferior belly) and hyoid bone.

Sternohyoid

- *Origin*—manubrium and clavicle (and posterior sternoclavicular ligament).
- *Insertion*—medial part of the hyoid bone.

Sternothyroid

- *Origin*—posterior surface of the manubrium sterni and first costal cartilage.
- *Insertion*—oblique line of the thyroid cartilage.

Etymology

- *Strap muscles*—with reference to the infrahyoid muscles because their long, flat shapes resemble a belt or strap.
- *Ansa*—from Latin, meaning 'loop' or 'handle'.
- *Omos*—with reference to omohyoid meaning 'shoulder', this refers to its origin at the superior border of the scapula.

Prevertebral muscles

See Fig. 5.16.

Anterior group

The four principal anterior group of prevertebral muscles, lying directly anterior to the cervical vertebrae and beneath the prevertebral layer of cervical fascia, are rectus capitis, rectus capitis lateralis, longus colli, and longus capitis.

- *Rectus capitis*—attached to the anterior surface of the lateral mass of the atlas and the basilar part of the occipital bone, anterior to the foramen magnum. Flexes the neck at the atlanto-occipital joint. Innervated by C1–C2.

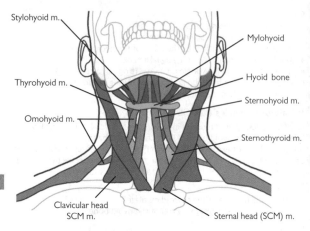

Fig. 5.14 Muscles of the neck, anterior view.
Reproduced courtesy of Daniel R. van Gijn.

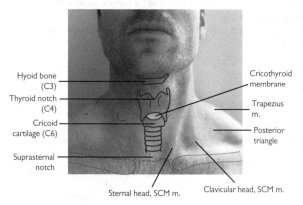

Fig. 5.15 Surface markings, anterior neck.
Reproduced courtesy of Daniel R. van Gijn.

- *Rectus capitis lateralis*—attached to the upper surface of the transverse process of the atlas and the jugular process of the occipital bone. Brings about lateral flexion of the neck and stabilizes the atlanto-occipital joint. Innervated by C1–C2.
- *Longus colli*—wide muscle with tapered ends that covers the anterior vertebral column from the atlas to the T3 vertebra. Consists of superior and inferior oblique and vertical parts. Originates from the transverse processes of C5–T3 vertebrae and inserts into the anterior arch of the atlas. Weak flexor of the neck. Innervated by C2–C6.

- *Longus capitis*—originates from the anterior tubercles of the transverse processes of C3–C6 vertebrae and inserts into the basilar part of the occipital bone lateral to the pharyngeal tubercle. Flexes the neck at the atlanto-occipital joint. Innervated by C1–C3.

Lateral group

The lateral group of prevertebral muscles are the scaleni anterior, medius, and posterior. Collectively, these three pairs of muscles elevate the first and second ribs and cause ipsilateral lateral flexion of the neck. Scalenus anterior serves as a cornerstone in the anatomy of the superior thoracic aperture or root of the neck.

- *Scalenus anterior*—originates from transverse processes of C3–C6 vertebrae and inserts onto the scalene tubercle of the first rib. Acts to raise the first rib during inspiration and assists in rotation and flexion of the neck. Blood supply is from the ascending cervical artery (from the thyrocervical trunk). Innervated by the anterior rami of C5–C6.
- *Scalenus medius*—largest of the scalene muscles. It originates from the transverse processes of most of the cervical vertebrae and inserts onto the posterior aspect of the first rib (separated from the scalenus anterior by the subclavian artery). Innervated by the anterior rami of C3–C8.
- *Scalenus posterior*—originates from the transverse processes of C5–C7 vertebrae and inserts into the outer surface of the second rib. Raises the second rib during respiration and assists in neck flexion, lateral flexion, and rotation.

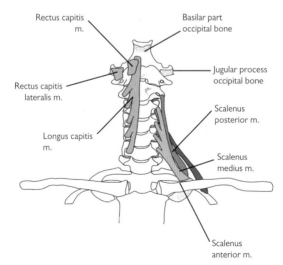

Fig. 5.16 Prevertebral muscles. Anterior group in yellow (longus colli not shown). Lateral group in grey.

Reproduced courtesy of Daniel R. van Gijn.

Osteology

The cervical spine supports the skull. It consists of seven cervical vertebrae and the intervening intervertebral discs (Fig. 5.17). While subtly different, C3–C6 are classed as typical cervical vertebrae (Fig. 5.18 and Fig. 5.19). C1 (atlas), C2 (axis), and C7 (vertebra prominens) have distinct anatomical features and are regarded as atypical.

C3–C6 vertebrae

Each has a small, oval vertebral body and a large, triangular vertebral foramen that is disproportionally large for the overall size of the bone. The typical cervical vertebrae have short, bifid, and inferiorly pointing spinous processes and foramina in their transverse processes (foramen transversarium) that house the vertebral arteries and veins. C7 is an atypical vertebra with a long, palpable spinous process.

Anterior components
- *Body.*
- *Pedicle.*
- *Uncinate processes (posterolateral lip).*
- *Anterior and posterior tubercles of transverse process.*
- *Transverse processes and foramina.*
- *Inferior articular processes.*

Posterior components
- *Lamina.*
- *Bifid spinous process.*
- *Superior and inferior articular processes.*

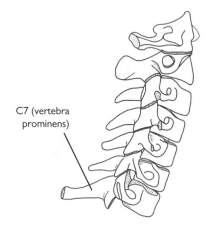

C7 (vertebra prominens)

Fig. 5.17 Cervical spine, lateral view.
Reproduced courtesy of Daniel R. van Gijn.

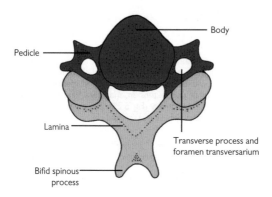

Fig. 5.18 A typical cervical vertebrae (C4), superior view. Anterior components, red; posterior components, yellow.

Reproduced courtesy of Daniel R. van Gijn.

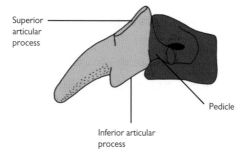

Fig. 5.19 A typical cervical vertebrae (C4), lateral view. Anterior components, red; posterior components, yellow.

Reproduced courtesy of Daniel R. van Gijn.

Atlas and axis

Atlas (C1)

See Fig. 5.20.

Named after the Greek Titan who bore the celestial heavens on his shoulders in punishment, the atlas is an atypical cervical vertebra that articulates superiorly with the occiput of the skull and inferiorly with the dens of the axis—allowing flexion, extension, and lateral flexion of the head and rotation of the head, respectively (Fig. 5.21). It consists of a short anterior and a long posterior arch, lateral masses, and paired transverse processes.

Anterior arch

- *Anterior tubercle*—attachment of anterior longitudinal ligament.
- *Upper and lower borders*—attachment of anterior atlanto-occipital membrane.
- *Posterior surface*—circular facet for articulation with dens of axis.

Posterior arch

Forms three-fifths of the circumference of the atlas.

- *Superior surface*—groove for the vertebral artery, first cervical nerve, and venous plexus (from anterior to posterior).
- *Superior border*—attachment of the posterior atlanto-occipital membrane.
- *Inferior border*—attachments of the ligamenta flava.

Lateral masses

Paired ovoid structures.

- *Superior articular facet*—concave, kidney-shaped facets that articulate with the occipital condyles.
- *Inferior articular facet*—flat, circular facet that articulates with the axis at the lateral atlanto-axial joints.
- *Medial surface*—tubercles for the attachment of the transverse ligament.

Transverse processes

Covered by costal lamellae (occasionally absent thus exposing the foramen transversarium anteriorly) and deeply palpable between the mastoid process and mandibular ramus.

- *Transverse foramina*—contain vertebral arteries and veins.

Vertebral canal

- Divided into two compartments by the transverse ligament, maintaining the dens of the axis in position against the anterior arch.
- *Anterior one-third*—occupied by dens.
- *Posterior two-thirds*—occupied by the cervical part of the spinal cord (one-third) and space (one-third).

Fractures of atlas

Jefferson fracture

A burst fracture of C1 involving a four-part fracture through the anterior and posterior arches, usually resulting from axial compression injuries such as diving or heavy objects falling atop the head. It is not normally associated with neurological injury. Named after the British neurosurgeon Geoffrey Jefferson (1920)

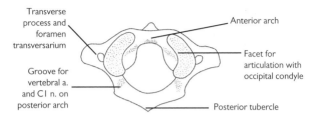

Fig. 5.20 Atlas (C1) vertebra, superior aspect.
Reproduced courtesy of Daniel R. van Gijn.

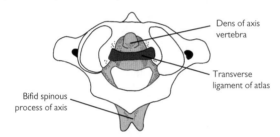

Fig. 5.21 Atlanto-axial joint, superior view.
Reproduced courtesy of Daniel R. van Gijn.

Fractures of axis

Hangman's fracture

Bilateral fractures of the pars interarticularis of the axis resulting in an inherently unstable traumatic spondylolysis. Caused by hyperextension injury of the cervical spine, classically by hanging. They can be classified from I to IV of the Levine and Edwards classification depending on the degree of displacement and angulation.

Axis (C2)

The second cervical vertebra is uniquely identifiable by the odontoid process (dens) (Fig. 5.22). Rotation of the head occurs at the *atlanto-axial joint*.

Anterior components

- *Dens*—conical and approximately 15 mm length. Bears a cartilage-covered groove on its posterior surface for the transverse ligament. The apical ligament is attached to its pointed apex and the alar ligaments are attached to its posterolateral surface.
- *Body*—synchondrosis between partly fused centra of axis and atlas.
- *Lateral mass.*
- *Transverse processes*—contain transverse foramina.
- *Superior and inferior articular facets*—articulate with the inferior articular facets of the atlas and the superior articular facets of C3 vertebra, respectively.

Posterior components
- *Pedicle (pars interarticularis)*—grooved anterolaterally by the vertebral artery. Large notch inferiorly for the posterior primary ramus of the third cervical nerve (C3).
- *Lamina*—attachment for ligamentum flavum.
- *Spinous process*—characteristically massive with bifid tip. Ligamentum nuchae is attached to the apical notch.

Atlanto-axial joint

See Fig. 5.23.

The atlanto-axial joint is a complex joint between the atlas and axis. It consists of three synovial joints, two lateral atlanto-axial joints between the atlas and axis and one median atlanto-axial joint.

Ligaments between the atlas and axis
- *Anterior longitudinal ligament*—thick band running from the anterior arch of the atlas to the body of the axis.
- *Posterior atlanto-occipital membrane*—continuation of the ligamentum flavum that extends from the lower border of the arch of the atlas and occipital bone to the laminae of axis.
- *Cruciform ligament*—consists of superior, inferior, and transverse components posterior to the dens of axis. These act to stabilize the dens to the lateral masses of atlas.

Ligaments between the axis and the occipital bone
- *Tectorial membrane*—a continuation of the posterior longitudinal ligament that extends from the body of the axis to the clivus, as far anteriorly as the spheno-occipital synchondrosis and laterally to the hypoglossal canals.
- Paired alar ligaments.
- Longitudinal part of the cruciform ligament.

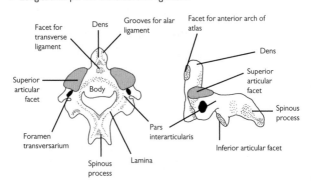

Fig. 5.22 Superior and lateral views of axis. Superior articular facets, yellow.
Reproduced courtesy of Daniel R. van Gijn.

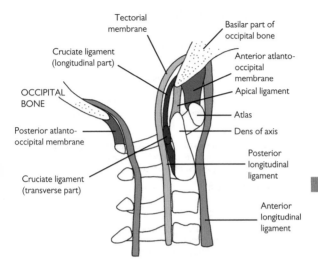

Fig. 5.23 Atlanto-axial joint and associated ligaments, sagittal view.
Reproduced courtesy of Daniel R. van Gijn.

Fasciae of the neck

The cervical fasciae of the neck represent an anatomical paradox. They provide an elegant example of surgical cleavage planes and organ insulation and an inconvenient and potentially catastrophic route for the spread of disease from neck to mediastinum. Cervical fasciae may be divided into superficial and deep layers. The former is an indistinct layer covering platysma and forming a loose connective tissue between dermis and deep fascia. The deep cervical fasciae are divided into four layers, namely the investing, pretracheal, and prevertebral layers and the carotid sheath.

Superficial fascia

- Extends from head and neck into thorax, shoulders, and axillae.
- Invests platysma and is continuous with the superficial muscular aponeurotic system (SMAS) of the face.

Deep cervical fascia

See Fig. 5.24.

Investing layer

- Completely encircles and 'invests' neck—covering trapezius and SCM; forms the roof of the posterior triangle. Encloses two muscles and two glands (parotid and submandibular) (Fig. 5.25).
- *Superior attachments*—superior nuchal line, mastoid process, and inferior border of mandible. Divides at insertion of masseter and covers medial pterygoid and masseter muscles, eventually attaching to the pterygoid plate and zygomatic arch.
- *Inferior attachments*—fuses with the periosteum of the acromion, clavicle, and manubrium sterni where it splits to form the suprasternal space of Burns (contains the inferior parts of anterior jugular vein anastomoses, the sternal heads of SCM, and a lymph node).

Pretracheal fascia

- Extends from the hyoid bone (via cricoid cartilage) and oblique line of the thyroid cartilage superiorly to the superior mediastinum inferiorly (fusing with the aortic arch and posterior pericardium). Encloses the thyroid gland (Fig. 5.26).
- Merges with the investing layer and carotid sheath laterally.
- *Ligament of Berry* arises from this layer, attaching the thyroid gland to the cricoid cartilage.
- *Contents*—infrahyoid strap muscles, thyroid gland, trachea and larynx, oesophagus, recurrent laryngeal nerve, and superior laryngeal nerves (internal and external branches).
- Continuous superiorly with the buccopharyngeal fascia.
- Trochlea of intermediate tendon of digastric muscle is thickening of pretracheal fascia.

Allan Burns (1781–1813)

Scottish anatomist and surgeon. Author of 'Observations on some of the most frequent and important diseases of the heart' (1809) and 'Observations on the surgical anatomy of the head and neck' (1811). A skilled dissector, he developed innovative methods of mummification and lends his name to the suprasternal space of Burns and to Burns' ligament (the superior horn of the falciform margin of the saphenous opening).

Prevertebral fascia
- Deepest layer of the deep cervical fascia.
- *Superior attachment*—skull base.
- *Inferior attachment*—descends into the superior mediastinum to blend with the anterior longitudinal ligament (vertebral column).
- Extends laterally inferior to the clavicle to form the axillary sheath— enclosing the axillary vessels and brachial plexus.
- Continuous with *Sibson's* suprapleural fascia covering the lung apices and the *transversalis fascia* in the abdomen.
- Separated from the buccopharyngeal fascia by the retropharyngeal space.
- *Contents*—include the vertebral column and associated vertebrae, discs, and ligaments, and the anterior vertebral and scalene muscles.
- Forms the floor of the posterior triangle of neck (neck dissection).

Carotid sheath
A roughly cylindrical space formed by the condensation of all three of the above layers of deep cervical fascia (Fig. 5.27).
- Extends from the skull base to the aortic arch.
- Encloses the CCA, ICA, IJV, cranial nerves IX–XII (and parts of ansa cervicalis), and cervical lymph node chain.
- Thicker surrounding the artery, allowing the IJV to expand.

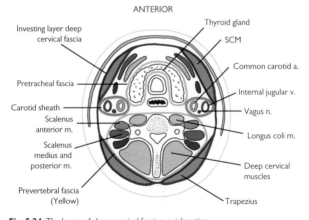

Fig. 5.24 The layers of deep cervical fasciae, axial section.
Reproduced courtesy of Daniel R. van Gijn.

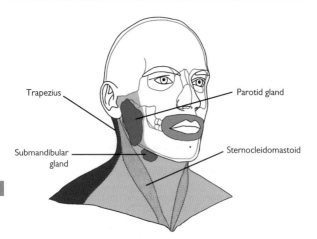

Fig. 5.25 The investing layer of deep cervical fascia—enclosing two muscles and two glands.
Reproduced courtesy of Daniel R. van Gijn.

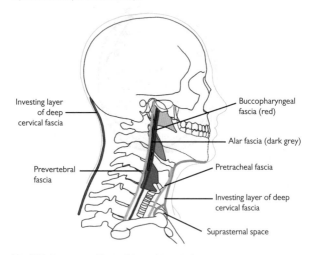

Fig. 5.26 Deep cervical fascia of the neck in sagittal section.
Reproduced courtesy of Daniel R. van Gijn.

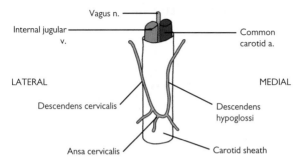

Fig. 5.27 The carotid sheath and ansa cervicalis.
Reproduced courtesy of Daniel R. van Gijn.

Fascial spaces of the face and neck

Knowledge of the fascial spaces of the face and neck and their contents and communications is critically important. It provides a tool by which to consolidate the three-dimensional understanding of these difficult regions and to appreciate the means by which pathology may pass from skull base to mediastinum. These spaces (or perhaps more accurately 'compartments') can be arbitrarily divided into spaces of the face (five), suprahyoid spaces (five), infrahyoid spaces, and spaces of the neck proper (five combined). There is inconsistency and confusion in these divisions. They exist only potentially—until parted by pus, blood, or a surgeon's finger.

Fascial spaces

Fascial spaces of the face
- Canine space.
- Buccal space.
- Parotid space.
- Infratemporal space.
- Periorbital space.

Suprahyoid spaces
- Masticator space (consisting of pterygomandibular, submasseteric, deep temporal, and superficial temporal spaces).
- Submandibular space.
- Submental space.
- Sublingual space.
- Lateral pharyngeal space (pre- and poststyloid).

Infrahyoid spaces
- Pretracheal (visceral) space.
- Prevertebral space.

Fascial spaces of the neck
- Carotid space.
- Retropharyngeal space.
- Danger space.

Grodinsky and Holyoke

Manuel Grodinsky and Edward Holyoke established the modern understanding of fascial spaces in the 1930s by defining five spaces (Fig. 5.28)—expanding on the pioneering work of Burns in 1811.
- *Space 1*: 'Within the fatty tissue superficial to the platysma as well as between the latter and the deep tissue.'
- *Space 2*: 'Between the superficial layer of deep fascia and the deep surface of sternothyroid fascia.'
- *Space 3*: 'Between the visceral fascia surrounding the thyroid gland, trachea and esophagus and the sternothyroid layer anteriorly.'
- *Space 3A*: 'Potential space within the carotid sheath.'
- *Space 4*: 'This is the most important space, often referred to as the danger space because of its relation to the posterior mediastinum.'

THE FASCIAE AND FASCIAL SPACES OF THE
HEAD, NECK AND ADJACENT REGIONS

MANUEL GRODINSKY AND EDWARD A. HOLYOKE
Department of Anatomy, College of Medicine, University of Nebraska, Omaha

TWENTY-ONE FIGURES

The fasciae of the head and neck have been a subject of controversy since their first description by Burns in 1811. Modern textbooks of anatomy and surgery, however, have treated them very briefly and inaccurately. This is partially due to the lack of sufficient interest, but chiefly to the fact that there are numerous discrepancies in observation, making the description of a fixed pattern difficult. This, in turn, is probably due to the inherent difficulties in dissecting these structures and the obvious artificiality of grouping them for descriptive purposes. Anatomically, fasciae are important in circumscribing and separating various structures such as muscle groups, blood vessels and nerves. Clinically, they are important in surgical orientation and in directing the course of infection.

Fig. 5.28 First page of Manuel Grodinsky and Edward Holyoke's article.

Reproduced from Grodinsky, Manuel, Holyoke, Edward A., The fasciae and fascial spaces of the head, neck and adjacent regions, The American Journal of Anatomy, 63:3, 1 Nov 1938, John Wiley and Sons.

Fascial spaces of the face

Canine (infraorbital) space
See Fig. 5.29.
- *Boundaries*—between levator anguli oris and levator labii superioris (superior and superficial), the bony maxilla (and canine fossa) at its deep surface, nasal cartilages (anterior), and buccal space (posterior).
- *Communications*—communicates with the buccal space posteriorly.
- *Contents*—angular artery and vein and infraorbital nerve.
- *Pathology*—from maxillary canine and first premolar, danger triangle.

Buccal (buccinator) space
See Fig. 5.29.
- *Boundaries*—lies deep to platysma and skin and superficial to buccinator and the overlying buccopharyngeal fascia. Bound anteriorly by the angle of the mouth and posteriorly by the pterygomandibular raphe, masseter, and the pterygoid muscles. Superiorly bound by the zygomatic process of the maxilla and zygomaticus muscles and inferiorly by the deep fascia attached to the body of the mandible.
- *Communications*—canine space superiorly, posteriorly communicates with submasseteric, pterygomandibular (and lateral pharyngeal), temporal spaces (masticator space) and submandibular space inferiorly.
- *Contents*—buccal fat pad, Stensen's duct, transverse facial artery and vein, and buccal branch of facial nerve.

Parotid space
Paired spaces enclosed by a continuation of the investing layer of deep cervical fascia (parotidomasseteric fascia).
- *Boundaries*—from the external auditory canal and mastoid superiorly to the angle of the mandible inferiorly.

- *Communications*—parapharyngeal space medially, masticator space anteriorly, and carotid space posteriorly.
- *Contents*—parotid gland, parotid lymph nodes (approximately 20, drain external auditory canal, auricle, and scalp), extracranial facial nerve, ECA, retromandibular vein.

Infratemporal space (postzygomatic/inferior part of deep temporal)
- *Boundaries*—superiorly, the infratemporal surface of the greater wing of the sphenoid and temporal bones; open inferiorly. Anteriorly by the posterior surface of the maxillary tuberosity and posteriorly by the TMJ and deep lobe of the parotid gland. Medial limit is the lateral pterygoid plate and lateral pterygoid muscle, lateral limit is the coronoid process of the mandible and attached temporalis.
- *Communications*—deep temporal space, buccal space, and pterygomandibular space (and orbital space by inferior orbital fissure).
- *Contents*—middle division of the maxillary artery, V_3, pterygoid venous plexus, and buccal fat pad.

Periorbital space (preseptal)
See Fig. 5.29.
- *Boundaries*—superiorly, inferiorly, laterally, and medially by the periosteal attachments of orbicularis oculi. The orbital septum limits posteriorly and the deep surface of orbicularis oculi lies anteriorly.
- *Communications*—canine space and orbital (postseptal) space.
- *Contents*—fat and areolar tissue.

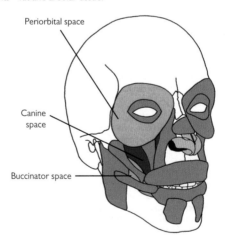

Fig. 5.29 The fascial spaces of the face.
Reproduced courtesy of Daniel R. van Gijn.

Suprahyoid spaces

Masticator space

The masticator space is a collective term for the four spaces defined and bound by the muscles of mastication and their respective deep cervical fascia (as the parotidomasseteric fascia laterally and investing layer of deep cervical fascia medially) (Fig. 5.30). The key pathological feature of the masticator spaces is trismus.

Submasseteric space

- *Boundaries*—zygomatic arch superiorly and inferior border of mandible inferiorly. Bound laterally by the parotidomasseteric fascia and medially/anteriorly/posteriorly by the ramus of the mandible.
- *Communications*—superficial temporal space superiorly, pterygomandibular space posteriorly, and buccal space anteriorly.
- *Contents*—masseter, masseteric artery (from maxillary artery), and vein.

Pterygomandibular space

- *Boundaries*—lateral pterygoid muscle superiorly and pterygomasseteric sling inferiorly. Laterally/anteriorly/posteriorly by the ramus of the mandible. Medially by superficial/investing layer of deep cervical fascia and medial pterygoid muscle.
- *Communications*—submasseteric space laterally, buccal space anteriorly, lateral pharyngeal and peritonsillar space medially, and deep temporal space superiorly.
- *Contents*—inferior alveolar neurovascular bundle, lingual nerve, and mylohyoid nerves.

Superficial temporal space

- *Boundaries*—temporal crest superiorly and zygomatic arch inferiorly, lateral orbital rim anteriorly and temporal crest posteriorly, temporalis muscle medially, and temporalis fascia laterally (note temporalis muscle divides temporal space into superficial and deep components).
- *Communications*—masseteric space inferiorly and deep temporal space.
- *Contents*—middle temporal artery and vein.

Deep temporal space

- *Boundaries*—temporalis muscle attachment at temporal crest superiorly and superior surface of lateral pterygoid muscle inferiorly, infratemporal surface maxilla and posterior surface orbit anteriorly, and temporalis muscle attachment posteriorly. Between the temporalis muscle laterally and greater wing of sphenoid/squamous temporal bone medially.
- *Communications*—pterygomandibular space, superficial temporal space, and infratemporal space.
- *Contents*—deep temporal artery and vein.

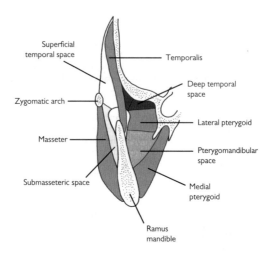

Fig. 5.30 The masticator space.
Reproduced courtesy of Daniel R. van Gijn.

Submandibular space

See Fig. 5.31.
- *Boundaries*—anterior and posterior bellies of digastric muscle. Limited superiorly by the lower border and lingual surface of the mandible and mylohyoid muscle, inferiorly by the investing fascia and digastric tendon. Platysma lies lateral and hyoglossus and mylohyoid lie medial.
- *Communications*—submental space, sublingual space, buccal space, and lateral pharyngeal space.
- *Contents*—facial artery and vein, marginal mandibular nerve, mylohyoid nerve and submandibular gland.

Submental space

- *Boundaries*—bound superiorly by the mylohyoid muscle and inferiorly by the investing layer of deep cervical fascia. Inferior border of mandible lies anteriorly and the hyoid bone posteriorly. The lateral boundaries are the anterior bellies of digastric.
- *Communications*—submandibular spaces.
- *Contents*—anterior jugular veins and lymph nodes.

Sublingual space

See Fig. 5.31.
- *Boundaries*—bound superiorly by the mucosa of the floor of the mouth and inferiorly by the mylohyoid muscle. The space is open posteriorly and limited by the mandible anteriorly. Tongue musculature lies medially and the lingual cortex of the mandible forms the lateral boundary.

- *Communications*—submandibular space and lateral pharyngeal space.
- *Contents*—sublingual gland and Wharton's duct, lingual nerve, hypoglossal nerve, and sublingual artery and vein.

Lateral pharyngeal (parapharyngeal) space
- *Boundaries*—lies between the muscles of mastication and the muscles of deglutition. The superior extent is the skull base and the inferior extent is the hyoid bone. Anterolaterally, it is bound by the investing layer of deep cervical fascia covering the medial pterygoid muscle anteriorly and the parotid gland laterally. Posteriorly bounded by prevertebral fascia and medially by pretracheal/ buccopharyngeal fascia.
- *Communications*—communicates with the masticator spaces, retropharyngeal space, carotid sheath, submandibular, and sublingual spaces.
- Can be further divided into anterior muscular (prestyloid) and posterior neurovascular (poststyloid) spaces by the styloid process and the stylopharyngeal fascia (the *aponeurosis of Zuckerkandl and Testut*), which is a fascial condensation between the styloid process and tensor veli palatini.
- *Contents*—fat, lymph nodes, and connective tissue (prestyloid). Cranial nerves IX, XI, XII, the carotid sheath, and sympathetic chain (poststyloid).

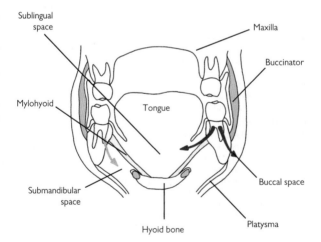

Fig. 5.31 The submandibular, sublingual, and buccal spaces, coronal section.
Reproduced courtesy of Daniel R. van Gijn.

Fascial space infection

Infections in the potential fascial spaces may be superficial or deep. Deep fascial space infections may lack external signs and can rapidly progress to sepsis, descending mediastinitis, jugular venous thrombosis, and airway collapse. Dental infections, trauma, salivary calculi/stasis, and upper respiratory tract infections may be responsible.

Deep fascial space infections may present with
- Odynophagia/dysphagia.
- Fever and neck pain.
- Swelling.
- Respiratory distress.

Commonest sites
- Submandibular space.
- Masticator space(s).
- Parapharyngeal space.
- Parotid space.
- Retropharyngeal space.

Infrahyoid spaces

Pretracheal (visceral) space

The pretracheal or visceral space (continuous with the buccopharyngeal fascia superiorly) is a cylindrical space in the anterior midline of the infrahyoid neck (Fig. 5.32). It is the largest space of the infrahyoid neck and extends from the hyoid bone to the posterior mediastinum.
- *Boundaries*—attachment of the infrahyoid muscles to the thyroid cartilage superiorly and superior mediastinum inferiorly. Bound anteriorly by the investing cervical fascia and posteriorly by the pretracheal/visceral cervical fascia and laterally by the carotid sheath.
- *Communications*—mediastinum and retropharyngeal spaces.
- *Contents*—thyroid gland, trachea, oesophagus, recurrent laryngeal nerves and strap muscles.

Perivertebral space

The *perivertebral space* is a cylindrical space surrounded by the prevertebral layer of deep cervical fascia. It can be divided into an anteriorly located prevertebral part and posterior paraspinal part by an extension of the deep cervical fascia to the transverse processes.
- *Boundaries*—bound superiorly by the base of the skull and extends inferiorly as far as the fourth thoracic vertebrae (or even to the coccyx) via the mediastinum. Posteriorly it is defined by the vertebral bodies and anteriorly by the deep layer of deep cervical fascia.
- *Communications*—the danger space and retropharyngeal space lie anteriorly.
- *Contents*— prevertebral muscles, vertebrae and associated discs/ ligaments, vertebral artery and vein, scalene muscles, phrenic nerve, and roots of the brachial plexus.

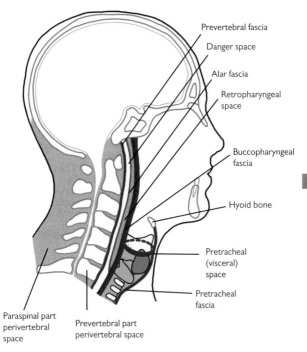

Prevertebral fascia

Danger space

Alar fascia

Retropharyngeal space

Buccopharyngeal fascia

Hyoid bone

Pretracheal (visceral) space

Pretracheal fascia

Paraspinal part perivertebral space

Prevertebral part perivertebral space

Fig. 5.32 Deep spaces of the neck.
Reproduced courtesy of Daniel R. van Gijn.

Fascial spaces of the neck

Carotid space

See Fig. 5.33.

Also known as the poststyloid parapharyngeal space or 'Lincoln's Highway' (Harris P. Mosher, 1929).

- *Boundaries*—extends from the skull base (jugular foramen) to the aortic arch. Formed by all three layers of the deep cervical fascia and confined anterolaterally by the SCM muscles.
- *Communications*— anteriorly with the masticator and lateral pharyngeal spaces, posteriorly with the perivertebral space, and laterally with the parotid space.
- *Contents*— the common/internal carotid and IJV, cranial nerves IX–XII, sympathetic nerves and deep cervical lymph nodes.

Retropharyngeal space (See Fig. 5.33, Space 3 Fig. 5.34)

- *Boundaries*—base of skull superiorly to the fusion of buccopharyngeal and alar fascia inferiorly (variable, approximately at level of tracheal bifurcation). Bound by the buccopharyngeal fascia anteriorly and alar fascia posteriorly. Continuous laterally with the lateral pharyngeal spaces (above hyoid) and carotid sheaths (below hyoid).
- *Communications*—lateral pharyngeal spaces, pretracheal space, carotid sheath space and mediastinum.
- *Contents*—connective tissue and lymphatics from Waldeyer's ring.

Danger space (See Fig. 5.33, Space 4 Fig. 5.34)

A midline space located behind the retropharyngeal space that owes its name to its communication inferiorly with the mediastinum and potential for necrotizing mediastinitis and purulent pericarditis.

- *Boundaries*—bound superiorly by the clivus of the skull base and inferiorly by the posterior mediastinum as far as the diaphragm. Bound anteriorly by the alar fascia and posteriorly by the prevertebral fascia (the layers are easily separated allowing for rapid spread of infection). Bound laterally by the fusion of both alar and prevertebral fascia at the transverse processes of the cervical vertebrae.
- *Communications*—retropharyngeal space, prevertebral space, and mediastinum.
- *Contents*—loose connective tissue.

> **Etymology**
> - *Lincoln's Highway (of the neck)*—a name given to the carotid space/ sheath by Harry Mosher in his address to the American Academy of Otology, reflecting its role in the spread of infections. The Lincoln Highway is one of the first transcontinental highway routes, running from Times Square in New York City to Lincoln Park in San Francisco.

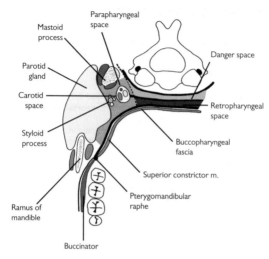

Fig. 5.33 The carotid, retropharyngeal, and danger spaces, transverse section.

Reproduced courtesy of Daniel R. van Gijn.

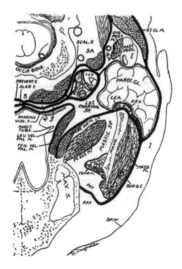

Fig. 5.34 Illustration from Grodinsky and Holyoke, 1938. 'Transverse section of adult cadaver at level of hard palate. Superior view.'

Reproduced from Grodinsky, Manuel, Holyoke, Edward A., The fasciae and fascial spaces of the head, neck and adjacent regions, The American Journal of Anatomy, 63:3, 1 Nov 1938, p378 John Wiley and Sons.

Common carotid artery

The principal blood supply to the head and neck is from the common, internal, and external carotid arteries (Fig. 5.35). The vertebral arteries, from the subclavian arteries, contribute the remainder (⊙ Fig. 5.36, p. 199).

Origin and course

See Fig. 5.35.

- Asymmetric paired structures that supply blood to the head and neck; the left originates directly from the arch of the aorta while the right arises from the right brachiocephalic trunk.
- The left CCA therefore has a thoracic component in addition to its cervical part cranial to the sternoclavicular joint.
- The right CCA only has a cervical component.
- Both arteries travel within the carotid sheath, medial to the IJV and separated by the vagus nerve.
- Both left and right CCAs pass obliquely upwards (separated by the trachea) to the upper border of the thyroid cartilage where they divide into external and internal branches at the level of the fourth cervical vertebra.
- The carotid pulsation can be felt against the prominent transverse process of the sixth cervical vertebrae—designated *Chassaignac's tubercle*.

Relations

- *Below omohyoid*—covered by SCM, sternohyoid, and sternothyroid.
- *Above omohyoid*—covered only by platysma and SCM.
- *Anteriorly*—crossed by SCM branch of superior thyroid artery, superior (and middle) thyroid vein and ansa cervicalis (and descendens hypoglossi and cervicalis).
- *Laterally*—IJV.
- *Medially*—trachea, oesophagus, larynx, pharynx, and thyroid gland.
- *Posteriorly*— four arteries (subclavian, vertebral, inferior thyroid, and ascending cervical), the sympathetic trunk, and the origin of scalenus anterior muscle. The thoracic duct lies posterior on the left.

Carotid sinus

Localized area of dilatation at the bifurcation of the CCA. It is innervated by carotid branches of the glossopharyngeal nerve and is a baroreceptor involved in the regulation of blood pressure in cerebral arteries.

Carotid body (glomus caroticum)

Subcentimetre oval structure on posteromedial surface of CCA, near its bifurcation. It acts as an arterial chemoreceptor and detects changes in oxygen and carbon dioxide partial pressures and pH, adjusting ventilatory volume and rate as required.

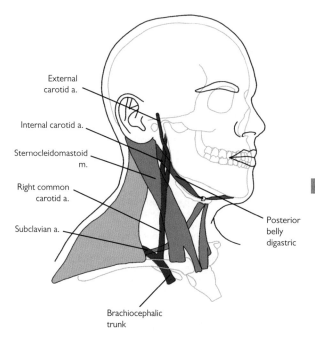

Fig. 5.35 Right common, internal, and external carotid arteries.
Reproduced courtesy of Daniel R. van Gijn.

External and internal carotid arteries

External carotid artery

Origin and course
See Fig. 5.37.
- Branch of the CCA supplying the neck, face, and base of skull. It begins at the upper border of the thyroid cartilage (C4 vertebra), passing anterosuperiorly through the carotid triangle before leaving it under the posterior belly of digastric to enter the parotid gland, where it gives rise to its terminal branches, the superficial temporal and maxillary arteries, behind the neck of the mandibular condyle.
- *Branches*—superior thyroid, lingual, facial (anterior surface), ascending pharyngeal (medial surface) occipital, posterior auricular (posterior surface), maxillary, and superficial temporal (terminal branches).

Relations
See Fig. 5.37 and Fig. 5.38.
- *Anterior relations*—crossed by the posterior belly of digastric. Above digastric it is crossed by the retromandibular vein and facial nerve (within the parotid gland). Below digastric it is crossed by the hypoglossal nerve (and the upper root of the ansa cervicalis) and the common facial and lingual veins.
- *Posterior relations*—three nerves (superior laryngeal and pharyngeal branches of vagus, glossopharyngeal); two muscles (stylopharyngeus and styloglossus), deep lobe of parotid, and pharyngeal wall.
- *Variations*—include common origins of some branches, linguofacial, thyrolingual, and thyrolinguofacial trunks.

Internal carotid artery

Origin and course
Supplies the majority of the ipsilateral cerebral hemisphere, orbit, forehead, and nose.

Ascends anterior to the first three cervical vertebrae and enters the intracranial cavity via the carotid canal of the petrous temporal bone - where it begins a series of 90° turns before terminating as the middle and anterior cerebral arteries.

Segments and branches
See Fig. 5.39.
The tortuous route of the ICA can be subclassified into its respective segments (Bouthillier classification):
- *C1: cervical*—no branches.
- *C2: petrous*—caroticotympanic and Vidian arteries.
- *C3: lacerum*—no branches.
- *C4: cavernous*—meningohypophysial and inferolateral trunk.
- *C5: clinoid*—no branches.
- *C6: ophthalmic*—ophthalmic and superior hypophysial arteries.
- *C7: communicating*—posterior communicating, anterior choroidal, anterior cerebral, and middle cerebral arteries.

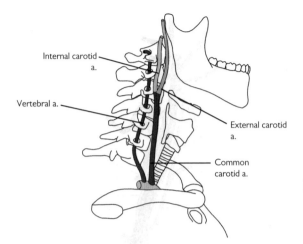

Fig. 5.36 The vertebral artery and common, internal, and external carotid arteries.
Reproduced courtesy of Daniel R. van Gijn.

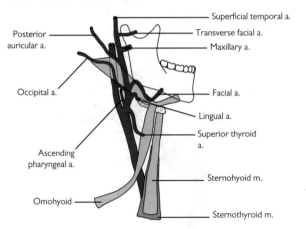

Fig. 5.37 Branches of the external carotid artery.
Reproduced courtesy of Daniel R. van Gijn.

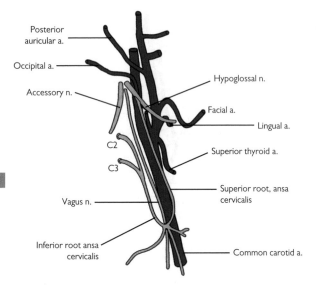

Fig. 5.38 Nervous relations of the common, internal, and external carotid arteries.
Reproduced courtesy of Daniel R. van Gijn.

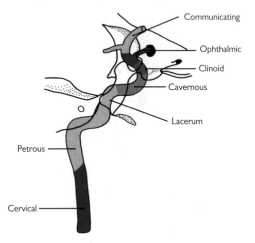

Fig. 5.39 The segments of the internal carotid artery.
Reproduced courtesy of Daniel R. van Gijn.

Subclavian artery

The left subclavian artery arises directly from the aorta while the right arises from the brachiocephalic artery/trunk. Both exit the thorax passing through the superior thoracic aperture arching over the cervical pleura and lung apices. It is separated from the latter by the suprapleural membrane (Sibson's fascia), a dense fascial layer attached to the first rib and costal cartilage anteriorly, C7 transverse process, and mediastinal pleura medially (Fig. 5.40).

Parts (and respective branches) (mnemonic 'VIT CD')

Split into three parts according to its relation with scalenus anterior (Fig. 5.41):
- *First part* (from origin to medial border of scalenus anterior)—vertebral artery, internal thoracic, and thyrocervical trunk. The latter divides into the inferior thyroid artery, suprascapular artery, ascending cervical artery, and transverse cervical artery.
- *Second part* (posterior to scalenus anterior)—costocervical trunk (divides into deep cervical and superior intercostal arteries) and dorsal scapular arteries.
- *Third part* (lateral border scalenus anterior to lateral border first rib)— no branches.

First part, relations

The first part of the subclavian artery is related to two nerves, two veins, and two muscles. The first part of the *left* subclavian artery is crossed by the thoracic duct and left phrenic nerve (⊛ Fig. 5.44, p. 209).
- *Two nerves*—vagus (and recurrent laryngeal nerve on right) and ansa subclavia (*Vieussens' ansa*).
- *Two veins*—IJV and vertebral vein.
- *Two muscles*—sternothyroid and sternohyoid.

Second part, relations

The second part of the subclavian artery lies posterior to scalenus anterior and the phrenic nerve. Posteriorly lie the lower trunk of the brachial plexus and the suprapleural membrane. Superiorly are the upper and middle trunks of the brachial plexus.

> **Etymology**
> - *Francis Sibson (1814–1876)*—British physician and anatomist.
> - *Raymond Vieussens (1635–1715)*—French anatomist. Credited as being the first physician to give accurate descriptions of the left ventricle and mitral stenosis.

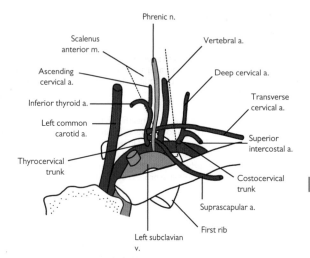

Fig. 5.40 The left subclavian artery, relations, and details (scalenus anterior is demonstrated by the dashed line).

Reproduced courtesy of Daniel R. van Gijn.

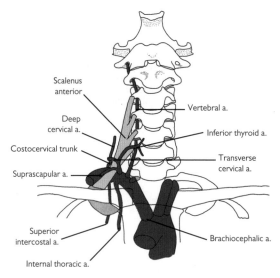

Fig. 5.41 Relationship of the subclavian artery to the first rib (yellow) and scalenus anterior.

Reproduced courtesy of Daniel R. van Gijn.

Vertebral artery

Origin and course

The paired vertebral arteries arise from the first part of their respective subclavian arteries and ascend in the neck posterior to the internal carotid arteries through the transverse foramina of the cervical vertebrae, ultimately joining their fellow to form the basilar artery and supply the posterior fossa and occipital lobes.

Segments

Can typically be divided into four segments (Fig. 5.42):

- *V1: preforaminal*—from origin to transverse foramen of C6 vertebra. Ascends between scalenus anterior and longus colli and is crossed by the inferior thyroid artery and thoracic duct (on left). The CCA and vertebral vein lie anteriorly. Posteriorly lie the ventral rami of spinal nerves C7 and C8, the transverse process of C7 vertebra, and inferior cervical ganglion.
- *V2: foraminal*—runs through the foramina of C6 to C1 vertebrae. Accompanied by the vertebral veins and sympathetic nerves.
- *V3: atlantic*—lies within the suboccipital triangle. Exits the foramen transversarium of C1 (atlas), passes behind the lateral mass of C1 and continues superomedially through the foramen magnum to pierce the dura and arachnoid mater. The tortuosity of the vessel allows length for movement during rotation at the atlantoaxial joints.
- *V4: intracranial*—lies inside the cranial cavity anterior to the roots of the hypoglossal nerve. Joins its contralateral counterpart at the lower border of the pons to become the basilar artery.

Branches

- *V1*—cervical muscular and spinal branches.
- *V2*—anterior meningeal and spinal branches.
- *V3*—muscular branches, posterior meningeal artery.
- *V4*—branches to the hindbrain and spinal cord: posterior inferior cerebellar artery (supplies inferior cerebellum, medulla, choroid plexus of the fourth ventricle), anterior and posterior spinal arteries, perforating branches to medulla oblongata.

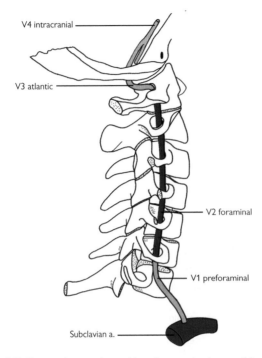

Fig. 5.42 The cervical spine and occipital bone demonstrating the parts of the vertebral artery, lateral view.
Reproduced courtesy of Daniel R. van Gijn.

Veins of the neck

External jugular vein

Origin and course

Drains the scalp, head, and face. Formed from the union of the posterior division of the retromandibular and posterior auricular veins at the angle of the mandible (Fig. 5.43). From here it travels, superficial to SCM, obliquely towards the midclavicular point. At the root of the neck it traverses the deep fascia and drains into the subclavian vein.

Tributaries

Receives the following tributaries:

- *Posterior EJV*—begins in the occipital scalp.
- *Transverse cervical vein.*
- *Suprascapular vein.*
- *Anterior jugular vein*—arises from the confluence of the superficial mandibular veins at the level of the hyoid bone, descending between the midline and anterior border of SCM. It joins the EJV above the sternum and its contralateral counterpart by the jugular arch.

Internal jugular vein

Origin and course

Initially dilated as the superior bulb, the IJV is a continuation of the sigmoid sinus, beginning at the posterior compartment of the jugular foramen and running downwards in the carotid sheath to join the subclavian vein (Fig. 5.43). It drains the skull, brain, superficial face, and neck.

Relations

- Lies lateral to the common and external carotid arteries, separated only by the posteriorly lying vagus nerve. At the skull base, the IJV lies posterior to the internal carotid artery from which it is separated by cranial nerves IX–XII lying in between.
- Crossed by the posterior belly of digastric superiorly and the inferior belly of omohyoid inferiorly.
- Crossed by the accessory nerve and inferior root of ansa cervicalis.

Tributaries

As follows. The IJV may communicate with the EJV.

- *Inferior petrosal*—joins the superior bulb.
- *Facial vein.*
- *Lingual.*
- *Pharyngeal.*
- *Superior and middle thyroid.*

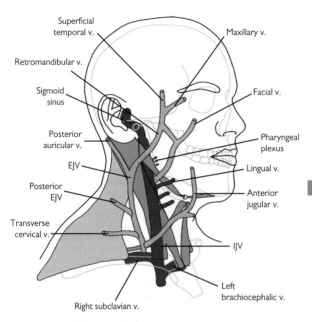

Fig. 5.43 Venous drainage of the head and neck. External jugular system, yellow. Internal jugular system, dark grey.

Reproduced courtesy of Daniel R. van Gijn.

Thoracic duct

The thoracic duct drains chyle from the small intestine and lymph from most of the body except the right side of the head, neck and heart, right upper limb, parts of the left and right lung and part of the convex surface of the liver.

Origin and course

- Originates as the *cisterna chyli* (cistern of Pecquet) under the right hemidiaphragm—entering the thorax via the aortic hiatus between the descending aorta and azygos vein before heading superiorly in the posterior mediastinum, to the left of the oesophagus.
- Passing laterally through the superior mediastinum, it exits the thoracic cavity via the thoracic inlet anterior to the phrenic nerve, scalenus anterior and the first part of the subclavian artery (Fig. 5.44).
- It terminates, with significant anatomical variation (40% of population), at the junction of the left IJV and subclavian vein.

Right lymphatic duct

Union of right jugular, subclavian, and mediastinal lymphatic trunks. It has a short 2 cm course (when a solitary trunk exists), terminating between the IJV and subclavian vein. More often the three trunks drain independently.

Chylous leak

Results from damage to the thoracic duct (left) or lymphatic duct (right). May be identified at the time of injury by the pooling of clear fluid, or as a milky fluid (in a feeding patient due to fat content) in the drain postoperatively. Ligation/oversewing of the duct may be attempted intraoperatively, although the tissues are friable. Management depends on output volume:

High output (>600 mL/24 hours)

- Generally needs surgical exploration and ligation/soft tissue flap cover of the leak. Oversewing, pressure dressings, and tissue adhesives have also been described.

Low output (<600 mL/24 hours)

- Can generally be treated non-operatively.
- Medium-chain triglyceride enteral feeding.
- Pressure dressings.
- Prescription of a somatostatin analogue (octreotide).
- Monitor fluid and electrolyte balance.

Etymology

- *Jean Pecquet (1622–1674)*—French scientist. Discovered the course of the lacteal vessels and the termination of the thoracic duct (the 'principal lacteal vessel') into the subclavian vein. He also studied the expansion of air, the nature of vision and psychology.
- *Chyle*—from the Greek, meaning 'juice'.

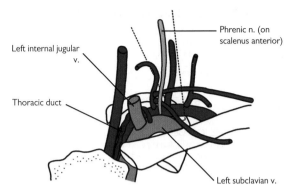

Fig. 5.44 Relations of thoracic duct left and subclavian vessels in root of neck.
Reproduced courtesy of Daniel R. van Gijn.

Nerves of the neck and relations

The structures of the neck (from skin to muscle to viscera) are innervated by cranial nerves IX, X, and XI, the cervical spinal nerves, and the cervical sympathetic trunk (Fig. 5.45 and Fig. 5.46).

Glossopharyngeal nerve

Origin and course

Emerges from the sides of the upper medulla and has motor, sensory, and autonomic components. Leaves the skull via the pars nervosa of the jugular foramen (anterior to the vagus and accessory nerves) and passes between the IJV and ICA. Descends on the ICA deep to the styloid process, curving forward on stylopharyngeus to enter the pharynx between the superior and middle pharyngeal constrictors. It continues medial and deep to hyoglossus to reach the fauces and tonsil, postsulcal tongue, and mucosa of the pharynx.

Ganglia

Situated on the glossopharyngeal nerve as it traverses the jugular foramen.
* *Superior (jugular) ganglion*—situated in groove where the nerve passes through the jugular foramen. Small and contains visceral sensory fibres from the pharynx, parotid gland, and middle ear.
* *Inferior (petrosal) ganglion*—larger and situated in the lower portion of the petrous temporal bone. Conveys information related to special and sensory information from the mucous membranes of the posterior one-third of the tongue and oropharynx, respectively.

Branches

* *Tympanic (Jacobsen's nerve)*—leaves the inferior ganglion and re-enters the skull through the inferior tympanic canaliculus where it contributes to the tympanic plexus within the middle ear. Becomes the lesser petrosal nerve.
* *Carotid (Hering's nerve)*—descends on the ICA. Contains afferent fibres from chemoreceptors in the carotid body and baroreceptors in the carotid sinus. Communicates with the pharyngeal branch of the vagus.
* *Pharyngeal*—three to four filaments that combine with the vagus and sympathetic nerves to form the pharyngeal plexus, perforating the pharynx to supply its mucous membranes.
* *Muscular*—supplies stylopharyngeus.
* *Tonsillar*—supplies the palatine tonsil directly and soft palate and fauces indirectly via a plexus (*circulus tonsillaris*). Communicates with the greater and lesser palatine nerves.
* *Lingual*—supplies the mucosa and vallate papillae of the base of tongue. Communicates with the lingual nerve.

Vagus nerve

Origin and course

The 'wandering' vagus is a complex mixed sensory, motor, and parasympathetic nerve that runs through the neck, thorax, and abdomen. It arises from the posterolateral medulla from four principal nuclei:
* *Nucleus ambiguus* (motor).
* *Dorsal nucleus of vagus* (parasympathetic).

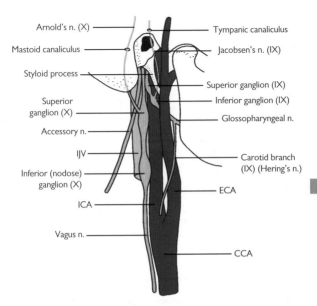

Fig. 5.45 The nerves of the neck and their relations to the common, internal, and external carotid arteries (hypoglossal nerve not shown).

Reproduced courtesy of Daniel R. van Gijn.

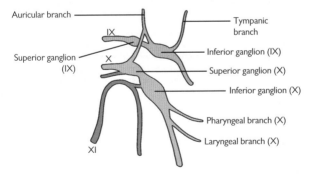

Fig. 5.46 Cranial nerves IX, X, and XI, schematic.

Reproduced courtesy of Daniel R. van Gijn.

- *Nucleus solitarius* (taste).
- *Spinal nucleus of trigeminal nerve* (general sensation).

The vagus nerve exits the skull through the pars vascularis of the jugular foramen to enter the carotid space, from where it descends vertically in the neck within the carotid sheath. The left and right nerves follow different paths *en route* to the thorax.

Branches and supply
See Fig. 5.47.
- *Meningeal*—from the superior vagal ganglion through the jugular foramen to the dura mater of the posterior cranial fossa.
- *Auricular (Arnold's/Alderman's nerve)*—from the superior vagal ganglion (and connections from the inferior ganglion of the glossopharyngeal nerve). Enters the mastoid canaliculus and traverses the temporal bone before supplying a branch to the facial nerve. Innervates the external auditory meatus—responsible for referred otalgia in laryngeal pathology.
- *Pharyngeal*—from the inferior vagal ('nodose') ganglion. The principal motor nerve of the pharynx. Forms part of the pharyngeal plexus (supplies all pharyngeal muscles except stylopharyngeus and all muscles of soft palate except tensor veli palatini).
- *Carotid body*—variable in number and origin.
- *Superior laryngeal*—from the inferior vagal ganglion, divides into external and internal branches.
- *Internal branch of superior laryngeal*—sensory to the laryngeal mucosa down to the level of the vocal folds. Pierces the thyrohyoid membrane above the superior laryngeal artery and divides into upper and lower branches. The former supplies the mucosa of the pharynx, epiglottis, and valleculae, and the latter supplies the mucosa of the arytenoid region.
- *External branch of superior laryngeal*—motor supply to cricothyroid. Gives branches to the pharyngeal plexus and inferior pharyngeal constrictor. Communicates with the superior cardiac nerve and superior cervical ganglion.
- *Recurrent laryngeal*—supplies all intrinsic muscles of the larynx except cricothyroid. Sensory to the larynx below the vocal cords. Curves around the subclavian artery on the right (closely related to the inferior thyroid artery near the thyroid gland) and the aortic arch (posterior to the ligamentum arteriosum) on the left. Both ascend within the tracheoesophageal groove.
- *Cardiac*.

Accessory nerve
Origin and course
While generally considered as a single nerve, the accessory nerve has two roots: a smaller cranial root arising from the nucleus ambiguus in the medulla oblongata and a spinal root arising from the upper five cervical segments of the spinal cord. The two roots briefly unite in the jugular foramen before again dividing (Fig. 5.48).
- *Cranial root*—joins the vagus nerve shortly after separating from the spinal root below the jugular foramen. Its fibres probably innervate pharyngeal/palatal muscles. May contribute to the recurrent laryngeal nerve.

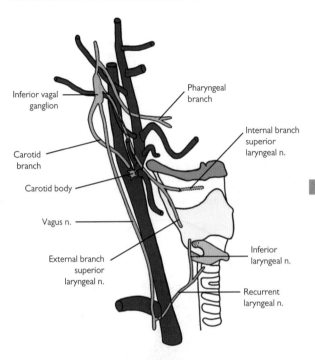

Fig. 5.47 Relations and branches of the right vagus nerve.
Reproduced courtesy of Daniel R. van Gijn.

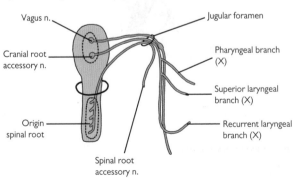

Fig. 5.48 The spinal accessory nerve. Note the cranial root joining (and 'accessory'
to) the vagus nerve.
Reproduced courtesy of Daniel R. van Gijn.

- *Spinal root*—fibres emerge laterally from the spinal cord between segments C1 and C5 before ascending through the foramen magnum. Exits the skull via the jugular foramen in a common dural sheath with the vagus. Descends deep to the IJV, running obliquely behind digastric and stylohyoid muscles to the upper part of SCM, and entering its deep surface. Emerges from the midpoint of the posterior border of the SCM and crosses the posterior triangle upon the prevertebral fascia to end in the deep surface of trapezius.

Branches supply
- SCM.
- Trapezius.

Clinical landmarks
Course corresponds to a line drawn on the side of the neck passing through the following points: tragus of ear, tip of transverse process of atlas, middle of posterior border of SCM, and anterior border of trapezius approximately 5 cm superior to the clavicle (Fig. 5.49).

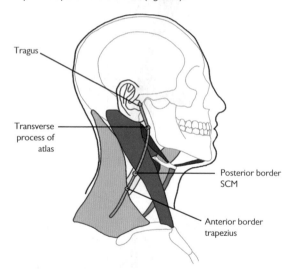

Tragus

Transverse process of atlas

Posterior border SCM

Anterior border trapezius

Fig. 5.49 Surface marking of the spinal accessory nerve.
Reproduced courtesy of Daniel R. van Gijn.

Accessory nerve injury
Incomplete denervation of SCM and trapezius following surgical sacrifice of the spinal accessory nerve during radical neck dissection suggests additional an additional motor contribution from the cervical plexus and thoracic roots, respectively. Intractable neuralgia may result from an unsupported shoulder and arm causing brachial plexus traction injury.

Hypoglossal nerve

The hypoglossal nerve supplies all of the extrinsic and intrinsic muscles of the tongue except palatoglossus (innervated by the vagus via the pharyngeal plexus). Receives fibres from the first cervical nerve.

Origin and course

Arises from the lateral medulla oblongata from a number of rootlets and exits the skull via the hypoglossal canal in the occipital bone before descending between the ICA and IJV anterior to the vagus nerve (Fig. 5.50). Below the posterior belly of digastric it curves forwards around the origin of the occipital artery, crossing the ICA and ECA and a loop of the lingual artery. It continues forward superficial to hyoglossus (the lingual artery passes deep to hyoglossus) before entering and supplying genioglossus.

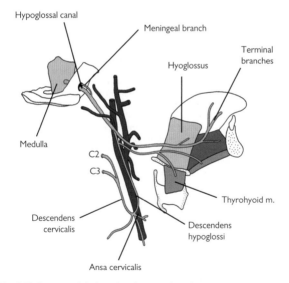

Fig. 5.50 Schematic of the hypoglossal nerve and its relations.
Reproduced courtesy of Daniel R. van Gijn.

Branches and supply
- *Meningeal*—leaves the nerve in the hypoglossal canal to supply the dura of the posterior cranial fossa and inferior petrosal sinus.
- *Descendens hypoglossi*—leaves the hypoglossal nerve when it curves around the occipital artery. Contains motor fibres from C1.
- *Muscular branches (to tongue, thyrohyoid, and geniohyoid)*—arise near the posterior border of hyoglossus.

Hypoglossal nerve injury

Lesions of the hypoglossal nerve (usually iatrogenic/traumatic) result in paralysis and atrophy of the ipsilateral tongue so that the tongue deviates towards the side of the lesion on protrusion. Paralysis of the hyoid depressors may result in contralateral deviation of the larynx upon swallowing.

Lesser-known triangles of the submandibular region

See Fig. 5.51.
- *Lesser's triangle*—named after Ladislaus Leon Lesser (1846–1925), German surgeon. Bound by the anterior and posterior bellies of the digastric muscle inferiorly and the hypoglossal nerve superiorly. Principal content is the lingual artery, found beneath hyoglossus, which forms its floor.
- *Pirogov's triangle*—named after Russian surgeon Nikolai Pirogov (1810–1881). It is the posterior part of Lesser's triangle and is bound by the hypoglossal nerve superiorly, the intermediate tendon of digastric inferoposteriorly, and the posterior border of mylohyoid muscle posteriorly. The lingual artery is consistently found in this triangle, deep to hyoglossus muscle.
- *Beclard's triangle*—named after the French anatomist Pierre Beclard (1785–1825). Bound by the posterior belly of the digastric muscle, the posterior border of hyoglossus muscle, and the greater cornu of the hyoid bone.

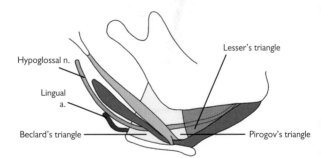

Fig. 5.51 Beclard's, Lesser's, and Pirogov's triangles in the right neck.
Reproduced courtesy of Daniel R. van Gijn.

Cervical plexus

Overview
Formed by the ventral rami of the upper four cervical nerves, and supplies some neck muscles, including most of the infrahyoid group, and areas of skin on the head, neck and chest (Fig. 5.52).

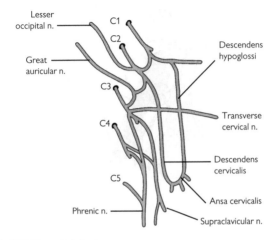

Fig. 5.52 The cervical plexus.
Reproduced courtesy of Daniel R. van Gijn.

Cutaneous (superficial) branches
Cutaneous branches emerge from a point approximately midway between the mastoid process and manubrium along the posterior border of SCM at the *punctum nervosum* (nerve point) of the neck. This is approximately at the junction of the superior one-third and inferior two-thirds of the SCM. The spinal accessory nerve can be found emerging approximately 1cm above the punctum nervosum (Fig. 5.53).

• *Lesser occipital (C2)*—innervates the skin of the neck and scalp superior and posterior to the auricle.
• *Great auricular (C2, C3)*—anterior facial branch supplies the skin over the parotid gland. The posterior mastoid branch supplies the skin over the mastoid process and concha, lobule, and posterior auricle.
• *Transverse cutaneous (C2, C3)*—superior (ascending) and inferior (descending) branches that pierce platysma. Supply the anterosuperior and inferolateral skin of the neck, respectively.
• *Lateral, intermediate, and medial supraclavicular (C3, C4)*—innervate the upper chest and shoulders.

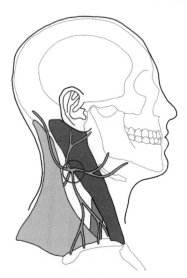

Fig. 5.53 The punctum nervosum of the neck—the point of emergence of the cutaneous branches of the cervical plexus (red circle).

Reproduced courtesy of Daniel R. van Gijn.

Muscular branches

- *Direct muscular branches*—to SCM, trapezius and the anterior and lateral muscles of the neck.
- *Ansa cervicalis*—nervous loop anterior to the carotid sheath with a superior root (descendens hypoglossi) and an inferior root (descendens cervicalis). Supplies all infrahyoid muscles except thyrohyoid.
- *Phrenic nerve (C3, C4, C5)*—mixed motor/sensory nerve that passes through the neck and thorax *en route* to supply the diaphragm. Descends over scalenus anterior (which separates it from the second part of the subclavian artery) beneath the prevertebral fascia. The left and right nerves follow different paths, closely skirting the pericardium before piercing their respective hemidiaphragms.

Etymology and Erb's point misnomer

Wilhelm Heinrich Erb (1840–1921)—German neurologist. Other neurological contributions include:

- *Erb–Duchenne palsy*—brachial plexus palsy caused during childbirth.
- *Erb–Westphal symptom*—an abnormal reflex seen in tabes dorsalis.
- *Erb–Goldflam disease*—myasthenia gravis. Described by Erb in 1878.

Erb's point misnomer

Erb's point is often, incorrectly, used interchangeably with the *punctum nervosum*: the terms are not synonymous. Erb originally described a superficial point 2–3 cm superior to the clavicle 'somewhat outside of the posterior border of SCM' at the level of the carotid tubercle (C6 vertebra).

Cervical sympathetic trunk

The cervical sympathetic trunks lie anterior to the transverse processes of the cervical vertebrae within the perivertebral space, posterior to the carotid sheaths. Each extends vertically from the base of the skull to the root of the neck and contains longitudinally arranged superior, middle and inferior ganglia: the middle ganglia may not be present (Fig. 5.54).

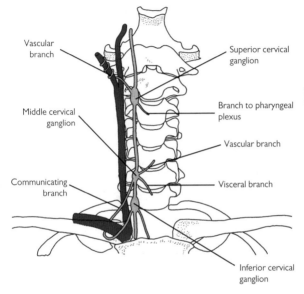

Fig. 5.54 Cervical sympathetic trunk demonstrating superior, middle, and inferior cervical ganglia and branches.

Reproduced courtesy of Daniel R. van Gijn.

Superior cervical ganglion

Lies opposite the second and third cervical vertebrae and consists of communicating, visceral, and vascular branches.

- *Communicating*—lateral branches to the upper four cervical spinal nerves. Branches to inferior vagal ganglion, hypoglossal nerve, superior jugular bulb, and meninges of the posterior cranial fossa.
- *Visceral*—to laryngopharynx (supplies carotid body, forms pharyngeal plexus with glossopharyngeal and vagus) and heart.
- *Vascular*—to common and external carotid arteries and branches of the latter.

Middle cervical ganglion

Smallest of the three ganglia and occasionally absent. Lies opposite the sixth cervical vertebra and anterior to the inferior thyroid artery. Has communicating, visceral, and vascular branches.

- *Communicating*—with fifth and sixth cervical nerves.
- *Visceral*—cardiac, parathyroid/thyroid/tracheal, and oesophageal branches. Communicates with superior cardiac, external laryngeal, and recurrent laryngeal nerves.
- *Vascular*—to inferior thyroid artery. Vasomotor to vessels in the thyroid and parathyroid glands.

Inferior (stellate) cervical ganglion

Lies superior to the neck of the first rib (posterior to the vertebral artery) and is separated from the cervical pleura inferiorly by Sibson's suprapleural membrane.

- *Communicating*—with seventh and eighth cervical nerves.
- *Visceral*—cardiac branch to deep cardiac plexus.
- *Vascular*—to subclavian and vertebral arteries (the latter forming a vertebral plexus).

Horner's syndrome

A syndrome consisting of ipsilateral ptosis, pupillary miosis, facial anhidrosis, and apparent enophthalmos. Occurs as a result of disruption to the oculosympathetic pathway. Ptosis occurs due to loss of innervation to the superior tarsal muscle ('Muller's muscle'). Pathology may affect the sympathetic pathway anywhere along its length and can be classified according to location into central, preganglionic, and postganglionic lesions. Postganglionic causes (third-order sympathetic neurons from the superior cervical ganglion to the cavernous sinus via the ICA) include ICA lesions (thrombi, aneurysms), mass lesions in the neck, or penetrating trauma.

Johann Friedrich Horner (1831–1886)

Although Swiss ophthalmologist, Johann Horner, is largely credited with the eponymous syndrome, it was the French physiologist Claude Bernard in 1854 who first described the syndrome, initially in animals and later in a soldier who had sustained a gunshot wound to the neck.

Lymph drainage of the head and neck

The lymphatics of the head and neck are located in superficial and deep layers, separated by the deep cervical fascia, and within a central compartment. The thoracic duct is discussed separately.

Superficial lymph nodes

Drain the superficial tissues of the head and neck, ie. the scalp, skin of forehead, upper face, and auricle. Can be described arbitrarily as forming a ring or pericervical collar from chin to occiput and ultimately draining into the deep cervical nodes (Fig. 5.55).

Four groups lie within the head:
- *Occipital*—one to three nodes. Drain the posterior scalp and posterior external ear.
- *Mastoid (postauricular)*—two nodes. Drain posterior neck, upper ear, and posterior external auditory meatus.
- *Parotid*—located above or below the parotidomasseteric fascia. Drain the anterior scalp, forehead, parotid, nose, nasal cavity, external auditory meatus and lateral borders of the orbit.
- *Facial*—drain the mucous membranes of the nose, cheek, eyelids, and conjunctiva.

Four groups lie within the neck:
- *Submandibular*—three to six nodes. Drain the upper lip, lateral lower lip, gingivae, and anterior tongue.
- *Submental*—superficial to mylohyoid. Drain the central lower lip, floor of mouth, and lower gingivae.
- *Anterior cervical*—drain the superficial surfaces of the anterior neck.
- *Superficial cervical*—drain the superficial surfaces of the neck.

Deep lymph nodes

Numerous nodes from the skull base to the neck lie along the carotid sheath, deep to SCM. They can be classified into superior and inferior groups divided by omohyoid (Fig. 5.56).
- *Superior (supra-omohyoid) group*—includes the jugulodigastric node (principal node of Kuttner) inferior to the posterior belly of digastric, which is a common site for metastases from carcinomas of the upper digestive tract (oral cavity, naso/oro/hypopharynx, supraglottic larynx) and the jugulo-omohyoid node (prominent inferior jugular group node, common site for metastases from papillary thyroid carcinoma).
- *Inferior (subomohyoid) group*—includes nodes from the spinal accessory chain to the jugular–subclavian vein junction, an inferior carotid group and a deep transverse cervical group (accompanies the transverse cervical artery, includes Virchow's node).

Central compartment nodes

Include the prelaryngeal, pretracheal, perithyroid, and paratracheal nodal groups (Fig. 5.57).
- *Prelaryngeal*.
- *Pretracheal (Delphian node)*—superior to the thyroid isthmus and anterior to the cricothyroid membrane within the pretracheal fascia. Involved in laryngeal and thyroid carcinomas and diffuse nodal involvement in head and neck SCC.

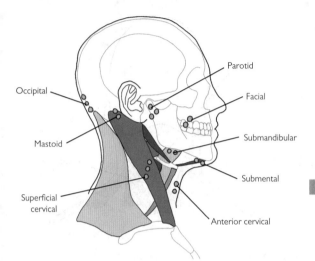

Fig. 5.55 Superficial lymph node groups.
Reproduced courtesy of Daniel R. van Gijn.

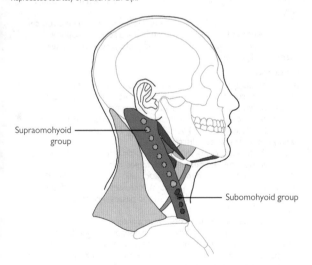

Fig. 5.56 Supra- and subomohyoid deep lymph node groups.
Reproduced courtesy of Daniel R. van Gijn.

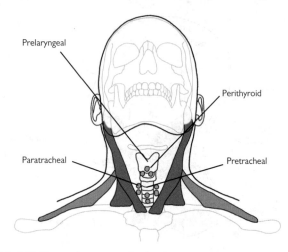

Fig. 5.57 The central compartment lymph nodes.
Reproduced courtesy of Daniel R. van Gijn.

- *Perithyroid*—nodes above/below thyroid fascia. Drain the thyroid and pretracheal group.
- *Paratracheal (recurrent laryngeal)*—numerous nodes along the course of the recurrent laryngeal nerve, within the tracheo-oesophageal gutter. Drain the infraglottic larynx and prelaryngeal, pretracheal, and perithyroid groups.

Thoracic duct

The main route by which chyle is returned to the venous system, the thoracic duct also conveys lymph from both lower limbs, the abdomen, left hemithorax, left upper limb, and left head and neck.

- Originates as a superior continuation of the cisterna chyli (cistern of Pecquet) adjacent to the L1 vertebral body. The cisterna chyli is not always very obvious as a discrete vessel.
- Enters the thoracic cavity through the aortic hiatus, passing posteriorly to the oesophagus and between the azygos vein and aorta.
- At or near the level of the transthoracic plane (of Ludwig, which divides the superior and inferior mediastinum), it crosses to the left of the midline.
- Traverses the superior mediastinum and passes through the thoracic inlet into the neck.
- In the space between longus colli, scalenus anterior and the suprapleural membrane, the duct usually arches 3–4 cm superior to the clavicle, crossing anterior to the vertebral vessels, the left sympathetic trunk, the vertebral sympathetic ganglion, the left thyrocervical trunk and the left phrenic nerve.
- Terminates by draining into the angle of the left IJV and left subclavian vein (this is subject to significant anatomical variation, including double thoracic ducts, multiple terminal channels, termination in left IJV, right IJV, azygos vein, or left subclavian vein).

Delphian node
From the 'Oracle of Delphi'—after the High Priestess of the Temple of Apollo at Delphi.

Sentinel lymph node biopsy
Identifies the first draining lymph node and used as a prognostic tool in the head and neck for cutaneous melanoma and mucosal squamous cell carcinoma of the oropharynx. Identification of the sentinel node is facilitated by injection of radioactive tracer at the site of the primary tumour which:
- *Produces a lymphoscintogram* that may be superimposed on a computed tomography (CT) positron emission tomography scan to give anatomically useful information.
- *Produces a radioactive count*—to guide location intraoperatively.

Blue dye is injected at the time of operative harvest, and the dye is visualized in the sentinel node.

In the head and neck, close proximity to the primary tumour site can give false radioactive readings ('shine through'), and complex anatomy, in particular for parotid bed nodes, can risk neurovascular injury. However, sentinel node harvest by head and neck trained surgeons has comparable morbidity to axilla and groin nodal basins.

Has an emerging role in midline oral cavity cancer in guiding management of the (bilateral) neck.

Clinical lymph nodal groups

Primarily for the purpose of staging squamous cell carcinoma of the head and neck, the cervical lymph nodes can be divided into six clinical levels (a seventh level representing lymph node groups in the superior mediastinum was previously used) (Fig. 5.58).

Level I: submental and submandibular group

• *Level Ia: submental group*—a triangular space bound by the anterior bellies of digastric and the hyoid bone. Drain the floor of mouth, anterior tongue, anterior mandibular alveolar ridge, and lower lip.
• *Level Ib: submandibular*—space bound by anterior and posterior bellies of digastric, stylohyoid, and inferior border mandible. Drain the oral cavity, anterior nasal cavity, midface, and submandibular gland.

Level II: upper jugular group

Lymph nodal group located around the upper third of the IJV. Bound superiorly by the skull base, inferiorly by the hyoid bone, medially by sternohyoid and stylohyoid, and laterally by the posterior border of SCM. Drains the oral and nasal cavities, naso-, oro-, and hypopharynx, larynx, and parotid gland.

• *Level IIa*—anterior to spinal accessory nerve.
• *Level IIb*—posterior to spinal accessory nerve.

Level III: middle jugular group

Lymph nodal group located around the middle third of the IJV; bound superiorly by the inferior border of the hyoid bone, inferiorly by the inferior border of the cricoid cartilage, medially by sternohyoid, and laterally by the posterior border of SCM. Drains the oral cavity and naso-, oro-, and hypopharynx.

Level IV: lower jugular group

Lymph nodal group located around the lower third of the IJV. Bound superiorly by the inferior border of the cricoid, inferiorly by the clavicle, medially by sternohyoid, and laterally by the posterior border of SCM. Drains the hypopharynx, cervical oesophagus, and larynx.

Level V: posterior triangle groups

Lymph nodal group located around the lower half of the spinal accessory nerve and transverse cervical artery. Bound superiorly by the junction of trapezius and SCM, inferiorly by the clavicle, medially by the posterior border of SCM, and laterally by the anterior border of trapezius. Levels Va and Vb are distinguished by an imaginary horizontal plane marked by the inferior border of the cricoid cartilage.

• *Level Va*—contains spinal accessory nodes.
• *Level Vb*—contains supraclavicular nodes and nodes located around the transverse cervical artery.

Level VI: anterior compartment group

Lymph nodal group including pre- and paratracheal nodes, perithyroid nodes, and precricoid (Delphian) node. Bound superiorly by the hyoid bone, inferiorly by the suprasternal notch, and laterally by the common carotid arteries. Drain the thyroid, larynx, piriform sinus and cervical oesophagus.

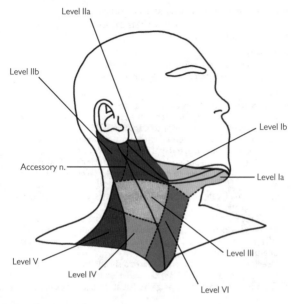

Fig. 5.58 Clinical lymph node levels.
Reproduced courtesy of Daniel R. van Gijn.

Neck dissection

Neck dissection describes excision of the investing layer of deep cervical fascia and the lymphatic tissue within for prophylactic or therapeutic regional control of malignancy. Various classifications have been described. A simple descriptive method is:
* *Selective* (sparing of one or more levels).
* *Comprehensive (levels I–V)*—structure-sparing or structure-sacrificing (spinal accessory nerve, SCM, IJV).
* *Extended*—other nodal basins also dissected such as parotid gland or postauricular nodes.

Selective neck dissection has been increasingly advocated for some malignancies as patterns of lymph node metastasis have been delineated to offer a less morbid procedure to achieve comparable regional control. For example, tongue malignancies requiring neck dissection drain to levels I–III, with some centres including level IV to account for skip lesions.

Neck dissection anatomy and complications

A detailed knowledge of anatomy assists dissection and can preclude in-advertent structural injury.

Boundaries
- *Superficial*—skin flap raised deep to platysma.
- *Deep*—posterior extent is prevertebral fascia.

Structures
- *Submandibular gland*—located in level Ib.
- *Greater auricular nerve*—located at the punctum nervosum, approximately 6.5 cm inferior to tragus on SCM.
- *Marginal mandibular nerve*—courses above the inferior border of the mandible and superficial to facial vessels in 80% of cases.
- *Level I–II boundary*—posterior belly of digastric is described as the 'resident's friend'. Deep to it are the hypoglossal nerve, ICA, ECA and IJV.
- *Levels II–IV*—located along the IJV, adjacent to CCA and vagus nerve, within carotid sheath.
- *Spinal accessory nerve*—divides level II and passes through level V. Its course is identified at the junction of the superior one-third and inferior two-thirds of SCM, and at the superior two-thirds to inferior one-third of trapezius.
- *Phrenic nerve*—posterolateral to carotid sheath, the only nerve travelling lateral to medial, at risk in level V.
- *Thoracic duct*—crosses from right to left at the inferior extent of level IV.

Dr Hayes Martin and his manoeuvre
Hayes Martin (1892–1977)
Chief of the head and neck service at Memorial Hospital. His book *Surgery of Head and Neck Tumours* (1957) became the standard textbook for those interested in head and neck surgery. One of the more famous of his 160 or more publications was 'Neck dissection' published in *Cancer* in 1951. In this he describes the technique for preserving the marginal mandibular branch of the facial nerve during neck dissection (Fig. 5.59 and Fig. 5.60):
  'After identification of the nerve the external maxillary artery and facial vein can be clamped, cut and ligated, after which the upper end of the vascular stump can be looped over the nerve and sutured to the upper skin flap for protection'.

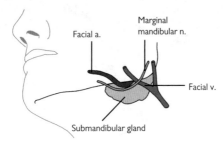

Fig. 5.59 The usual relationship of the facial vessels to the marginal mandibular nerve.

Reproduced courtesy of Daniel R. van Gijn.

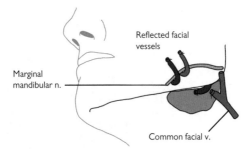

Fig. 5.60 Ligation of the facial vessels and their superior reflection to protect the marginal mandibular nerve.

Reproduced courtesy of Daniel R. van Gijn.

Viscera of the neck

Introduction

The shield-like thyroid is a superficially located (and thus clinically identifiable) endocrine gland in the anterior lower neck. Its principal responsi-
bilities lie in the production of triiodothyronine, tetraiodothyronine, and
calcitonin, involved in the control of basal metabolic rate and calcium
homeostasis.

The small (usually) paired, and inconsistent parathyroid glands lie behind
the lobes of the thyroid gland. They measure 6 mm by 4 mm by 2 mm and
are ordinarily four in number, two superior and two inferior. They are involved in the careful regulation of the body's calcium levels.

Thyroid gland

The thyroid gland is a symmetrical H-shaped endocrine structure in the lower neck. It consists of two lobes, each extending from the oblique line of the thyroid cartilage above to the sixth tracheal ring below—united by a median isthmus covered by the anterior jugular veins. See Figs. 6.1–6.3.

Features

- *Lobes*—each measuring approximately 5 cm (superoinferiorly) by 3 cm (transverse) by 2 cm (anteroposterior). Attached at their posteromedial aspects to the cricoid cartilage by a lateral thyroid ligament (of Berry).
- *Isthmus*—anterior to second and third tracheal cartilages and measuring a little over a centimetre squared.
- *Pyramidal lobe*—an occasional conical projection from the isthmus marking the inferior extent of the embryonic thyroglossal duct. The tip is sometimes connected to the body of the hyoid bone by either a ligament or elevator muscle (also in the path of the thyroglossal duct).

Surfaces

The thyroid gland has three surfaces and respective relations:

Lateral (superficial) surface
- Convex and covered by the pretracheal fascia (see later in topic) and four muscles: SCM, sternothyroid (attached to oblique thyroid line), superior belly of omohyoid, and sternohyoid (Fig. 6.3).

Medial surface
See Fig. 6.1.
- *Superior relations*—inferior constrictor muscle, external laryngeal nerve, and cricothyroid muscle.
- *Inferior relations*—trachea, oesophagus, and recurrent laryngeal nerve.

Posterior surface
See Fig. 6.2.
- Related to the superior and inferior parathyroid glands and the superior and inferior thyroid arteries.
- Overlaps the CCA.

Blood supply

Three principal arteries supply the thyroid gland and share multiple anastomoses (Fig. 6.4):
- *Superior thyroid artery*—from external carotid artery. It divides into anterior and posterior branches after piercing the thyroid fascia. Closely related to the external laryngeal nerve.
- *Inferior thyroid artery*—arises from thyrocervical trunk. Divides into superior ascending and inferior branches. Important relationship with the recurrent laryngeal nerve.
- *Thyroidea ima artery*—variable. Arises from the arch of the aorta.

Venous drainage

The venous drainage of the thyroid gland is via the superior, middle, and inferior thyroid veins which together form a pretracheal plexus.

- *Superior thyroid vein*—travels with the superior thyroid artery. Drains into the IJV.
- *Middle thyroid vein*—emerges from the lateral surface of the gland. Drains into the IJV.
- *Inferior thyroid vein*—drains into the brachiocephalic vein.

Lymphatic drainage

The thyroid gland drains into the prelaryngeal, pretracheal, lower deep cervical (via vessels travelling with superior thyroid vein) and paratracheal lymph nodes. May drain directly to thoracic duct.

Innervation

The thyroid gland receives its autonomic innervation from the superior, middle, and inferior cervical sympathetic ganglia. A plexus from the inferior cervical ganglion travels alongside the inferior thyroid artery to the thyroid gland and communicates with the recurrent and external laryngeal nerves. The relationships between the superior thyroid gland and external laryngeal nerve and the inferior thyroid artery and recurrent laryngeal nerve are of clinical significance.

Capsule

The thyroid capsule is invested by an inner true capsule and an outer false capsule.

- *True capsule*—thin and closely adherent to the gland. Venous plexus lies within true capsule.
- *False capsule*—thicker and formed from the pretracheal layer of deep cervical fascia. The ligament of Berry is a condensation of the false capsule and both anchors the thyroid gland to the cricoid cartilage and is intimately related to the recurrent laryngeal nerve, inferior thyroid artery, superior parathyroid gland, and tubercle of Zuckerkandl.

Zuckerkandl tubercle

A (variable) bilateral pyramidal extension of the thyroid gland (Fig. 6.2) and important surgical landmark owing to its relations as described previously.

> *Emil Zuckerkandl (1849–1910)* Professor of anatomy at the University of Vienna.
>
> *Sir James Berry (1860–1946)* British surgeon born in Kingston, Ontario, and educated at St Bartholomew's Hospital, London.

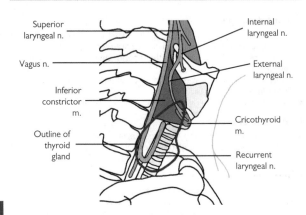

Fig. 6.1 Relations of the medial surface of the thyroid gland.
Reproduced courtesy of Daniel R. van Gijn.

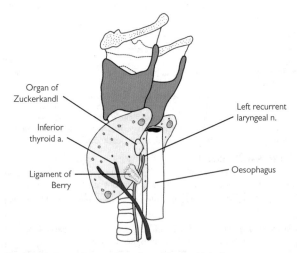

Fig. 6.2 Relations of the posterior surface of the thyroid gland.
Reproduced courtesy of Daniel R. van Gijn.

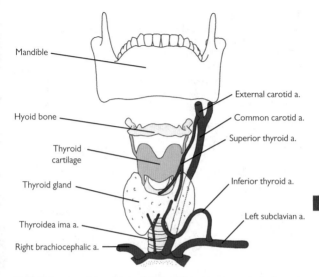

Fig. 6.3 Overview of the relations of the thyroid gland (transverse section).
Reproduced courtesy of Daniel R. van Gijn.

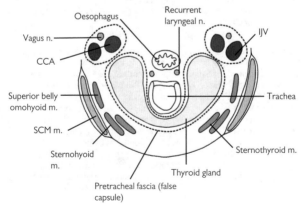

Fig. 6.4 Arterial supply of the thyroid gland.
Reproduced courtesy of Daniel R. van Gijn.

Thyroidectomy

Indications include tumour, diffuse enlargement causing compression of adjacent structures, and overactivity where other treatments have failed. Patients should be euthyroid preoperatively to avoid a thyroid crisis.

Surgical technique

- Neck in extended position, and horizontal incision made through skin, fat, and platysma.
- Investing fascia is incised vertically and the gland mobilized from adherent tissue.
- Superior thyroid artery ligated close to gland to avoid injuring the external laryngeal nerve.
- Inferior thyroid artery ligated distal to gland to avoid injuring the recurrent laryngeal nerve.
- Closed in layers—platysma and skin.

Complications

- Bleeding.
- External laryngeal and recurrent laryngeal nerve injury—leading to a change in pitch, hoarseness (weakness), or complete loss of voice (aphonia).
- Parathyroid gland excision or injury causing hypocalcaemia.

Thyroid tumours

Benign

- Adenomas—common and often multiple.
- May cause hyperthyroidism and necessitate surgery if failure to control medically.

Malignant

- *Papillary* (70%)—the commonest malignant tumour with many being thyroid-stimulating hormone dependent and multifocal, frequently occurring in young patients with a history of irradiation, and many metastasize to cervical lymph nodes. Pathology is characteristically 'Orphan Annie' nuclei (pale and empty).
- *Follicular* (20%)—a solitary tumour of glandular tissue, may spread via lymphatics to lymph nodes or via haematogenous spread.
- *Anaplastic* (<5%)—older patients and carries the worst prognosis. Spreads to regional lymph nodes and adjacent tissues.
- *Medullary* (5%)—tumour of calcitonin secreting cells and may metastasize to regional lymph nodes and via haematogenous spread. It is associated with multiple endocrine neoplasia type 2 syndromes.

Thyroid gland examination

Examination should form part of a head and neck examination, in addition to systemic features of hypothyroidism and hyperthyroidism.

Patient seated in a chair, with neck exposed to clavicles

- *Inspection*—from in front and side, assess scars and lumps.
- *Sip of water and swallow*—assess for lump moving superiorly (thyroglossal cyst).
- *Palpation*—assess any lump for site, size, shape, surface, consistency, borders, mobility or tethering, punctum, fluctuance, and transillumination.
- Assess cervical lymph nodes, and midline position of trachea, thyroid, and larynx.
- *Percussion*—for retrosternal extension.
- *Auscultation*—listen for thyroid bruit.

Parathyroid glands

The small (usually) paired, and inconsistent parathyroid glands lie behind the lobes of the thyroid gland. They measure 6 mm by 4 mm by 2 mm and are ordinarily four in number, two superior and two inferior. They are involved in the careful regulation of the body's calcium levels (Fig. 6.5).

Superior parathyroids

- More consistent in location.
- Termed 'parathyroid IV'; develop from the fourth pharyngeal pouch.
- Found within the pretracheal fascia.
- Found midway along the posterior borders of the thyroid gland.

Inferior parathyroids

- Inconsistent location.
- Termed 'parathyroid III'; develop from the third pharyngeal pouch. They are pushed caudally by the developing thymus, hence their inconsistent location.
- May be found within the thyroid fascia (below inferior thyroid arteries), outside (above inferior thyroid arteries), or within the thyroid gland itself.

Blood supply

Both superior and inferior glands are ordinarily supplied by the inferior thyroid artery. Drainage is into the venous plexus on the anterior surface of the thyroid gland.

Innervation

Sympathetic vasoconstrictor activity comes from the superior and middle cervical ganglia. Generally speaking, the postganglionic sympathetic nerves travel with the arterial supply.

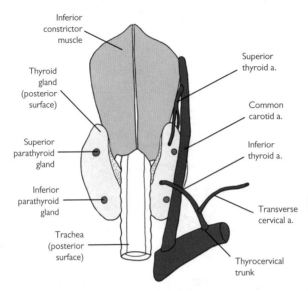

Fig. 6.5 Posterior view of thyroid gland and parathyroid glands.
Reproduced courtesy of Daniel R. van Gijn.

Chapter 7

The pharynx

Introduction

The pharynx is the cranial limit of the alimentary tract and lies behind the nasal (nasopharynx), oral (oropharynx), and laryngeal (laryngopharynx) cavities, extending from the skull base above to the level of the sixth cervical vertebra below, at the commencement of the oesophagus (Fig. 7.1).

The pharynx consists of a thick muscular tube formed from the three constrictor muscles, stylopharyngeus, palatopharyngeus, and salpingopharyngeus; it is lined by the pharyngobasilar fascia internally and buccopharyngeal fascia externally.

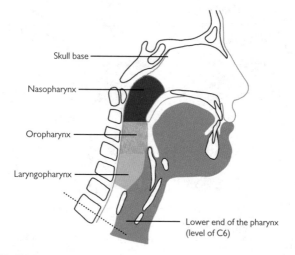

Fig. 7.1 The parts of the pharynx.
Reproduced courtesy of Daniel R. van Gijn.

Nasopharynx

The nasopharynx lies anterior to the first and second cervical vertebrae, communicating with the nasal cavity anteriorly via the posterior nasal apertures and laterally with the middle ear via the Eustachian tubes (Fig. 7.2).

Boundaries

- *Anterior*—postnasal choanae.
- *Posterior*—atlas and axis (C1 and C2 vertebrae).
- *Superior*—called the 'fornix'; formed by basiocciput/basisphenoid. The mucosa is attached to pharyngobasilar fascia.
- *Inferior*—upper surface of soft palate and pharyngeal isthmus, separating nasopharynx from oropharynx.

Features

- *Pharyngeal recess*—a depression behind the tubal elevation known as the fossa of Rosenmüller. It is situated behind the ostium of the Eustachian tube and contains the retropharyngeal lymph node (node of Rouviere). Immediately deep to the mucosa in this region is the deficiency in the pharyngobasilar fascia, the *sinus of Morgagni*.
- *Eustachian tube*—the tubal eminence (nasal end of the cartilaginous auditory tube) lies anteriorly on the lateral wall just superior to the soft palate. The opening of the auditory tube lies approximately 1 cm posterior to the posterior part of the inferior meatus.
- *Tubal elevation*—bounds the opening of the auditory tube from above and behind.
- *Salpingopharyngeal fold*—extends downwards from the tubal elevation and contains salpingopharyngeal muscle.
- *Nasopharyngeal tonsil*—a mass of lymphoid tissue embedded in the mucous membrane of the posterior wall of the nasopharynx. Termed adenoids when enlarged and can contribute to respiratory obstruction in children.

Blood supply

- *Ascending pharyngeal artery* (branch of ECA).
- *Ascending palatine branch of facial artery.*
- *Ascending cervical artery* (branch of thyrocervical trunk).
- *Maxillary artery.*

Sensory innervation

- The pharyngeal branch (of the maxillary division of the trigeminal nerve) via the pterygopalatine ganglion.
- The nerve leaves the pterygopalatine fossa to enter the nasopharynx via the palatovaginal canal.

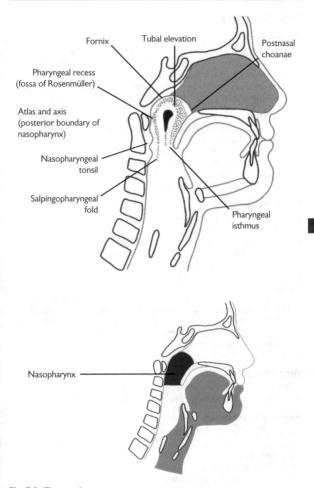

Fig. 7.2. The nasopharynx.
Reproduced courtesy of Daniel R. van Gijn.

Oropharynx

Overview

Extends from the soft palate superiorly to the superior border of the epiglottis below, communicating with the nasopharynx superiorly via the pharyngeal isthmus and with the oral cavity anteriorly via the oropharyngeal isthmus. It is characterized by *Waldeyer's* lymphatic ring, which is composed of the nasopharyngeal, tubal, palatine, and lingual tonsils (Fig. 7.3).

Boundaries

- *Anterior*—a vertical line running through the junction of the hard and soft palates, anterior tonsillar pillars, and circumvallate papillae.
- *Posterior*—posterior pharyngeal wall.
- *Superior*—level of the free edge of the soft palate.
- *Inferior*—level of the hyoid bone/superior edge of the epiglottis.
- *Lateral*—the tonsillar fossae and pillars.

Features/contents

- The posterior third (pharyngeal part) of the tongue and lingual tonsils (continuous with palatine tonsils).
- The palatine tonsils and the anterior and posterior tonsillar pillars (the palatoglossal and palatopharyngeal folds, respectively).
- The inferior surface of the soft palate.
- The posterior pharyngeal wall.
- Uvula.
- Valleculae—paired spaces between the posterior tongue and epiglottis. They are separated from one another by the median glossoepiglottic fold and bound laterally by the lateral glossoepiglottic folds. The mucous membrane of the epiglottis is reflected onto the tongue base and lateral walls of pharynx.
- Glossotonsillar sulci.

Blood supply

- Ascending palatine branch of the facial artery.
- Ascending pharyngeal artery (smallest branch of the ECA).

Sensory innervation

Predominantly by the glossopharyngeal nerve.

> **Etymology**
> - *Uvula*—meaning 'little grape'.
> - *Vallecula*—meaning 'small valley'.

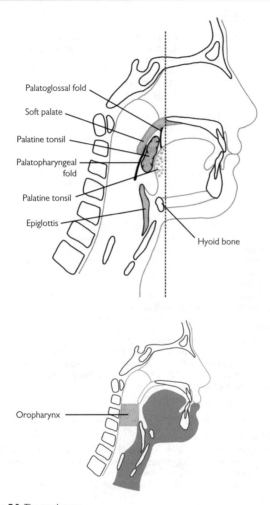

Fig. 7.3 The oropharynx.
Reproduced courtesy of Daniel R. van Gijn.

Hypopharynx

The hypopharynx (or laryngopharynx) is the continuation of the oropharynx superiorly and extends from the epiglottis to the lower border of the cricoid cartilage, where it continues as the cervical oesophagus. Its anterior wall is formed by the inlet of the larynx superiorly and by the posterior part of the cricoid cartilage inferiorly (Fig. 7.4).

Boundaries

- *Anterior*—postcricoid mucosa (area behind cricoid and arytenoid cartilages; at level of pharyngo-oesophageal junction).
- *Posterior*—middle and inferior constrictor muscles, posterior pharyngeal mucosa supported by the vertebral bodies of C4–C6, prevertebral fascia, and the retropharyngeal space.
- *Superior*—hyoid bone and glossoepiglottic and pharyngoepiglottic folds.
- *Inferior*—cricoid cartilage and cricopharyngeus muscle.

Features/subsites

The following components of the hypopharynx are collectively important subsites in the staging of malignancy in the region.
- *Piriform fossae (sinuses)*—formed by the invagination of the larynx within the hypopharynx. A pear-shaped depression posterolateral to each side of the laryngeal opening from the level of the pharyngoepiglottic fold to the upper end of the oesophagus. Bound between the aryepiglottic fold medially and mucous membrane lining the inner surface of the thyroid cartilage laterally. The mucous membrane is intimately related to the branches of the internal laryngeal nerve.
- *Postcricoid region*—comprises the mucosa and submucosa of the anterior wall of the hypopharynx and extends from the inferior aspect of the arytenoids to the inferior border of the cricoid cartilage. Its lateral margins are continuous with the medial wall of the piriform sinus.
- *Posterior pharyngeal wall*—from within outward consists of the mucous membrane, pharyngobasilar fascia, muscles of the pharynx, and the buccopharyngeal fascia.

Sensory innervation

Predominantly from the (internal branch of) the vagus nerve.

Killian's dehiscence

A triangular area in the posterior wall of the pharynx without muscular cover, between thyropharyngeus and cricopharyngeus (parts of the inferior pharyngeal constrictor muscle). It represents a potentially weak area where a pouch or pharyngoesophageal (Zenker's) diverticulum is more likely to occur.

Gustav Killian (1860–1921)
- German professor of laryngology and founder of bronchoscopy.

Friedrich Albert von Zenker (1825–1898)
- German pathologist and physician.

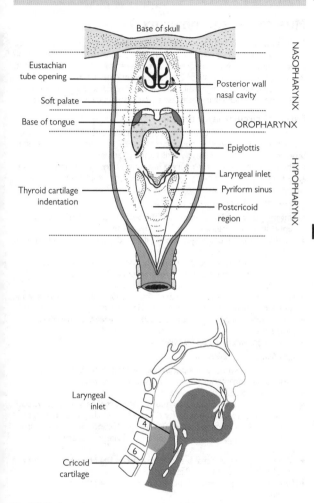

Fig. 7.4 The hypopharynx.
Reproduced courtesy of Daniel R. van Gijn.

Muscles of the pharynx

The wall of the pharynx is principally composed of two layers of striated muscle: an external circular layer of the three constrictor muscles and an inner longitudinal layer composed of three paired muscles. From within out, the pharyngeal wall consists of a mucous membrane spanning the length of the pharynx, the pharyngobasilar fascia, the external and internal muscular layers, and the buccopharyngeal fascia which covers their outer surface.

External circular layer muscles

The superior, middle, and inferior constrictor muscles of the pharynx are stacked within one another and are continuous posteriorly at a median fibrous raphe which extends upwards to the pharyngeal tubercle. As a rule of thumb, all muscles of the pharynx are supplied by the cranial root of the accessory nerve via the pharyngeal plexus except stylopharyngeus, which is supplied by the glossopharyngeal nerve (Figs. 7.5–7.8).

Superior pharyngeal constrictor
- *Origin*—pterygoid hamulus, posterior border of pterygomandibular raphe, and the posterior end of mylohyoid line.
- *Insertion*—median pharyngeal raphe (attached to pharyngeal tubercle on the basilar part of the occipital bone).
- *Relations*—free upper border related to levator veli palatini muscle and the Eustachian tube. The lower border is related to the glossopharyngeal nerve and stylopharyngeus muscle.
- *Blood supply*—pharyngeal branch of the ascending pharyngeal artery and tonsillar branch of the facial artery (➲ Fig. 7.12, p. 259).
- *Innervation*—cranial root of the accessory nerve via the pharyngeal plexus.
- *Action*—constricts the upper pharynx.

Middle pharyngeal constrictor
- *Origin*—lesser cornu and upper border of the greater cornu of the hyoid bone and inferior part of the stylohyoid ligament.
- *Insertion*—median pharyngeal raphe.
- *Relations*—the stylopharyngeus muscle and glossopharyngeal nerve pass between the middle and superior constrictor muscles. The pharyngeal plexus, internal laryngeal nerve, and laryngeal branch of the superior thyroid artery pass between the middle and inferior constrictor muscles.
- *Blood supply*—pharyngeal branch of the ascending pharyngeal artery and tonsillar branch of the facial artery.
- *Innervation*—cranial root of the accessory nerve via the pharyngeal plexus.
- *Action*—participates in swallowing.

> *Gustav Philip Passavant (1815–1893)*
> - German surgeon based in Frankfurt—first noted a pad on the posterior pharyngeal wall in a patient with unrepaired cleft palate.
> - Remains an anatomically and functionally poorly understood structure.

Inferior pharyngeal constrictor

- *Origin*—oblique line of the thyroid cartilage and lateral aspect of the cricoid cartilage (thyropharyngeus and cricopharyngeus parts of the inferior pharyngeal constrictor, respectively).
- *Insertion*—median pharyngeal raphe.
- *Relations*—the internal laryngeal nerve and superior laryngeal artery pass between the middle and inferior constrictors. The recurrent laryngeal nerve and inferior laryngeal artery pass deep to the lower border of the inferior constrictor muscle.
- *Blood supply*—ascending pharyngeal artery.
- *Innervation*—pharyngeal plexus.
- *Action*—participates in swallowing.

Internal longitudinal layer muscles

The laryngopharyngeal elevators consist of three paired muscles that insert into the pharyngeal wall and thyroid cartilage (Figs. 7.5, 7.6, and 7.8).

Palatopharyngeus

- *Origin*—palatine aponeurosis and hard palate.
- *Insertion*—upper border of the thyroid cartilage. Blends with the fibres of the superior constrictor muscle.
- *Blood supply*—facial artery.
- *Innervation*—pharyngeal branch of the facial nerve.
- *Action*—elevates the larynx and pharynx.

Stylopharyngeus

- *Origin*—medial aspect of the styloid process of the temporal bone.
- *Insertion*—posterior border of the thyroid cartilage and lateral glossoepiglottic fold.
- *Relations*—passes between the superior and middle constrictor muscles.
- *Blood supply*—pharyngeal branch of the ascending pharyngeal artery.
- *Innervation*—glossopharyngeal nerve.
- *Action*—elevates the larynx and pharynx and participates in swallowing.

Salpingopharyngeus

- *Origin*—arises from the superior border of the medial cartilage of the Eustachian (pharyngotympanic) tube.
- *Insertion*—merges with fibres of palatopharyngeus muscle.
- *Innervation*—vagus nerve via the pharyngeal plexus.
- *Action*—participates in speech and swallowing by elevating the larynx and shortening the pharynx respectively. Opens the nasopharyngeal orifice of the pharyngotympanic (Eustachian) tube.

Passavant's ridge (palatopharyngeal sphincter)

Horizontal upper fibres of palatopharyngeus run and merge on the deep surface of the superior constrictor muscles. On contraction, this forms a ridge on the posterior pharyngeal wall called *Passavant's ridge*—a ledge that the elevated soft palate meets to close the nasopharyngeal isthmus.

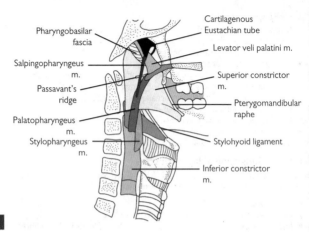

Fig. 7.5 Arrangement and relationships of the longitudinal and circular muscles of the pharynx, internal (lateral) view.
Reproduced courtesy of Daniel R. van Gijn.

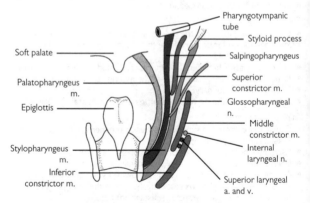

Fig. 7.6 Arrangement and relationships of the longitudinal and circular muscles of the pharynx, posterior (coronal) view.
Reproduced courtesy of Daniel R. van Gijn.

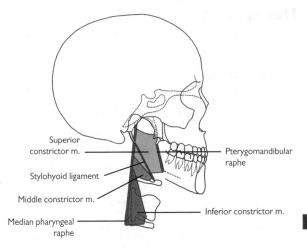

Fig. 7.7 The constrictor muscles of the pharynx and ligaments of pharynx, lateral view.
Reproduced courtesy of Daniel R. van Gijn.

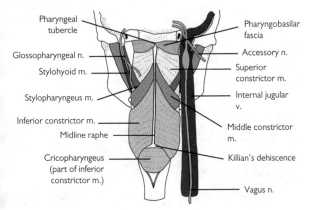

Fig. 7.8 The pharynx, posterior view.
Reproduced courtesy of Daniel R. van Gijn.

Pharyngeal fascia

The pharyngeal fascia forms part of the pretracheal (middle) layer of the deep cervical fascia and consists of two parts: the pharyngobasilar fascia and the buccopharyngeal fascia (Fig. 7.9).

Pharyngobasilar fascia

The pharyngobasilar fascia may be considered an aponeurotic extension of the pharyngeal constrictor muscles and their internal epimysium; it completes the space between the free superior edge of the superior constrictor muscle and the base of the skull (Fig. 7.10).

Features
* *Sinus of Morgagni*—a defect in the anterior aspect of the pharyngobasilar fascia containing the levator veli palatini muscle and Eustachian tube.

Attachments
* *Superiorly*—basilar part of the petrous bone and petrous temporal bone.
* *Inferiorly*—superior pharyngeal constrictor muscle.
* *Anteriorly*—posterior free edge of the medial pterygoid plate bilaterally.
* *Posteriorly*—median pharyngeal raphe (midline).

Buccopharyngeal fascia

The thinner external component of the pharyngeal fascia, covering the pharyngeal constrictor muscles and extending anteriorly to invest buccinator muscle. Related loosely by areolar tissue to the prevertebral fascia: the intervening space is the retropharyngeal space.

Features
* May be considered part of the visceral (middle) layer of the deep cervical fascia.
* Blends laterally with the carotid sheath on either side.
* Blends inferiorly with the fibrous pericardium.

Trotter's syndrome

A combination of signs and symptoms relating to advanced nasopharyngeal carcinoma in the region of the sinus of Morgagni. Symptoms and signs include:
* Unilateral conductive hearing loss secondary to middle ear effusion.
* Pain and anaesthesia in the distribution of the mandibular division of the trigeminal nerve.
* Immobility of the soft palate secondary to palatal muscle infiltration.

Wilfred Trotter (1872–1939)
* British general surgeon with an interest in neurosurgery.
* Sociologist and author of *Instincts of the Herds in Peace and War* among others on the behaviour of man.

Giovanni Batista Morgagni (1682–1771)
* Professor of anatomy, University of Padua, Italy.

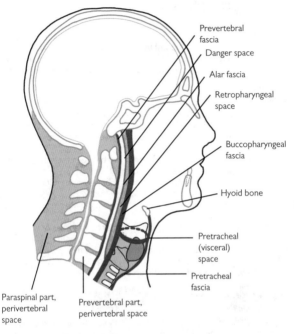

Fig. 7.9 Pharyngeal fascia and associated spaces, sagittal view.
Reproduced courtesy of Daniel R. van Gijn.

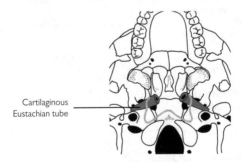

Fig. 7.10 Superior attachment of the pharyngeal fascia (yellow outline).
Reproduced courtesy of Daniel R. van Gijn.

Pharyngeal plexus

The pharyngeal plexus is a network of nerve fibres lying mainly posterior
to the middle constrictor muscle in the retropharyngeal space, within the
buccopharyngeal fascia. It contributes the principal motor and sensory
nerve supply to the muscles of the pharynx and soft palate and allows for
the co-ordination of both speech and swallowing (Fig. 7.11 and Fig. 7.12).

Features

- The pharyngeal plexus is formed from the pharyngeal branches of the
vagus, glossopharyngeal, and cervical sympathetic nerves.
- Its branches extend dorsolaterally over the pharyngeal constrictor
muscles, branching between the muscular layer and mucosa of the
pharynx.
- Some branches extend superiorly, onto and between the superior and
middle pharyngeal constrictor muscles.
- Some branches extend inferiorly, onto and between the middle and
inferior pharyngeal constrictor muscles.
- The motor nerve supply is predominantly from the pharyngeal branches
of the vagus nerve.
- The sensory nerve supply is from the pharyngeal branches of the
glossopharyngeal nerve.
- All muscles of the pharynx and soft palate receive their motor supply
from the pharyngeal plexus, *except* for stylopharyngeus muscle which is
supplied by the glossopharyngeal nerve.

Jugular foramen syndromes

Vernet's syndrome

A combination of signs and symptoms, mainly resulting from compressive
pathology at the jugular foramen. Compression of the vagus, glossopha-
ryngeal, and accessory nerves give rise to the following symptoms:
- Loss of sensation on the posterior one-third of the tongue.
- SCM and trapezius paresis.
- Deviation of the uvula away from the side of the lesion.
- Loss of gag reflex.
- Hoarse voice.
- Causes include glomus tumours, schwannomas, trauma (including
fractures of the occipital bone), and infection.
  Other syndromes affecting cranial nerves IX, X and XI include:

Collett–Sicard syndrome

(Frederic Collett and Jean-Athanase Sicard.)
- Ipsilateral palsy of cranial nerves IX, X, XI, and XII. Initially described
in a soldier shot in World War I, it is essentially Vernet's syndrome
with an additional hypoglossal nerve palsy.

Villaret's syndrome

(Maurice Villaret, 1877–1947, French neurologist.)
- Ipsilateral palsy of cranial nerves IX, X, XI, XII and cervical
sympathetic nerves causing Horner's syndrome. Caused by lesions in
the retroparotid space.

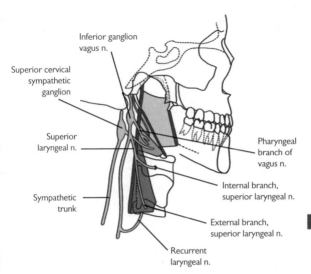

Fig. 7.11 Contributions to the pharyngeal plexus.
Reproduced courtesy of Daniel R. van Gijn.

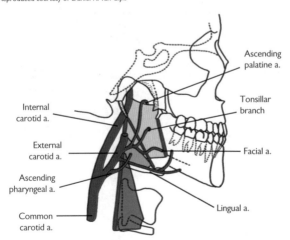

Fig. 7.12 Blood supply to the pharynx.
Reproduced courtesy of Daniel R. van Gijn.

The larynx

Introduction

The larynx, trachea, and bronchi develop embryologically from the foregut in the form of an outpouching during the 4th week of gestation. The larynx bridges the interval from the base of the tongue superiorly to the trachea inferiorly, lying within the hypopharynx and spanning the distance from the third to the sixth cervical vertebrae. It is a complex respiratory organ composed of a cartilaginous framework, associated ligaments and intrinsic and extrinsic muscles, and lined by an epithelial mucous membrane that is continuous superiorly with the pharynx and inferiorly with the trachea.

Its primary function is to protect the lower respiratory tract against aspiration. It allows the generation of a high intrathoracic pressure required for coughing, straining, and lifting (*Valsalva* manoeuvre) and phonation.

The anatomy of the larynx can be considered according to its surgical subdivisions into supraglottis, glottis, and subglottis that are important in the consideration of cancer spread, or according to its constituent parts of cartilagenous framework, ligaments, membranes, muscles, and mucous membranes. The spaces around the larynx are filled with loose connective tissue and fat and are fundamental to the understanding of tumours within the larynx.

There are anatomical differences between the paediatric and adult larynx (⊃ p. 272) and the male and female larynx. The infant larynx is more funnel-shaped, a third of the adult size, and narrowest in the subglottis (whereas the glottis is narrowest in the adult), which means that even slight swellings in this area can lead to respiratory obstruction. After puberty, the antero-posterior diameter almost doubles to reach approximately 36 mm (men) and 26 mm (women). Male vocal cord length is 17–25 mm and 12.5–17.5 mm in women. These differences in dimensions contribute to the prominent 'Adam's apple' (laryngeal prominence) and lower vocal pitch of the male (the increased anteroposterior dimension produces longer vocal folds).

The larynx consists of three unpaired and three paired cartilages and is suspended from the hyoid bone at the level of the third cervical vertebra. The unpaired cartilages are the shield-like thyroid cartilage, the epiglottis (situated upon the base of the tongue as per its name), and the cricoid cartilage, the latter forming the only complete (signet-shaped) ring of the larynx.

Surgical anatomy of the larynx

The anatomy of the larynx may be broadly divided into supraglottic, glottic, and subglottic regions (Fig. 8.1).

Supraglottis—'laryngeal structures above the vocal cords'

- Extends from the free margin of the epiglottis and the aryepiglottic folds to a line drawn tangentially across the superior margin of the vocal cords.
- Consists of the epiglottis, the aryepiglottic folds, the arytenoids, and the false cords (ventricular bands).

Glottis

- Consists of the vocal cords (composed of the vocal folds anteriorly and the bodies and vocal processes of the arytenoid cartilages posteriorly), and the anterior and posterior commissures.

Subglottis—'undersurface' of the vocal cords

- An area 5–10 mm below the vocal cords.
- Becomes the trachea at the lower border of the cricoid cartilage.

Constituent parts

- *Laryngeal framework (skeleton)*—hyoid bone and cartilages.
- *Ligaments and membranes*— extrinsic ligaments connect the cartilages to the hyoid bone and trachea; intrinsic ligaments connect the cartilages; fibroelastic membranes are suspended from the laryngeal skeleton.
- *Muscles*—extrinsic muscles attach the larynx to neighbouring structures and maintain the position of the larynx in the neck. Intrinsic muscles move the cartilages within the larynx.
- *Vocal cords* (true cords).
- *Mucous membranes*—the lining of the larynx.

Antonio Maria Valsalva (1666–1723)

Italian anatomist and contemporary of Sir Isaac Newton and Johann Sebastian Bach. In addition to coining the term 'Eustachian tube', Valsalva lends his name to his eponymous manoeuvre, which involves a forced expiration against a closed glottis. This is achieved by pinching one's nose, closing one's mouth, and attempting to expel air. The manoeuvre has multiple everyday applications in medicine and surgery, from checking haemostasis (by increasing stroke volume and cardiac output and observing for bleeding sources previously not seen), determining if an oroantral communication exists following the removal of a maxillary molar tooth, and in the management of supraventricular tachycardias.

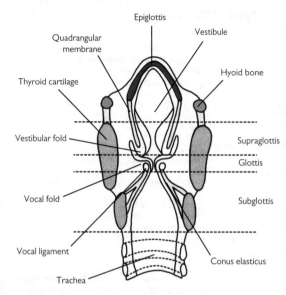

Fig. 8.1 Constituent parts of the larynx, coronal section.
Reproduced courtesy of Daniel R. van Gijn.

Laryngeal framework

Hyoid bone

A U-shaped bone providing the superior attachment for many of the laryngeal extrinsic muscles. Consists of an anterior midline body from which the greater horns (cornua) project backwards on each side and two lesser horns (cornua) which arise from the upper part of the body of the hyoid (Fig. 8.2).
- Muscles attached to superior aspect of hyoid (suprahyoid)—mylohyoid, geniohyoid, stylohyoid, digastric, middle constrictor, hyoglossus.
- Muscles attached to inferior aspect of hyoid (infrahyoid)—thyrohyoid, sternohyoid, omohyoid.

Thyroid cartilage

Composed of two laminae fused anteriorly in the midline (with an angle of approximately 90° in men and 120° in women). The posterior border extends above and below to form the superior and inferior cornua, respectively (Fig. 8.3).
- The superior cornu is attached at its conical extremity to the lateral thyroid ligament and helps support the thyrohyoid membrane.
- The inferior cornu bears a small, oval facet inferomedially for articulation with the cricoid cartilage at the cricothyroid joint).

Muscles attaching to the thyroid cartilage
See Fig. 8.4.
- *External aspect*—thyrohyoid, sternothyroid, and inferior pharyngeal constrictor. Attachment is marked by the oblique line on the external surface of each lamina.
- *Internal aspect*—thyroarytenoid, thyroepiglottic, and vocalis muscles.

Ligaments and membranes
- *Internal aspect*—midline superiorly, the thyroepiglottic ligament. Just inferior to this attachment, and on either side of the midline, the vestibular and vocal ligaments (the fusion of their anterior ends produces the anterior commissure tendon).
- Superior border of each lamina—thyrohyoid ligament.
- Inferomedial border—cricothyroid ligament.

Epiglottis

- A thin, leaf-shaped sheet of fibroelastic cartilage that projects upwards behind the tongue (Fig. 8.5).
- Attached inferiorly to the thyroid cartilage by the thyroepiglottic ligament and anteriorly to the hyoid bone by the hyoepiglottic ligament (Fig. 8.6).
- The pre-epiglottic space lies between the thyro- and hyo-epiglottic ligaments.
- Aryepiglottic folds extend from the sides of the epiglottis to the apices of the arytenoid cartilages.
- The mucosa covering the lingual surface of the epiglottis extends superiorly to form the posterior wall of each vallecula: it is reflected onto the tongue base forming the midline glosso-epiglottic fold and the two lateral glosso-epiglottic folds (Fig. 8.7).

During ingestion of a food bolus, the epiglottis is passively folded down over the laryngeal inlet.

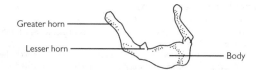

Fig. 8.2 The hyoid bone.
Reproduced courtesy of Daniel R. van Gijn.

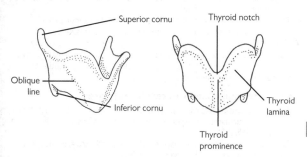

Fig. 8.3 The thyroid cartilage.
Reproduced courtesy of Daniel R. van Gijn.

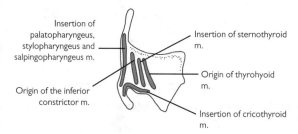

Fig. 8.4 Muscles attached to the thyroid lamina, lateral view.
Reproduced courtesy of Daniel R. van Gijn.

Cricoid cartilage

See Figs. 8.8–8.12.
- The only complete cartilaginous ring (resembling a signet ring in shape) in the airway (Fig. 8.8 and Fig. 8.9).
- Narrow arch anteriorly.
- Broad lamina posteriorly with sloping shoulders that bear facets for articulations with the arytenoid cartilages and the inferior cornua of the thyroid cartilage.
- A vertical posterior midline ridge on the lamina gives attachment to the longitudinal muscle of the oesophagus.

Arytenoid cartilages (paired)

- Three-sided, pyramidal cartilages (Fig. 8.8 and Fig. 8.10).
- Each contains an anterior projection, the vocal process, to which the vocal fold is attached.
- Each contains a lateral projection, the muscular process, to which the lateral cricothyroid and posterior arytenoid muscles are attached.
- Between the vocal and muscular processes the anterolateral surface is divided into two triangular fossae: the vestibular ligament is attached to the superior fossa and vocalis and lateral cricoarytenoid muscles are attached to the inferior fossa.
- The apex of each arytenoid cartilage curves posteromedially and articulates at a synovial joint with the corniculate cartilage.
- The posterior surface of each arytenoid cartilage is covered by the transverse arytenoid muscle. The base of each cartilage articulates with the cricoid cartilage via a synovial joint that allows rotary, medial and lateral gliding movements during phonation.

Corniculate and cuneiform cartilages (paired)

- The corniculate cartilages lie in the posterior part of the aryepiglottic fold. Each articulates via a synovial joint with the apices of the arytenoid cartilages (Fig. 8.8).
- The cuneiform cartilages are two small, elongated cartilaginous chips found in the margin of the aryepiglottic fold.

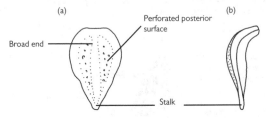

(a)   Perforated posterior surface   (b)

Broad end

Stalk

Fig. 8.5 The epiglottis, posterior view (a) and lateral view (b).
Reproduced courtesy of Daniel R. van Gijn.

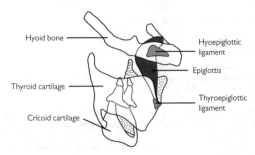

Hyoid bone

Hyoepiglottic ligament

Epiglottis

Thyroid cartilage

Thyroepiglottic ligament

Cricoid cartilage

Fig. 8.6 Laryngeal framework. Hyo- and thyroepiglottic ligaments and pre-epiglottic space, oblique view.
Reproduced courtesy of Daniel R. van Gijn.

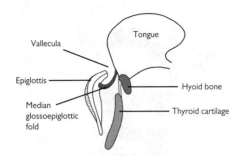

Fig. 8.7 The relationship between epiglottis and tongue, lateral view.
Reproduced courtesy of Daniel R. van Gijn.

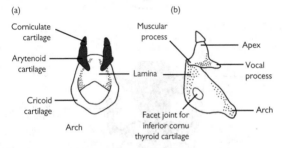

Fig. 8.8 Cricoid, arytenoid, and corniculate cartilages, anterior view (a) and lateral view (b).
Reproduced courtesy of Daniel R. van Gijn.

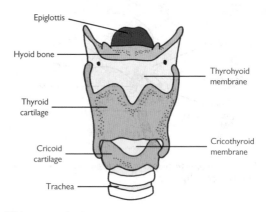

Fig. 8.9 Larynx, anterior view.
Reproduced courtesy of Daniel R. van Gijn.

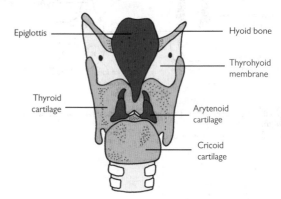

Fig. 8.10 Larynx, posterior view.
Reproduced courtesy of Daniel R. van Gijn.

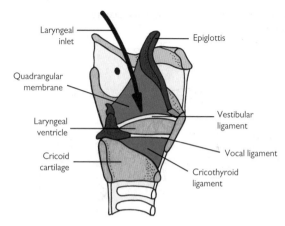

Fig. 8.11 Larynx, lateral (internal) view.
Reproduced courtesy of Daniel R. van Gijn.

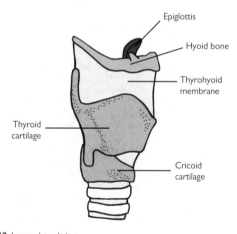

Fig. 8.12 Larynx, lateral view.
Reproduced courtesy of Daniel R. van Gijn.

Differences between adult and paediatric larynxes and airways

See Fig. 8.13 and Table 8.1.

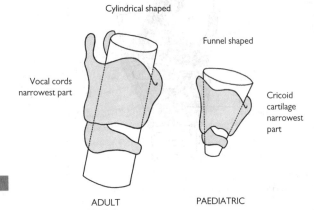

Fig. 8.13 The difference between adult and paediatric larynxes/airways.
Reproduced courtesy of Daniel R. van Gijn.

Table 8.1 Key airway differences between adults and children

Anatomy	Adult	Child
Tongue	Relatively smaller	Relatively larger
Epiglottis	Leaf-shaped, floppy Opposite C5/C6 vertebrae	Omega-shaped, stiffer Opposite C3/C4 vertebrae
Trachea	Wider and longer (20–25 mm by 10–16 cm)	Narrower and shorter (4 mm by 4–5 cm)
Shape of larynx	Funnel-shaped	Cylindrical
Vocal cords	Horizontal	Shorter, concave
Narrowest point	Vocal cords	Cricoid cartilage
Mucosa/submucosa	Adherent	Less adherent and prone to oedema and swelling

Laryngeal ligaments

Extrinsic ligaments and membranes

These ligaments attach the cartilagenous components of the larynx to the hyoid bone superiorly and the trachea inferiorly (Fig. 8.14).

Thyrohyoid membrane and median and lateral thyrohyoid ligaments

- Between the superior aspect of the thyroid cartilage and the posterior surface of the body and greater cornua of the hyoid bone.
- Composed of fibroelastic tissue reinforced in the midline by a fibrous thickening, the median thyrohyoid ligament, and posterolaterally by the thinner lateral thyrohyoid ligaments.
- The lateral thyrohyoid ligaments are pierced by the superior laryngeal vessels and the internal laryngeal nerve.

Thyroepiglottic ligament

- Connects the narrow stem of the epiglottis to the internal angle between the thyroid laminae.

Hyoepiglottic ligament

- Connects the hyoid bone to the anterior aspect of the epiglottis.

Cricotracheal ligament

- Connects the inferior border of the cricoid cartilage to the first tracheal ring.

Intrinsic ligaments and membranes

Form a broad sheet of fibroelastic tissue that lies directly below the mucous membrane of the larynx and internally hold the cartilages of the larynx together as a functional unit.

The fibroelastic membrane is divided into an upper quadrilateral part and lower cricothyroid part by the laryngeal ventricle, which is a fusiform fossa situated between the vestibular and vocal folds on either side (Fig. 8.15).

Quadrangular ligament

- Extends between the arytenoid cartilages and the lateral border of the epiglottis; its upper margin forms the framework of the aryepiglottic fold.
- The lower free edge forms the vestibular folds (false cords).

Cricothyroid ligament

- Extends from its attachment to the superior border of the cricoid cartilage, anteriorly to the laryngeal prominence of the thyroid cartilage and posteriorly to the vocal process of the arytenoid cartilage.
- The free upper margin becomes the vocal ligament, which is the framework of the true vocal cord.
- *Laryngeal ventricles*— pouches between the true and false cords on either side; each has a further outpouching beyond the lower quadrangular membrane (the saccule) lined with mucinous glands that lubricate the glottis during phonation.
- The laryngeal ventricles and saccules are encompassed by the paraglottic space, which in turn is in direct continuity medially with the pre-epiglottic space.

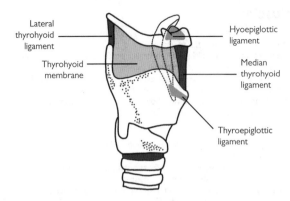

Fig. 8.14 Extrinsic ligaments of the larynx.
Reproduced courtesy of Daniel R. van Gijn.

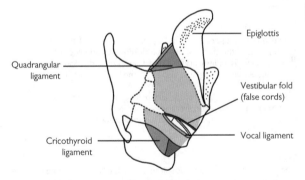

Fig. 8.15 Intrinsic ligaments and membranes of the larynx.
Reproduced courtesy of Daniel R. van Gijn.

Muscles

The muscles of the larynx can be divided into extrinsic and intrinsic groups. The extrinsic muscles act to elevate or depress the larynx during swallowing: elevation and tilting of the larynx protects the airway as the epiglottis is opposed to the contracted
aryepiglottic folds, thereby encouraging the food bolus to pass into the lateral food channels (piriform fossae of the hypopharynx). The intrinsic muscles act to move the individual components of the larynx and play vital roles in breathing and phonation. See Table 8.22.

Extrinsic muscles

- Composed of the suprahyoid and infrahyoid groups and stylopharyngeus.
- In general, the suprahyoid muscles and stylopharyngeus elevate the larynx, and the infrahyoid muscles depress the larynx.
- The suprahyoid and infrahyoid muscle groups are all attached to the hyoid bone (see page 172 and 173).
- Stylopharyngeus arises from the medial aspect of the styloid process and is inserted into the posterior border of the lamina of the thyroid cartilage.

Intrinsic muscles

- The intrinsic muscles act on individual components of the larynx.
- They control the shape of the rima glottidis (an opening between the vocal folds and the arytenoid cartilages) by abduction (opening) and adduction (closing) and also affect the length and tension of the vocal folds.
- All the intrinsic muscles of the larynx (except the cricothyroid) are innervated by the recurrent laryngeal nerve.
- Cricothyroid is innervated by the external branch of the superior laryngeal nerve.

Cricothyroid
See Fig. 8.16.
- Stretches and tenses the vocal ligaments by pulling the thyroid cartilage forwards, acting on the cricothyroid joint. Important for speech projection.
- Has a role in altering the tone of voice (with the thyroarytenoid muscle), hence its colloquial name of the 'singer's muscle'.
- Arises from the anterolateral aspect of the cricoid cartilage and is attached to the inferior margin and inferior cornu of the thyroid cartilage.

Thyroarytenoid (vocalis)
Shortens and thickens the vocal ligament allowing for a softer voice. Originates from the inferoposterior aspect of the angle of the thyroid cartilage and attaches to the anterolateral part of the arytenoid cartilage. Some authors regard vocalis as a medial part of thyroarytenoid and others consider it to be a separate muscle.

Posterior cricoarytenoid

The sole abductor of the vocal folds because it is the only muscle capable of widening the rima glottidis. Originates from the posterior surface of the cricoid cartilage and is attached to the muscular process of the arytenoid cartilage (Fig. 8.17 and Fig. 8.18).

Lateral cricoarytenoid

The major adductor of the vocal folds, narrowing the rima glottidis, modulating the tone and volume of speech. Originates from the arch of the cricoid cartilage and is attached to the muscular process of the arytenoid cartilage (Fig. 8.17 and Fig. 8.18).

Transverse and oblique arytenoids

- Collectively, these muscles span the arytenoid cartilages. On contraction they adduct the cartilages, closing the posterior portion of the rima glottidis and narrowing the laryngeal inlet. (Fig. 8.19 and Fig. 8.20).
- The aryepiglotticus muscle is a continuation of the oblique arytenoid muscle and is thought to help to protect the vocal tract during swallowing.

Vocal cords

- Composed of the vocal folds anteriorly (2/3) and the vocal processes of arytenoids posteriorly (1/3) (Fig. 8.21).
- The folds extend from the anterior commissure (the middle of the angle of the internal aspect of the thyroid cartilage) to the vocal processes of the arytenoid cartilages.
- Each fold is a layered structure composed of a superficial layer of non-keratinizing stratified squamous epithelium beneath which is the three-layered lamina propria. The superficial layer, *Reinke's space*, contains a gelatinous substance; the intermediate layer contains elastin fibres; the deep layer contains collagen fibres (the intermediate and deep layers make up the vocal ligament). Beneath the lamina propria is the vocalis muscle (thyroarytenoid) which forms the main body of the vocal cord (Fig. 8.22).

Mucous membranes of the larynx

- Most of the larynx is lined by a pseudostratified ciliated columnar 'respiratory type' epithelium.
- The vocal folds, the upper half of the laryngeal surface of the epiglottis, and the upper part of the aryepiglottic fold are lined by a non-keratinizing stratified squamous epithelium.
- Mucous glands are freely distributed throughout the larynx except that the vocal folds are devoid of glands, relying on lubrication by the glands in the laryngeal saccules.

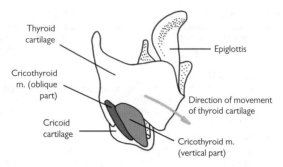

Fig. 8.16 Larynx, lateral view.
Reproduced courtesy of Daniel R. van Gijn.

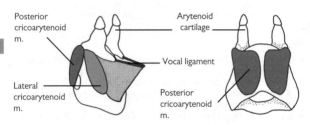

Fig. 8.17 Larynx, lateral view (a) and posterior view (b)
Reproduced courtesy of Daniel R. van Gijn.

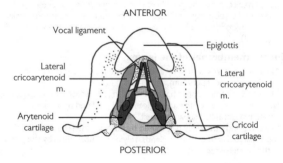

Fig. 8.18 Larynx, superior view.
Reproduced courtesy of Daniel R. van Gijn.

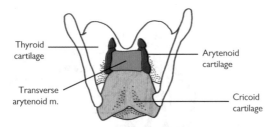

Fig. 8.19 Larynx, posterior view.
Reproduced courtesy of Daniel R. van Gijn.

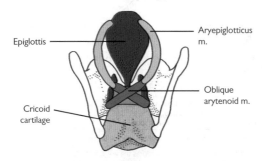

Fig. 8.20 Larynx, posterior view.
Reproduced courtesy of Daniel R. van Gijn.

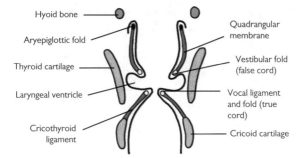

Fig. 8.21 Larynx, coronal section.
Reproduced courtesy of Daniel R. van Gijn.

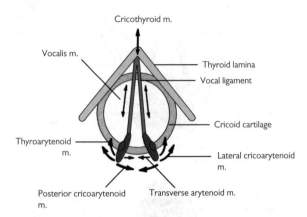

Fig. 8.22 Laryngeal muscle function, schematic. Arrows indicate direction of movement.

Reproduced courtesy of Daniel R. van Gijn.

Table 8.2 Summary table of laryngeal muscle function

Muscle	Function
Cricothyroid, thyroarytenoid	Tighten the vocal cord
Posterior cricoarytenoid	Abducts the vocal folds. Opens/widens the rima glottidis
Lateral cricoarytenoid	Adducts the vocal folds. Closes the rima glottidis
Transverse arytenoid, thyroarytenoid	Adduct the vocal folds. Close the rima glottidis

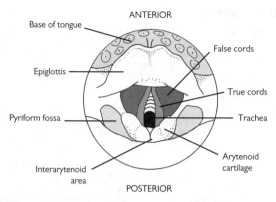

Fig. 8.23 Superior view of the larynx seen at fibreoptic nasendoscopy.
Reproduced courtesy of Daniel R. van Gijn.

Fibreoptic nasendoscopy

Nasendoscopy is a procedure that involves the insertion of a flexible fibreoptic camera through the nose of an awake patient to examine the laryngopharynx and upper airways. It is regularly used by head and neck surgeons to assess the anatomy of the airway (Fig. 8.23), the function of the vocal cords (especially prior to any surgery that may injure their nerve supply), and to exclude malignant disease in the face of hoarse voice (dysphonia) and painful (odynophagia) or difficult (dysphagia) swallowing.

Nerve supply

The vagus supplies both motor and sensory via the superior and recurrent laryngeal nerves and their branches (Figs. 8.24–8.26). The vocal fold itself receives dual innervation from branches of both nerves. All of the intrinsic laryngeal muscles except cricothyroid are innervated by the recurrent laryngeal nerve. Cricothyroid is innervated by the superior laryngeal nerve.

Superior laryngeal nerve

Arises from the middle of the inferior ganglion of the vagus nerve. It descends lateral to the pharynx, posterior to the ICA, and divides into two branches at the level of the greater cornu of the hyoid bone. It supplies sensation to the larynx above the vocal cords and innervates the cricothyroid muscles. Its branches are:

- *Internal laryngeal nerve* (sensory)—pierces the thyrohyoid membrane (in company with the superior laryngeal artery) and divides into its two main sensory and secretomotor branches that supply the mucosa of the hypopharynx, larynx, and the vocal folds; a filament descends beneath the mucous membrane on the inner surface of the thyroid cartilage and joins the recurrent laryngeal nerve.
- Supplies sensory innervation to the larynx superior to the vocal folds.
- *External laryngeal nerve* (motor)—descends on the larynx and passes beneath the sternothyroid muscle to supply the cricothyroid muscle.

Recurrent laryngeal nerve

- The right and left nerves are not identical in their initial trajectories. The left nerve loops under the aortic arch lateral to the ligamentum arteriosum, and the right nerve loops under the right subclavian artery. Both nerves subsequently ascend in the trachea-oesophageal grooves, and accompanied by a branch of the inferior thyroid artery, pass deep to the lower border of the inferior pharyngeal constrictor and enter the larynx just posterior to the cricothyroid joints. The right recurrent laryngeal nerve may be non-recurrent.
- The recurrent laryngeal nerves supply sensation to the larynx below the vocal cords, give cardiac branches to the deep cardiac plexus, and to the trachea, oesophagus, and the inferior pharyngeal constrictor muscles.

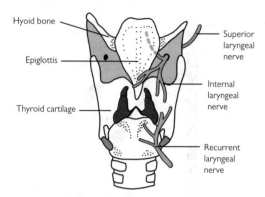

Fig. 8.24 Nerves of the larynx, internal view.
Reproduced courtesy of Daniel R. van Gijn.

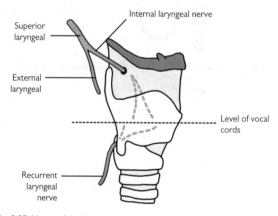

Fig. 8.25 Nerves of the larynx, external view.
Reproduced courtesy of Daniel R. van Gijn.

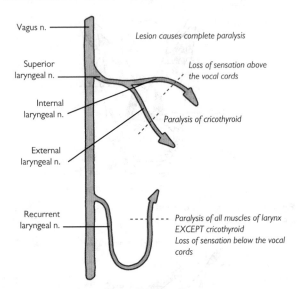

Fig. 8.26 Laryngeal branches of the vagus nerve and consequences of individual lesions (red dashed lines), schematic.

Reproduced courtesy of Daniel R. van Gijn.

Blood supply and lymphatic drainage

Arterial

The arterial supply to the larynx is derived from the superior and inferior laryngeal arteries (Fig. 8.27).

Superior laryngeal artery
- A branch of the superior thyroid artery (derived from the ECA).
- It follows the internal branch of the superior laryngeal nerve into the larynx, passing deep to the thyrohyoid muscle, and pierces the thyrohyoid membrane.

Inferior laryngeal artery
- A branch of the inferior thyroid artery (derived from the thyrocervical trunk).
- It arises from the inferior thyroid artery at the inferior border of the thyroid gland and ascends with the recurrent laryngeal nerve into the larynx.
- The relationship between the artery and the recurrent laryngeal nerve is variable. The nerve may pass anterior or posterior or between the terminal branches of the artery. On the right, it has an equal chance of any of the three aforementioned locations. On the left, it is more likely to lie posterior to the artery.

Venous
- Venous drainage is by the superior and inferior laryngeal veins.
- The superior laryngeal vein drains to the IJV via the superior thyroid vein.
- The inferior laryngeal vein drains to the left brachiocephalic vein via the inferior thyroid vein.

Lymphatic drainage
- Separated into upper and lower drainage groups by the vocal folds (Fig. 8.28).
- Above the folds, drainage is via lymphatics that accompany the superior laryngeal vein and empty into the upper jugular chain lymph nodes.
- Below the folds, drainage is to the lower jugular chain through the prelaryngeal and pretracheal nodes.
- The vocal folds are firmly bound to the underlying vocal ligament and have no lymphatic drainage.

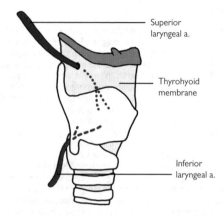

Fig. 8.27 Arteries of the larynx, lateral view.
Reproduced courtesy of Daniel R. van Gijn.

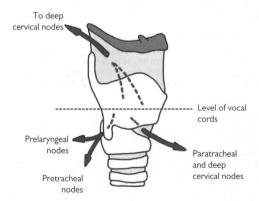

Fig. 8.28 Lymphatic drainage of the larynx, lateral view.
Reproduced courtesy of Daniel R. van Gijn.

Trachea

The trachea is a cartilagenous and fibromuscular tube, lined internally by mucosa. It extends from the lower border of the cricoid cartilage to the carina, where it bifurcates into left and right main bronchi approximately at the level of T5 vertebra posteriorly and the manubriosternal angle anteriorly (Fig. 8.29). The adult trachea has an inner diameter of about 1.5–2 cm and a length of about 11 cm. The anterior and lateral surfaces of the trachea consist of 16–20 superimposed and incomplete D-shaped 'rings' of hyaline cartilage and intervening fibroelastic anular ligaments.

- The trachealis muscle connects the ends of the incomplete rings posteriorly: it contracts during coughing, reducing the size of the lumen of the trachea to increase the rate of air flow.
- The oesophagus lies posterior to the trachea.
- The trachea is lined with a layer of pseudostratified ciliated columnar epithelium. The epithelium contains goblet cells, which secrete mucins, the main component of mucus, and an integral part of the mucosal barrier to infection. Viscous mucus coats the mucosal surfaces, moistening and protecting the airways by trapping inhaled foreign particles. Ciliary action wafts the mucus towards the larynx and pharynx where the trapped particles and mucus can be either swallowed or expelled as phlegm: this self-clearing mechanism is termed mucociliary clearance.

Tracheal innervation

- Both recurrent laryngeal nerves supply parasympathetic secretomotor fibres to the secretory glands, and sensation and motor innervation to the trachealis (smooth muscle). Postganglionic sympathetic nerves from the cervical ganglia mediate bronchodilation and reduced secretion.

Tracheal vasculature

Arteries

- Predominantly via the superior and inferior thyroid arteries. The thoracic trachea is supplied by the bronchial arteries.
- There are three bronchial arteries (two on the left and one on the right). The left arises from the anterior aspect of the descending thoracic aorta. The right is more variable, arising from the aorta, the first or third intercostal artery, the internal thoracic (mammary) artery, or the subclavian artery.

Veins

The tracheal veins drain upwards to the thyroid venous plexus.

Lymphatic drainage

Arise in a plexus beneath the mucous membrane and drain into the pretracheal and paratracheal groups of lymph nodes.

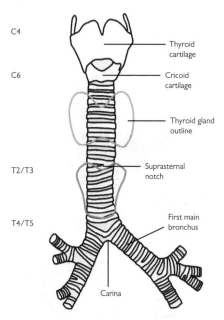

C4

C6

T2/T3

T4/T5

Thyroid cartilage

Cricoid cartilage

Thyroid gland outline

Suprasternal notch

First main bronchus

Carina

Fig. 8.29 The trachea, relations, and vertebral levels (on left).
Reproduced courtesy of Daniel R. van Gijn.

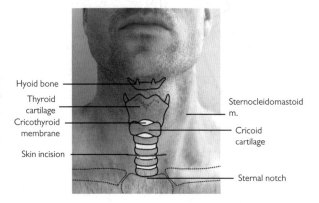

Hyoid bone

Thyroid cartilage

Cricothyroid membrane

Skin incision

Sternocleidomastoid m.

Cricoid cartilage

Sternal notch

Fig. 8.30 Surface marking for tracheostomy. Incision (red) is placed approximately half-way between cricoid cartilage and suprasternal notch. Yellow dashed line marks site of tracheal stoma.
Reproduced courtesy of Daniel R. van Gijn.

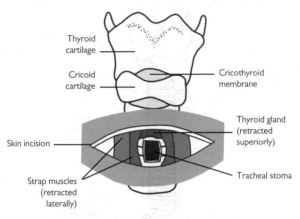

Fig. 8.31 Anterior view of tracheal stoma through skin incision.
Reproduced courtesy of Daniel R. van Gijn.

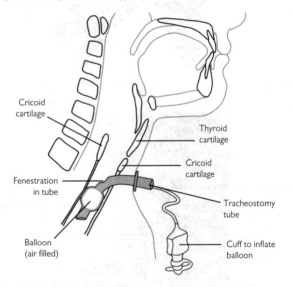

Fig. 8.32 Sagittal view of laryngopharynx demonstrating position of tracheostomy.
Reproduced courtesy of Daniel R. van Gijn.

Tracheostomy

Introduction

Tracheostomies are thought to have been performed as early as 3600 BCE. Alexander the Great was said to have used his sword to open the trachea of a soldier suffocating on a bone.

Indications

Tracheostomy involves the insertion of a plastic tube into the trachea below the level of the vocal cord. It is indicated in upper airway obstruction, pending upper airway obstruction, prolonged intubation requiring mechanical ventilation, and prophylactically in major head and neck surgery.

Procedure

An approximately 4 cm skin incision is made halfway between the sternal notch and the cricoid cartilage (Fig. 8.30). Subcutaneous fat and the investing layer of deep cervical fascia are incised and the strap muscles beneath retracted laterally. Anterior jugular veins and the thyroid gland may be encountered. The former can be safely ligated while the latter can either be divided at its midline isthmus or retracted superiorly. The trachea is exposed and a stoma or alternative incision is made before inserting and securing a tracheostomy tube (Fig. 8.31 and Fig. 8.32).

The face, scalp, and temporal region

Introduction

The anatomy of the face and its clinical relevance are arguably the most important components of this book—particularly in relation to the facial plastic surgeon and the potentially catastrophic sequelae of injury and the deformity and disability that follow it. The face conveys our conscious and subconscious emotions, provides reassurance to those who recognize and rely on its gross symmetry, and projects vulnerability in disfigurement.

Functionally, the face encompasses the muscles that surround our eyes, nose, and mouth, contributing to the sphincters and dilators that allow the fine motor control of our eyelids, nostrils, and lips, and indeed the remaining muscles that allow for the infinite expressions imparted by the face.

An intimate knowledge of the elegant interplay of skin, soft tissue, bony foundations of the skull, and the nervous, vascular, and glandular tissues interposed between them, is essential for the surgeon attempting to restore both structure and function of the face while preventing further, iatrogenic, injury.

Facial aesthetics

From the beginnings of what we know as man we have embraced reflections, icons, paintings, and sculptures that hint, taunt, and celebrate the *beauty* of the face. While a unifying and subjective definition of beauty varies depending on generation, gender, era, and indeed the eye of the beholder (see following subsection), there have been scientific attempts to objectify beauty and attractiveness—with the common themes perhaps being harmony and symmetry. It is these values, along with meticulous facial analysis, aesthetic principles, reference planes, and mathematics, that are considered and addressed in facial analysis. Da Vinci's *Vitruvian* man perhaps best exemplifies this blend of art, science, and proportion.

Divine proportion and the golden ratio

The golden ratio is a mathematical ratio of 1.618 to 1 and consistently appears in things deemed beautiful throughout life (Fig. 9.1). A proportion described by Euclid in 300 BCE, it accounts for the perfectly proportioned and subconsciously appealing appearances found throughout nature, art, architecture, and mathematics, including:

- Leonardo's *Mona Lisa*.
- Fibonacci's sequence.
- Phidias' Parthenon (accounting for the Greek letter *phi* ascribed to the number 1.618).
- Pentagons.
- The logarithmic spiral of the nautilus shell.

Clinical relevance

The divine proportion can be seen throughout the face. Extrapolating the golden ratio from pentagon to decagon matrices and beyond, Dr Stephen Marquardt, an American oral and maxillofacial surgeon, arrived at a facial overlay 'golden mask', the archetype for the ideal human face and intended as a tool for clinicians to perform objective facial analysis (Fig. 9.2 and Fig. 9.3).

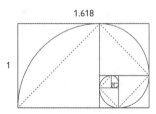

Fig. 9.1 Phi.

Reproduced courtesy of Daniel R. van Gijn.

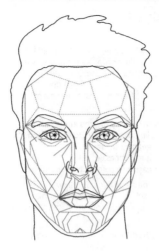

Fig. 9.2 Marquardt's 'golden mask'.
Reproduced courtesy of Daniel R. van Gijn.

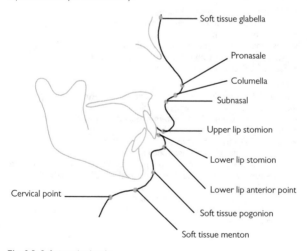

Fig. 9.3 Soft tissue landmarks.
Reproduced courtesy of Daniel R. van Gijn.

Facial analysis

Overview

The key to successful outcomes in aesthetic and deformity surgery of the face is a systematic evaluation of its proportions and their discrepancy or adherence to recognized and reproducible 'ideals'. Examination is best achieved with the head in a neutral position in natural light and involves assessment of the face from the front (vertical proportions) and in profile.

Vertical proportions

The face can be conveniently divided into thirds (Fig. 9.4):

- *Upper face*—hairline to glabella (flat area of bone between eyebrows, from 'glabellus' meaning smooth).
- *Midface*—glabella to subnasale.
- *Lower face*—subnasale to soft tissue menton.

The lower face can be subdivided as follows:

- *Upper one-third*—subnasale to upper lip stomion.
- *Lower two-thirds*—lower lip stomion to soft tissue menton.

Transverse proportions

The rule of facial fifths describes the *ideal* transverse proportions of the face to comprise approximately equal fifths, each the width of one eye (Fig. 9.5).

- Intercanthal distance, alar base width, palpebral fissure, and intercanine widths should be equal.

Additional ideal anatomical relationships of note:

- Interpupillary width is equal to width of mouth.
- Nasal dorsum is one-half of intercanthal width.
- Nasal lobule is two-thirds of intercanthal width.
- Nasal length (radix to tip) equal to stomion to menton.
- Facial, nasal, chin, lip, and dental midlines should be coincident.

Lateral view

Most useful in assessing the nose, lips, and anteroposterior discrepancies in the positions of the maxilla and mandible.

- Alar base should be slightly anterior to medial canthus.
- Upper lip is slightly anterior to lower lip.
- Lower lip slightly anterior to chin.
- Radix corresponds with nasofrontal angle.
- Nasolabial angle (angle formed by lines drawn through the anterior and posterior ends of nostril and vertical plane): 90–95° in males; 95–100° in females.
- Maxilla may be normal, prominent, or hypoplastic.
- Mandible may be normal, prognathic, or retrognathic (or -genic if referring to the chin).

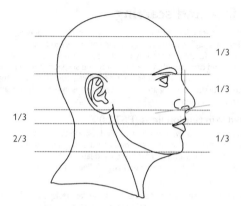

Fig. 9.4 Facial thirds and nasolabial angle (yellow lines).
Reproduced courtesy of Daniel R. van Gijn.

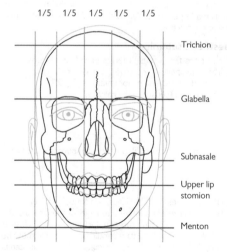

Fig. 9.5 Facial fifths (yellow vertical lines) and thirds (red horizontal lines).
Reproduced courtesy of Daniel R. van Gijn.

The face and scarring

Any full-thickness injury of the skin, be it acquired or iatrogenic, will result in scar formation. The ultimate appearance of an individual scar depends on a multitude of factors, some beyond the control (especially those caused by trauma) and others within the control of the surgeon. An understanding of skin tension lines and facial aesthetic subunits, combined with the basic principles of tissue handling and suture techniques, means a favourable scar can often be achieved.

Relaxed skin tension lines (RSTLs)

RSTLs are lines roughly coincident to the facial rhytids (skin wrinkles) seen in the ageing face and lie at right angles to the long axis of the underlying muscle. Initially described by Dupuytren and later by Langer, whose name is attached to their alternative name, 'Langer's lines' (Fig. 9.6).

Clinical relevance

Surgical incisions, elliptical excisions, and local flap designs should lie parallel to RSTLs in order to reduce tension across the wound and in turn minimize the width of the resultant scar. It follows that placement of incisions within skin rhytids will generally result in aesthetic scars that are well camouflaged within the natural skin creases. The converse is also true in that incisions and wounds made perpendicular to the RSTLs will result in maximal and unsightly scar contraction.

Facial aesthetic subunits

The surface of the face varies in terms of colour, texture, thickness, and mobility. These properties, however, are generally consistent within an area, or unit, of the face. The major units are (Fig. 9.7):

- Forehead and scalp (separated by hairline).
- Eyes.
- Nose (dorsal, lateral, tip, alar).
- Lips.
- Chin.
- Cheek (zygomatic, infraorbital, preauricular, buccomandibular).
- Ears.
- Neck.

Clinical relevance

Fixed junction lines, essentially ridges, shadows, and creases, bound the major units of the face. The aesthetic subunits of the face are of significant importance to the facial plastic surgeon. Incisions, wound closure, and the planning and placement of local flaps should be situated at these boundaries in order to optimize favourable scar formation. Major units can be further divided into aesthetic subunits. Excision of the complete subunit should be considered in the treatment of skin lesions or soft tissue deformity.

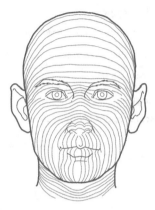

Fig. 9.6 Langer's lines of relaxed skin tension.
Reproduced courtesy of Daniel R. van Gijn.

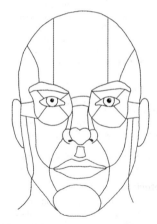

Fig. 9.7 Facial aesthetic subunits.
Reproduced courtesy of Daniel R. van Gijn.

Botulinum toxin and non-surgical rejuvenation

- Botulinum toxin is produced by *Clostridium botulinum* and inhibits presynaptic release of acetylcholine at the neuromuscular junction.
- Causes muscle relaxation and is used in facial rejuvenation to treat rhytids, which lie perpendicular to the direction of muscle contraction.
- Many areas are targeted: horizontal forehead rhytids, glabellar complex, crow's feet (lateral orbital rhytids), bunny lines (superior nasal side wall), perioral region, chin dimple, and platysmal bands.

Layers of the face

The face forms the anterior part of the head medial to the ears and between the hairline superiorly and the chin inferiorly. It comprises everything that lies between what is visible anteriorly and laterally. The face consists of four recognizable tissue planes: skin, a subcutaneous layer of fibroadipose tissue (held responsible for some of the changes of the ageing face), the superficial muscular aponeurotic system (SMAS, of considerable importance to the aesthetic surgeon), and the parotidomasseteric fascia (Fig. 9.8).

Superficial muscular aponeurotic system

Deep to skin and subcutaneous tissue, the SMAS forms a crucial support structure of the face and neck enveloping the lateral facial musculature and forming the superficial fascia of the face.

Characteristics

- Deep to skin and subcutaneous fat.
- Comprises the attachments of the facial muscles to dermis.
- Interdigitates anteriorly with inferior orbicularis oculi, the levators and depressors of the lips, and orbicularis oris.
- Continuous superolaterally with the temporoparietal fascia and superficial to the temporalis fascia covering temporalis here. (Note that the temporoparietal fascia attaches to the zygomatic arch while the temporalis muscle fascia passes deep to it).
- Continuous superoanteriorly with frontalis and therefore indirectly with the galea aponeurosis and occipitalis muscle posteriorly.
- Superficial to the parotidomasseteric fascia laterally.
- Continuous with platysma inferiorly.

Neurovascular relationships to SMAS

- Parotid region: the facial nerve lies deep to the parotidomasseteric fascia, which is deep to SMAS.
- Branches of the facial nerve become progressively superficial at the anterior border of the parotid gland and are immediately deep to SMAS.
- Facial artery and vein lie deep to SMAS; perforators pass through SMAS.

Parotidomasseteric fascia

The parotid gland is engulfed by the parotidomasseteric fascia, a superior continuation of the investing layer of the deep cervical fascia from below which divides into superficial and deep slips around the parotid gland and extends superiorly as the temporalis fascia. The fascia at the deep surface of the parotid attaches to the skull base superiorly.

Characteristics

- Continuous with the investing layer of the deep cervical fascia inferiorly (which invests trapezius, SCM, and the submandibular gland).
- Attached superiorly to the lower border of the zygomatic arch.
- Continuous with the temporalis fascia superiorly.
- Lies deep to SMAS.
- Is supplied by the great auricular nerve (C2).
- The fascia deep to the parotid gland contributes to the stylomandibular ligament separating masseter from the medial pterygoid muscle.

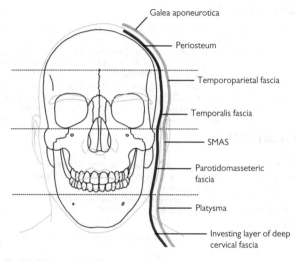

Fig. 9.8 The layers of the face.
Reproduced courtesy of Daniel R. van Gijn.

The SMAS

- First described by Vladimir Mitz and Martine Peyronie in 1976, the SMAS has been successfully used by plastic, oral, maxillofacial and ENT surgeons as the foundation for different face lift techniques.
- Mitz V and Peyronie M. The superficial musculo-aponeurotic system (SMAS) in the parotid and cheek area. *Plast Reconstr Surg* 1976;58(1):80–88.

Scalp and forehead

The scalp forms the soft tissue envelope of the cranial vault. The triad it forms with the forehead anteriorly and the temporal regions laterally should be considered as a continuum rather than three separate entities (Fig. 9.9). The forehead forms the upper third of the face and is bound between the hairline (variable) superiorly, the supraorbital rims inferiorly, and extends to the temporal lines bilaterally. The scalp consists of five layers easily remembered by the acronym 'SCALP' (Fig. 9.10). The first three layers, however, should be considered as a single unit which glides freely over the periosteum via the loose areolar tissue, a fact with clinical sequelae.

Layers ('SCALP')

Skin

- Forms the thickest layer, particularly over the occipital area.
- Contains the hair follicles and, through fibrous septa, is intimately connected to the galea aponeurosis.
- Richly supplied with sebaceous glands, which accounts for the propensity of sebaceous cysts found in the scalp.

Connective tissue (subcutaneous)

- Houses the arteries, veins, nerves, and lymphatics of the scalp within tough fibrous septa.

Aponeurosis (galea aponeurotica)

- The keystone of the scalp. Connects the frontalis anteriorly and the occipitalis posteriorly (aponeurosis of occipitofrontalis).
- Continuous with the temporoparietal fascia laterally.
- Attached to the zygomatic arches inferiorly.

Loose areolar tissue

- Comprises the potential (danger) space between the epicranial muscles superiorly and underlying periosteum.
- Traversed by numerous emissary veins which communicate directly with the diploic veins between the tables of the skull and thence with the intracranial venous sinuses.

Pericranium

- Contributes minimal vascular supply to the skull bones it covers (unlike periosteum elsewhere) and can therefore be detached or stripped without undue concern for subsequent bony necrosis.
- The majority of the blood supply to the bone comes from the middle meningeal artery, a branch of the first part of the maxillary artery.

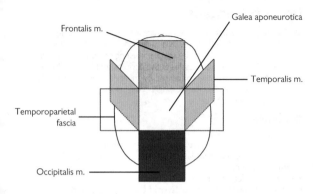

Fig. 9.9 Scalp, superior view.
Reproduced courtesy of Daniel R. van Gijn.

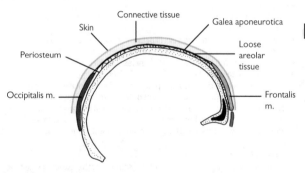

Fig. 9.10 The layers of scalp, sagittal section.
Reproduced courtesy of Daniel R. van Gijn.

Occipitofrontalis

Occipitofrontalis is part of the epicranius with temporoparietalis (a variable muscle situated between frontalis and the anterior and superior auricular muscles). It is the muscle of the scalp, consisting of occipitalis and frontalis, two pairs of quadrilateral muscles at the occipital and frontal aspects of the skull, respectively that are connected by the galea aponeurotica. Laterally the aponeurosis blends with the fascia covering the temporalis muscle superior to the zygomatic arch.

Occipitalis

See Fig. 9.11.
- *Origin*—external occipital protuberance, superior nuchal line of the occipital bone, and as far laterally as the mastoid process of the temporal bone.
- *Insertion*—galea aponeurotica.
- *Action*—draws the superficial layer of the scalp posteriorly.
- *Innervation*—posterior auricular branch of the facial nerve.

Frontalis

See Fig. 9.11.
- *Origin*—anterior aspect of the galea aponeurotica, anterior to the coronal suture.
- *Insertion*—blends with orbicularis oculi, adjacent the procerus and corrugator supercilii muscles and skin of the brow.
- *Action*—raises the eyebrows and wrinkles the skin of the forehead.
- *Innervation*—temporal branches of the facial nerve.
- The accumulation of blood and pus in the subgaleal plane (i.e. within the loose areolar tissue) will be restrained by the attachments of occipitalis posteriorly and by the temporalis muscle fascia at the zygomatic arches laterally, but may pass forward into the orbit and upper and lower lids anteriorly due to the lack of any bony attachment for frontalis.

Scalping

Scalping is the tearing or cutting of the human scalp, either in part or whole, from the head. While now commonly resulting from traumatic avulsion in industrial and road traffic incidents, it was historically part of a broader cultural practice involved with the taking of human parts as trophies, particularly in the American Indian Wars (Fig. 9.12).

Loose areolar tissue

The loose areolar tissue (or subgaleal) layer provides a convenient cleavage plane, whether breached by a stone flint, the surgeon's scalpel, or by pus. If blood and pus accumulate in the subgaleal plane they will be restrained by the attachments of occipitalis posteriorly and by temporalis fascia at the zygomatic arches laterally. They will, however, pass anteroinferiorly into the orbit and upper and lower eyelids because frontalis has no bony attachment.

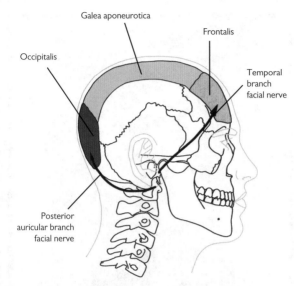

Fig. 9.11 Occipitofrontalis. Occipitalis (red), frontalis (yellow).
Reproduced courtesy of Daniel R. van Gijn.

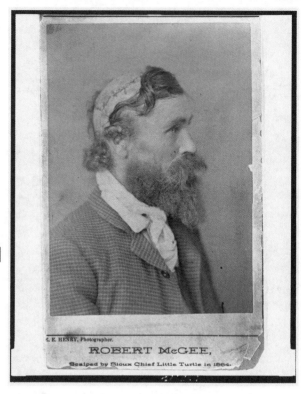

Fig. 9.12 Robert McGee—scalped by Sioux Chief Little Turtle in 1864.

Photographed by Henry, E. E., 1826–1917. Reproduced from the Library of Congress, http://hdl.loc.gov/loc.pnp/cph.3c05942.

Neurovascular supply to the scalp

Within the subcutaneous connective tissue layer, the scalp has a rich blood supply, derived from branches of the ECA and indirectly from branches of the ICA, with rich anastomoses between these branches. The location of neurovascular structures in this layer allows for the raising of subgaleal scalp flaps, either in the closure of defects or for access to the craniofacial skeleton, without compromise to the blood and nervous supply. Conversely, the tough fibrous septa that surround the vessels prevent their contraction and contribute to the significant bleeding that occurs with scalp lacerations.

Arterial supply

There are five pairs of arteries that supply the scalp: three arise anterior to the auricle and two arise posteriorly (Fig. 9.13). The venous drainage of the scalp follows that of the arteries (Table 9.1).

Preauricular vessels
- *Supratrochlear artery*—terminal branch of ophthalmic artery, from the ICA.
- *Supraorbital artery*—branch of the ophthalmic artery, from the ICA.
- *Superficial temporal artery*—one of the two terminal branches of the ECA.

Postauricular vessels
- *Posterior auricular*—from the ECA.
- *Occipital artery*—from the ECA.

Nerve supply

Ten pairs of nerves supply the scalp. As with the arterial supply, they can be divided into pre- and postauricular groups (Fig. 9.13). Each group has one motor nerve (from the facial nerve) with the remainder providing sensation (from all divisions of the trigeminal nerve) to the scalp.

Preauricular nerves (from anterior to posterior)
- *Supratrochlear*—ophthalmic division of the trigeminal nerve (V_1).
- *Supraorbital*—ophthalmic division of the trigeminal nerve (V_1).
- *Zygomaticotemporal*—maxillary division of the trigeminal nerve (V_2).
- *Temporal branch of the facial nerve* (motor).
- *Auriculotemporal*—mandibular division of the trigeminal nerve (V_3).

Postauricular nerves
- *Posterior branch of the great auricular nerve*—C2, C3 (cervical plexus).
- *Posterior auricular branch of the facial nerve*.
- *Lesser occipital nerve*—C2, C3 (cervical plexus).
- *Greater occipital nerve*—dorsal ramus, C2.
- *Third occipital nerve*—dorsal ramus, C3.

Table 9.1 Venous drainage of the scalp.

Vein	Drainage/comments
Supratrochlear and supraorbital veins	Form the angular vein in the region of the medial canthus and run obliquely across the face to form the facial vein
Superficial temporal vein	Enters the parotid gland, joins the maxillary vein to form the retromandibular vein (RMV). The anterior division of the RMV joins the facial vein to become the common facial vein which ultimately drains into the IJV
Posterior auricular vein	Joins the posterior division of the retromandibular vein to form the EJV (which ultimately drains into the subclavian vein)
Occipital vein	Terminates in the suboccipital venous plexus

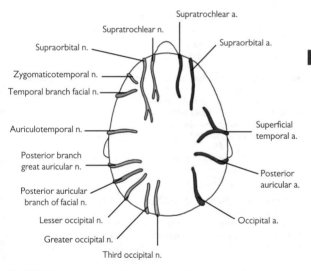

Fig. 9.13 Neurovascular supply to scalp, superior view.
Reproduced courtesy of Daniel R. van Gijn.

The temporoparietal region

The temporoparietal region and its layers are a common area of confusion confounded by terminological inconsistencies. It is an area of interest to the facial plastic, maxillofacial, and neurosurgeon, where a sound understanding of the relationships of the neurovascular structures to their respective fascial layers, in particular the topographical anatomy of the temporal branch of the facial nerve, justifies dedicating a section of this book to this important region.

Layers of the temporoparietal region

The layers of the temporoparietal region are continuous with the corresponding layers of the face inferiorly and scalp proper superiorly. The additional layer in this region (compared to the scalp) is the temporalis muscle and its related fascia (Fig. 9.14 and Fig. 9.15).

Skin and subcutaneous connective tissue (S and C of SCALP)
- Continuous with the skin and subcutaneous tissue of the scalp and forehead.
- Variably hair-bearing and affected by male pattern baldness.

Temporoparietal fascia (superficial temporal fascia) ('A' of SCALP)
- Deep and closely adherent to skin and subcutaneous tissue.
- Attached to the zygomatic arch.
- Contains loose areolar tissue and temporoparietal fat pad beneath.
- Continuous with the galea aponeurotica superiorly (above superior temporal line).
- Continuous with the SMAS inferiorly.
- Continuous with frontalis anteriorly.
- Continuous with occipitalis posteriorly.
- Intimately related to the temporal branch of the facial nerve, which lies deep to it (Fig. 9.16).
- Contains the superficial temporal vessels and the auriculotemporal nerve and its branches (from V_3).

Loose areolar tissue ('L' of SCALP)

Temporalis muscle fascia ('P' of SCALP) (deep temporal fascia)
- Covers the temporalis muscle.
- A dense aponeurotic layer, deep to temporoparietal fascia and its fat pad.
- Cranial extension of the parotidomasseteric fascia and deep cervical fascia.
- Laterally, lies deep to:
  The anterior and superior auricular muscles.
  Galea aponeurotica.
  Part of orbicularis oculi muscle.
- Blends with the periosteum of the skull superior to the superior temporal line.
- Splits into deep and superficial layers, which attach to the lateral and medial borders of the zygomatic arch, respectively. The space between these layers contains the superficial temporal fat pad.

- The superficial temporal fat pad contains the zygomaticotemporal branch of the maxillary nerve and the zygomatico-orbital branch of the superficial temporal artery.
- Deep to the deep layer of the temporalis muscle fascia is the deep temporal fat pad, which lies between this layer and the temporalis muscle and is considered a cranial extension of the buccal fat pad.

Temporalis muscle

The temporalis muscle is a fan-shaped muscle of mastication and occupies the entirety of the temporal fossa from the inferior temporal line; it lies upon the deep surface of the temporalis fascia.

- Originates from the infratemporal crest of the greater wing of the sphenoid.
- Its fibres become tendinous and traverse a gap between the zygomatic arch and the lateral surface of the skull.
- Converges towards and is inserted onto the whole medial surface and apex of the coronoid process and ramus of the mandible, almost as far inferiorly as the third mandibular molar tooth.

Etymology

There are numerous, all equally romantic, proposed sources of the word 'temporal' (some say the temple of the head was so called because by observing the pulsating, tortuous vessels in this region one could determine the *temperament* of a person):

- *Tempus*—the most obvious association is with 'time'. Relating either to the appearance of grey hairs in the temporal region with the passage of time, or to the pulsation of the superficial temporal artery beneath, rhythmically counting out our remaining time.
- *Temnien*—meaning 'to wound in battle', which presumably refers to the vulnerability of the area of the pterion and its relationship with the middle meningeal artery.

- *Ivor Pitanguy (1923–2016)*—celebrity pioneering Brazilian plastic surgeon based in Rio de Janeiro. Described 'Pitanguy's line' which is the classic reference line for the general path of the frontal branch of the facial nerve within the temporal region (Fig. 9.16).

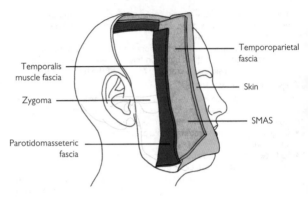

Fig. 9.14 Layers of the temporoparietal region.
Reproduced courtesy of Daniel R. van Gijn.

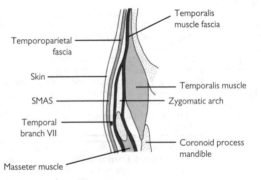

Fig. 9.15 Layers of the temporoparietal region, coronal section.
Reproduced courtesy of Daniel R. van Gijn.

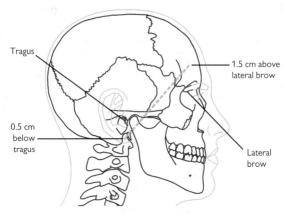

Tragus

1.5 cm above
lateral brow

0.5 cm
below
tragus

Lateral
brow

Fig. 9.16 Pitanguy's line. Surface marking of the frontal branch of the facial nerve.
Reproduced courtesy of Daniel R. van Gijn.

Rhytidectomy (facelift)

Literally meaning the removal/excision of wrinkles. Early management of
facial ageing initially addressed the skin only, however, other structures
are also attenuated with time. Relocating SMAS and altering its vector of
pull are crucial to the aesthetic result. The approach must consider nerve
branches: the greater auricular nerve is most frequently damaged.

Operative planning
- Facial assessment to determine skin excess and required change in
  facial vectors to address ageing and ptosis.
- Incision—temporal, preauricular, and postauricular components.
- Skin flap elevation—avoid disruption of orbital retaining ligament and
  nasolabial fold.
- SMAS—can address by excision and suture; plication, which also
  augments facial volume; sub-SMAS dissection and elevation, which
  may improve elevation, however there is a greater risk of facial nerve
  injury.
- Subperiosteal or supraperiosteal dissection is an alternative method
  that has been described and that avoids facial nerve injury.

Muscles of the craniofacial skeleton

Derived from the second branchial arch and innervated by the facial nerve, the muscles of the face and scalp differ from muscles in other regions of the body in that they arise from bone (or fascia) and are embedded in the superficial fascia of the face as the cutaneous muscles. Their subsequent actions on the skin are as functional sphincters and dilators of the orifices, while the by-product of conveying emotion has given rise to their alternative (and slightly erroneous) name as the 'muscles of facial expression'. Morphologically akin to the *panniculus carnosus* (see later) of lower mammals, their action is achieved through the contraction of muscle groups rather than through the contraction of a single muscle, conveyed by the SMAS to the skin. The efficiency of the conveyed message, from muscle to SMAS and thence to skin, is reduced as the elastic fibres of the SMAS attenuate with age. The groups of muscles of the craniofacial skeleton can be divided and discussed according to their location and function (Fig. 9.17):

- Muscles of the eyes and eyelids (circumorbital and palpebral).
- Muscles of the nose and nostrils (nasal).
- Muscles of the cheek and lips (buccolabial).
- Muscles of the external ear (auricular) (discussed in Chapter 14, ➔ Auricular muscles, p. 501).
- Muscles of the scalp and forehead (epicranial).

Panniculus carnosus

Principally observed, and significantly better established, in other mammals, the panniculus carnosus represents a muscular sheath or layer found within the superficial fascia. The flickering and shivering of the skin seen among horses and cattle to dislodge bothersome flies is a function of the panniculus carnosus, producing the independent movement of the skin over the deeper musculature. Vestigial and significantly less hair-bearing examples in the human are the platysma and muscles of facial expression, the dartos muscle of the scrotum, the palmaris brevis, and subareolar muscle around the nipple.

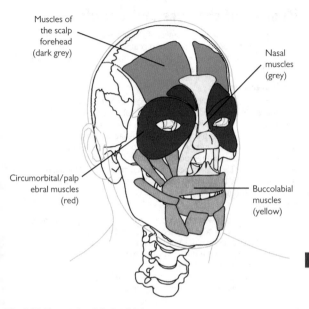

Muscles of the scalp forehead (dark grey)

Nasal muscles (grey)

Circumorbital/palpebral muscles (red)

Buccolabial muscles (yellow)

Fig. 9.17 The muscles of the facial skeleton, overview.
Reproduced courtesy of Daniel R. van Gijn.

Muscles of the eyes and eyelids

The muscles concerned with control of the aperture of the palpebral fissure are the sphincter *orbicularis oculi*, *corrugator supercilii*, and *levator palpebrae superioris*. The latter, and a description of the eyelid proper, will be discussed further in **Ə** Chapter 10.

Orbicularis oculi

Orbicularis oculi is the predominant muscle acting to constrict the palpebral fissure and close the eye; its action as a sphincter is opposed by levator palpebrae superioris. It has a broad base surrounding the orbital rim and consists of orbital and palpebral parts. The latter component can be subdivided into preseptal and pretarsal components. It is supplied by branches of the facial, superficial temporal, maxillary (infraorbital artery; ECA), and ophthalmic arteries (supratrochlear, supraorbital, medial, and lateral palpebral arteries). The relationship and involvement of the SMAS and orbicularis oculi is unclear (Fig. 9.18).

Orbital part
- *Origin and insertion*—frontal process of the maxilla, the nasal component of the frontal bone, and the medial palpebral ligament, encircling the bony orbit with continuous concentric fibres.
- Superiorly, blends with the corrugator supercilii and the frontalis muscles of the forehead.
- Medially, may blend with the muscles involved in raising the upper lip, zygomaticus minor, levator labii superioris, and levator labii superioris alaeque nasi.
- *Action*—voluntary forced closure of the eye; the attachments to the skin of the eyebrow (depressor supercilii) act to bring the brow medially and inferiorly to create a furrow of frustration and shield the eye from sunlight.

Palpebral part—preseptal
- *Origin*—from the bifurcation of the medial palpebral ligament and its adjacent bony surfaces.
- *Insertion*—courses over the eyelids superficial to the orbital septum and ultimately converges at the weaker lateral palpebral raphe.
- *Action*—involuntary (blinking).
- Fibres that pass close to the free edge of the eyelid posterior to the eyelashes are termed the ciliary bundle of Riolan and form the 'grey line', a useful surgical landmark in transconjunctival approaches to the orbit, for example.
- *Innervation*—temporal and zygomatic branches of the facial nerve (entering from the deep surface of the muscle).

Palpebral part—pretarsal
- Lacrimal component at its medial origin is known as Horner's muscle.
- *Origin*—arises from the lacrimal crest, lying posterior to the lacrimal sac and medial palpebral ligament.
- *Insertion*—adherent to the upper and lower tarsal plates of the eyelids; continues laterally deep to the lateral palpebral raphe, converging at the lateral canthal tendon.

- *Action*—thought to assist in the flow of tears into the nasolacrimal duct by compressing the lacrimal sac.
- *Innervation*—temporal and zygomatic branches of the facial nerve.

Corrugator supercilii

- Paired, small, narrow, and pyramidal muscles of the medial brow; deep to and blending with the frontalis and orbicularis oculi bilaterally.
- *Origin*—arises from the medial aspect of the bony superciliary arch.
- *Insertion*—skin superior to the supraorbital margin.
- *Action*—together with orbicularis oculi, assists in frowning by bringing the brow medially and inferiorly. Of interest to the aesthetic physician and plastic surgeon in administering botulinum toxin.
- *Innervation*—temporal and zygomatic branches of the facial nerve.

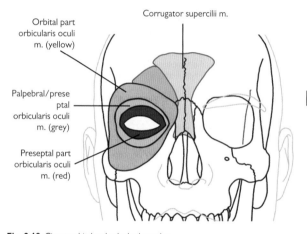

Corrugator supercilii m.

Orbital part orbicularis oculi m. (yellow)

Palpebral/preseptal orbicularis oculi m. (grey)

Preseptal part orbicularis oculi m. (red)

Fig. 9.18 Circumorbital and palpebral muscles.
Reproduced courtesy of Daniel R. van Gijn.

Muscles of the nose and nostrils

The muscles acting on and around the nose and nostrils are primarily in-volved in elements of facial expression, assistance in respiration, and, in conjunction with orbicularis oris, the production of certain sounds. They are incorporated into nasal SMAS and consist of two principal opposing groups (Fig. 9.19): the elevators and depressor and the dilators and compressor (Fig. 9.19).

Elevators (procerus and levator labii superioris alaeque nasi)

Procerus

- An unpaired, pyramidal, vertically orientated slip of muscle.
- *Origin*—arises from the lower end of the nasal bone and superior aspect of the upper lateral cartilages.
- *Insertion*—courses superiorly over the root of the nose to insert into the skin of the glabellar region (between the eyebrows) to blend with frontalis.
- *Action*—draws the medial eyebrows inferiorly and forms the horizontal wrinkles over the nasal bridge associated with concentration.
- *Innervation*—temporal, zygomatic, and possibly buccal branches of the facial nerve.
- *Blood supply*—branches from the supraorbital branch of the ophthalmic artery.

Depressor (depressor septi)

Depressor septi

- *Origin*—incisive fossa of the maxillary periosteum.
- *Insertion*—passes superiorly deep to the mucous membranes of the upper lip, where it blends with orbicularis oris and inserts into the columella and mobile nasal septum.
- *Action*—brings the columella (and indirectly the nasal tip) and septum downwards.
- *Innervation*—buccal branch of the facial nerve.
- *Blood supply*—lateral nasal and septal branches of the superior labial branch of the facial artery.

Dilators (dilator naris anterior and posterior)

Dilator naris anterior

- *Origin*—upper lateral cartilage and alar component of nasalis.
- *Insertion*—lateral alar crus.
- *Action*—dilator of the nostril. Prevents collapse of the nasal valve during inspiration.
- *Innervation*—buccal branch of the facial nerve.

Dilator naris posterior (or alar component of nasalis)

- *Origin*—arises medial to compressor nares from maxilla, superior to the lateral incisor tooth.
- *Insertion*—attaches to the upper lateral cartilage.
- *Action*—encircles nares and opposes the action of compressor naris. Dilates nostrils.
- *Innervation*—buccal branch of the facial nerve.

Compressor (compressor naris)

Compressor naris (transverse component of nasalis)

Nasalis consists of compressor (transverse) and dilator (alar) components. Both parts are supplied by branches of the facial and infraorbital arteries.

Compressor naris

- *Origin*—attaches to the maxilla superolateral to the incisive fossa.
- *Insertion*—symmetrical muscle in continuity with the contralateral muscle via its aponeurosis. Blends with the aponeurosis of procerus.
- *Action*—compresses the nostrils.
- *Innervation*—buccal branch of the facial nerve.
- *Blood supply*—lateral nasal branch of the superior labial branch of the facial artery.

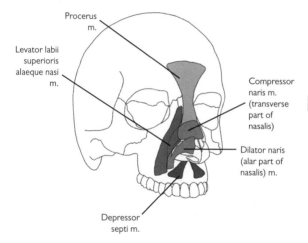

Fig. 9.19 Muscles of the external nose and nostrils.
Reproduced courtesy of Daniel R. van Gijn.

Muscles of the perioral region

Responsible for both the subtleties and coarseness of actions associated with feeding, speech, sounds, and the conveyance of the full spectrum of emotion. The versatility of this region relies upon the three-dimensional mobility of the *modioli*, the convergence points lateral to the buccal angle for the sphincters and paired dilator and buccinator muscles. The levator and depressor muscles surround orbicularis oris, acting upon the angles of the lips (*anguli oris*) or the upper and lower lip proper (direct labial tractors).

Direct labial retractors

The levators and depressors pass directly into the tissues of the lip perpendicular to the oral fissure and bypassing the modioli. They blend with the fibres of orbicularis oris, rather like the spokes of a bicycle wheel around a central hub, where they are insert into the dermis of the vermilion zone, submucosa, and periglandular connective tissue. From medial to lateral (Fig. 9.20 and Fig. 9.21):

Levator labii superioris alaeque nasi
- The most medial of the lip elevators.
- *Origin*—superior aspect of the frontal process of the maxilla; overlapped by orbicularis oculi.
- *Insertion*—courses inferolaterally, dividing into two slips which either insert into the greater alar cartilage and skin (medial slip) or blend with levator labii superioris and the dermis of the upper nasolabial fold (lateral slip).
- *Action*—elevates the upper lip and dilates the ala of the nose.
- *Innervation*—buccal branch of the facial nerve.

Levator labii superioris
- *Origin*—maxilla above the infraorbital foramen.
- *Insertion*—lateral substance of the upper lip, lateral to levator labii superioris alaeque nasi.
- *Action*—elevates and everts the upper lip and adjusts the nasolabial furrow.
- *Blood supply*—facial and infraorbital arteries (maxillary artery).
- *Innervation*—buccal branch of the facial nerve.

Zygomaticus minor
- *Origin*—posterior to the zygomaticomaxillary suture on the zygomatic bone (anteromedial to zygomaticus major).
- *Insertion*—passes obliquely downwards to the skin and muscle of upper lip.
- *Action*—elevates the upper lip, displaying the maxillary teeth as in a smile.
- *Blood supply*—superior labial branch of the facial artery.
- *Innervation*—buccal branch of facial nerve.

> ### Etymology
> - *Levator labii superioris alaeque nasi*—literally meaning the lifter of the upper lip and ala/wing of the nose. Colloquially referred to as Elvis's muscle in reference to the snarl made famous by Elvis Presley.

Depressor labii inferioris

- A quadrilateral muscle continuous with platysma.
- *Origin*—oblique line of the mandible.
- *Insertion*—converges with the opposite depressor and merges with the skin and mucosa of the lower lip and orbicularis oris.
- *Action*—everts and draws the lower lip inferiorly and laterally as in the portrayal of doubt.
- *Innervation*—marginal mandibular branch of the facial nerve.

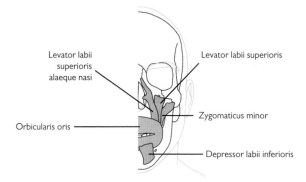

Fig. 9.20 Direct labial retractor muscles, anterior view.
Reproduced courtesy of Daniel R. van Gijn.

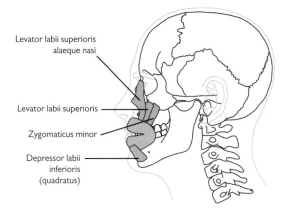

Fig. 9.21 Direct labial retractor muscles, lateral view.
Reproduced courtesy of Daniel R. van Gijn.

Muscles acting on the angle of the lip and modiolus

Zygomaticus major
See Fig. 9.22 and Fig. 9.23.
- *Origin*—anterior to the zygomaticotemporal suture on the zygomatic bone.
- *Insertion*—modiolus at angle of mouth (blends with fibres of levator anguli oris and orbicularis oculi).
- *Action*—more lateral insertion than that of zygomaticus minor, so that it draws the angle of the mouth laterally as well as superiorly.
- *Blood supply*—superior labial branch of the facial artery.
- *Innervation*—buccal and zygomatic branches of the facial nerve.

Levator anguli oris
- *Origin*—below infraorbital foramen from the canine fossa.
- *Insertion*—modiolus at angle of mouth.
- *Action*—elevates the angle of the mouth. Shapes and deepens the nasolabial fold in conjunction with levator labii superioris alaeque nasi, levator labii superioris, and zygomaticus minor (collectively known as the *quadratus labii superioris*).
- *Blood supply*—facial and infraorbital arteries (maxillary artery).
- *Innervation*—buccal branches of the facial nerve via its superficial surface.

Risorius
- An inconsistent muscle.
- *Origin*—as far posteriorly as the parotidomasseteric fascia.
- *Insertion*—modiolus and skin at the angle of the mouth.
- *Action*—displaces the corners of the mouth laterally and the skin of the cheek backwards. Contributes to the formation of dimples.
- *Blood supply*—is from the superior labial branch of the facial artery.
- *Innervation*—from the facial nerve, either via one of the buccal branches or the marginal mandibular branch; possibly both sources.

Depressor anguli oris
- Triangular muscle.
- *Origin*—broad origin from the oblique line of the mandible (continuous with platysma, cervical fascia, and its contralateral counterpart forming a 'mental sling' that converge as a narrow fasciculus).
- *Insertion*—modiolus at angle of mouth.
- *Action*—depresses the angle of the mouth and opposes the action of levator anguli oris and zygomaticus major.
- *Blood supply*—inferior labial branch of the facial artery.
- *Innervation*—marginal mandibular and buccal branches of the facial nerve.

Etymology
- *Risorius*—from 'risus' meaning to be 'laughed at'.
- *Risus sardonicus*—a fixed, sarcastic, mocking grimace. Caused by abnormal sustained spasm of the muscles of facial expression. Characteristic of tetanus and strychnine poisoning.
- *Sardonic*—thought to relate to the country Sardinia and an ancient belief that a local plant with neurotoxic properties used in ritual killings, the Hemlock water dropwort, resulted in a victim's sardonic grin prior to their death.

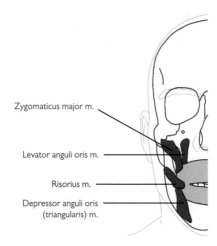

Fig. 9.22 Muscles acting on the angle of the lip and modiolus, anterior view.
Reproduced courtesy of Daniel R. van Gijn.

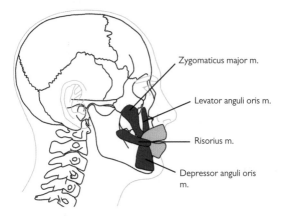

Fig. 9.23 Muscles acting on the angle of the lip and modiolus, lateral view.
Reproduced courtesy of Daniel R. van Gijn.

Orbicularis oris

Orbicularis oris is a multilayered muscular complex that takes contributions from surrounding muscles and is attached to the dermis of the upper and lower lips via the SMAS. It has peripheral and marginal components that originate either directly from the midline maxilla or mandible (the intrinsic incisive slips), by the modiolus itself, or by extension from the surrounding buccolabial muscles (Fig. 9.24 and Fig. 9.25). From each modiolus a large *pars peripheralis* and a smaller *pars marginalis* pass to both upper and lower lips, meeting along the length of the vermilion border. The complex is supplied by the buccal branches of the facial nerve and receives its blood supply from the superior and inferior labial branches of the facial artery (Fig. 9.26), the mental and infraorbital branches of the maxillary artery, and the transverse facial branch of the superficial temporal artery.

Pars peripheralis
- Forms the muscle underlying the skin of the lips.
- Fibres originate both from the modiolus directly and indirectly from buccinator and the depressors and elevators of the angle of the mouth.
- Fibres of the upper lip run close to and blend with the nasolabial sulcus, ala, and septum, and similarly with the mentolabial sulcus of the lower lip.
- The majority of fibres continue medially, where they meet their contralateral counterparts, and interdigitate across the midline with their dermal insertions, potentially contributing to the philtrum of the lip.

Pars marginalis
- Give rise to the muscle of the lips proper.
- Deepest component of the modiolus; the fibres in each quadrant pass from lateral to medial to meet and blend with their contralateral counterparts a little beyond the midline, and adherent to the dermis of the vermilion border.

Incisivus labii
- Accessory muscles of orbicularis oris in both upper and lower lips.
- Bony origins from the incisive fossae of the maxilla and mandible respectively, deep to the pars peripheralis of orbicularis oris.
- Fibres travel laterally and blend with the modiolus and fibres of the pars peripheralis.

Platysma

Platysma, although a muscle of the neck, will be discussed here briefly in relation to its association with orbicularis oris via its mandibular, modiolar, and labial constituents.
- *Pars mandibularis*—attached to the inferior border of the mandible.
- *Pars labialis*—fibres from platysma that act as direct labial tractors of the lower lip lie in the same plane and between the depressors of the angle of the mouth and the depressors of the lip proper.
- *Platysma pars modiolaris*—passes deep to risorius and lateral to depressor anguli *en route* to the modiolus.
- Contraction of platysma, e.g. while shaving to tighten the neck and facilitate close hair removal, brings the corners of the mouth inferiorly.

Mentalis

- Paired muscles originating from the incisive fossae, either side of the frenulum of the lower lip; they descend to insert into the skin of the chin.
- Evert and protrude the lower lip, while producing wrinkles on the skin of the chin, as in a demonstration of uncertainty or contempt.
- *Blood supply*—mental branch of the inferior alveolar artery (maxillary artery).
- *Innervation*—marginal mandibular branch of the facial nerve.

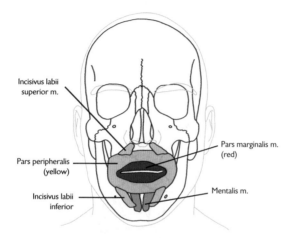

Fig. 9.24 Orbicularis oris and contributing muscles.
Reproduced courtesy of Daniel R. van Gijn.

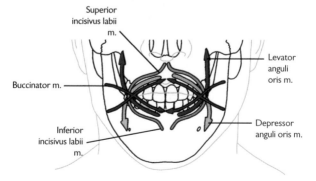

Fig. 9.25 The contributions from surrounding buccolabial muscles to orbicularis oris.
Reproduced courtesy of Daniel R. van Gijn.

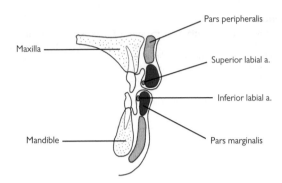

Fig. 9.26 The components of orbicularis oris and respective location of the superior and inferior labial arteries.

Reproduced courtesy of Daniel R. van Gijn.

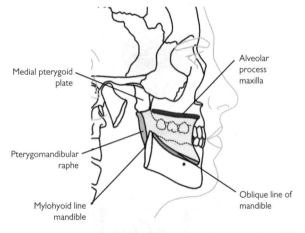

Fig. 9.27 Origin of the buccinator muscle (ramus and coronoid process of mandible and lateral pterygoid plate have all been removed).

Reproduced courtesy of Daniel R. van Gijn.

Layers of facial musculature

The muscles of facial expression can be divided arbitrarily into four layers, where layer four is clinically unique in that its muscles receive their innervation from their superficial surfaces. The remaining three layers are all supplied from their deep surfaces.

Layers of facial muscles
- *Layer 1*—depressor anguli oris, zygomaticus minor, orbicularis oculi.
- *Layer 2*—depressor labii inferioris, risorius, platysma, zygomaticus major, levator labii superioris alaeque nasi.
- *Layer 3*—orbicularis oris, levator labii superioris.
- *Layer 4*—mentalis, levator anguli oris, buccinator.

Buccinator

Buccinator forms the fundamental framework of the cheek (more specifically, it is the trumpeter's muscle). It is an important keystone structure with several clinically (and surgically) important relationships, amalgamating multiple anatomical regions such as the skin, oral cavity, parotid gland, maxilla, and pharynx.

Characteristics
- Quadrilateral muscle anterior to masseter and superior to platysma.
- *Origin*—anterior edge of pterygomandibular raphe (superior pharyngeal constrictor muscle takes its origin posteriorly); outer surface of the alveolar process of the maxilla; outer surface of the alveolar process of the mandible along the oblique line of mandible (Fig. 9.27).
- *Insertion*—progresses anteriorly within the submucosa of the cheek and lips to reach the modiolus near the angle of the mouth.
- *Action*—contracts and tenses the cheek (e.g. in the expulsion of air); keeps the cheek against the underlying dentition and gums to aid mastication.
- Lies internal to the ramus of the mandible, from which it is separated only by the buccal fat pad and temporalis.
- Contributes to the lateral wall of the mouth.
- The uppermost (maxillary) and lowermost (mandibular) fibres continue to serve their respective lips while the central fibres decussate, those from above entering the lower lip and those from below entering the upper lip (Fig. 9.28).
- Within the oral cavity, buccinator is covered by the buccopharyngeal fascia and the mucous membranes of the mouth.
- Anteriorly, it is covered by the four angular muscles of the mouth and is crossed and supplied by the facial vessels and branches of the long buccal (proprioception via V_3) and facial nerves (Fig. 9.29).
- Buccinator and the buccal fat pad superficial to it are pierced by the parotid duct, which enters the superficial surface of buccinator obliquely, opposite the third upper molar, and marks its presence in the oral cavity as the parotid papilla, facing the second upper molar.
- *Blood supply*—buccal branch of the maxillary artery and branches of the facial artery.
- *Innervation*—lower buccal branches of the facial nerve.

Pterygomandibular raphe
- A tendinous band extending between the hamulus of the medial pterygoid plate superiorly and the posterior end of the mylohyoid line of the mandible inferiorly.
- Its posterior border provides attachment for the superior pharyngeal constrictor; buccinator originates from its anterior border.

Pterygomaxillary ligament
- A fibrous band that extends between the hamulus of the medial pterygoid plate and the maxillary tuberosity, from which buccinator partially arises. The tendon of tensor veli palatini passes superior to its superior free border

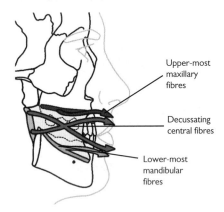

Upper-most maxillary fibres

Decussating central fibres

Lower-most mandibular fibres

Fig. 9.28 The decussation of fibres of buccinator muscle.
Reproduced courtesy of Daniel R. van Gijn.

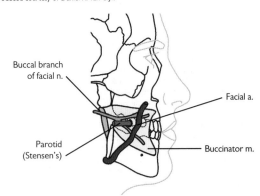

Buccal branch of facial n.

Facial a.

Parotid (Stensen's)

Buccinator m.

Fig. 9.29 Relations of buccinator muscle.
Reproduced courtesy of Daniel R. van Gijn.

Blood supply to the face

The face has an extensive blood supply arising primarily from branches of the ECA—via the facial, superficial temporal, maxillary, occipital, and posterior auricular arteries (Fig. 9.30). These anastomose freely with their contralateral counterparts and with contributions from the ICA via the ophthalmic artery (Table 9.2). This rich blood supply allows for the viability of ambitious skin flap design at the expense of significant bleeding in the event of penetrating trauma.

Facial artery

The facial artery runs a remarkably tortuous course from its point of first contact at the inferior border of the mandible just anterior to the masseter muscle at the antegonial notch (where it may be palpated and avoided). It continues towards the medial angle of the eye as the angular artery. One explanation for this tortuosity is to allow for the significant movements of the mandible and entire buccolabial complex. Through its various branches in the neck and face, it supplies structures of the superficial face. Its full course can be divided into cervical and facial components:

Cervical course

- Arises as the third anterior branch of the ECA within the carotid triangle, in close relation to the greater cornu of the hyoid bone.
- Quickly heads deep to the posterior belly of digastric and via the lateral aspect of the superior constrictor muscle (which separates it from the palatine tonsils) and continues towards the medial surface of the ramus of the mandible.
- In a sinusoidal fashion, it proceeds up and over the submandibular gland and underneath the inferior border of the mandible—grooving first the posterior and then lateral aspects of the submandibular gland to reach the lateral mandible.
- Deep to platysma.

Branches of the cervical part of the facial artery

- Ascending palatine artery.
- Tonsillar artery.
- Submental artery.
- Glandular branches (to submandibular gland and surroundings).

Facial course

- Begins its facial course proper at the anterior lower border of masseter where its pulsation is palpable.
- Continuing its tortuous tendencies, it weaves deep to the skin, fat, and the muscles acting at the angle of the mouth becoming superficial over buccinator and the levators of the upper lip and finally terminating at the medial eye as the *angular artery* within levator labii superioris alaeque nasi where it anastomoses with the dorsal nasal branch of the ophthalmic artery (internal carotid).

Branches of the facial part of facial artery
- *Premasseteric artery.*
- *Inferior labial artery*—supplies the muscles and associated structures of the lower lip and anastomoses with the mental branch of the inferior alveolar artery.
- *Superior labial artery*—passes between labial mucosa and orbicularis oris and anastomoses with its contralateral fellow. It supplies the upper lip and nasal septum via a *septal* branch.
- *Lateral nasal artery.*

Anastomoses

In addition to the anastomoses of the labial arteries mentioned previously, the facial artery anastomoses with the following arteries:
- Transverse facial artery (superficial temporal branch).
- Buccal branch (internal maxillary artery).
- Mental branch of inferior alveolar artery.
- Infraorbital artery (internal maxillary artery).

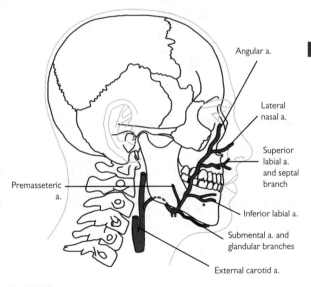

Fig. 9.30 Facial artery and its branches.
Reproduced courtesy of Daniel R. van Gijn.

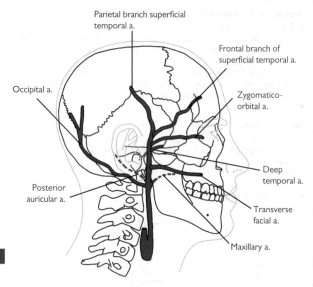

Fig. 9.31 Blood supply to the face (facial artery not shown).
Reproduced courtesy of Daniel R. van Gijn.

Blood supply and nasal reconstruction

Knowledge of the blood supply of the face is pivotal to successful reconstruction.

- May utilize either the axial supply of the supratrochlear or supraorbital arteries for nasal reconstruction of the external soft tissue.
- Supratrochlear artery within 1.5 cm radius of medial brow.
- Typically, flap is raised superficial to muscle in distal third, deep to frontal belly of occipitofrontalis in middle third, and deep to periosteum in proximal third (to incorporate artery).

Superficial temporal artery

The superficial temporal artery is one of two terminal branches of the ECA, passing superiorly along a similar trajectory. In addition to supplying the lateral face and scalp, it contributes to the vascular supply of the parotid gland and TMJs. It originates within the substance of the parotid gland behind the neck of the mandible and continues ever more superficially where it becomes readily palpable over the posterior root of the zygomatic process of the temporal bone. It lies within the temporoparietal fascia. It is crossed by the uppermost two branches of the facial nerve within the parotid gland and lies superficial to the auriculotemporal nerve.

Table 9.2 Sites of internal and external carotid anastomoses

External carotid contribution	Internal carotid contribution	Other anastomoses
Superior labial artery (facial)	Anterior ethmoidal artery (ophthalmic artery)	Contralateral artery
Inferior labial artery (facial)	Nil	Contralateral artery
Lateral nasal (facial)	External nasal (from anterior ethmoidal/ophthalmic artery)	Contralateral artery
Transverse facial artery (superficial temporal)	Lacrimal artery (ophthalmic artery)	Infraorbital (maxillary), facial, masseteric, buccal arteries
Zygomatico-orbital artery (superficial temporal)	Lacrimal and medial palzpebral branches of ophthalmic artery	Medial palpebral with supraorbital artery
Middle temporal artery (superficial temporal)	Nil	Deep temporal of maxillary artery
Frontal branch (from superficial temporal)	Supraorbital and supratrochlear branches of ophthalmic	Contralateral artery
Parietal branch (from superficial temporal)	Nil	Contralateral artery. Posterior auricular and occipital arteries from external carotid
Buccal artery (from maxillary artery)	Nil	Infraorbital and facial arteries
Infraorbital artery (from maxillary artery)	Ophthalmic branches (dorsal nasal artery)	Transverse facial and buccal arteries
	Supratrochlear artery (ophthalmic)	Supraorbital and contralateral arteries
Deep temporal artery (maxillary)	Lacrimal (ophthalmic)	Transverse facial artery
Angular artery	Dorsal nasal artery	

Branches
See Fig. 9.31 and Fig. 9.32.

Transverse facial artery
- Largest branch of the superficial temporal artery.
- Supplies the parotid gland and duct, masseter, and overlying skin.
- Leaves the superficial temporal artery within the parotid gland and proceeds horizontally across the masseter approximately parallel and inferior to the zygomatic arch.

- In instances where the facial artery fails to continue beyond the angle of the mouth, an enlarged transverse facial artery may appropriate the territory.
- Accompanied along its course by branches of the facial nerve.

Auricular artery
- Supplies the lateral auricle, lobe of the ear, and external acoustic meatus.

Zygomatico-orbital artery
- Passes between the deep and superficial layers of the temporalis fascia (superior to the zygomatic arch after the temporalis fascia splits), passing towards the eye where it supplies orbicularis oculi.

Middle temporal artery
- Arises above the zygomatic arch.
- Pierces the deep layer of the temporalis fascia to pass within the deep temporal fat pad.

Frontal branch
- Supplies frontalis, pericranium, and skin overlying region.
- Anastomoses with contralateral, supratrochlear, and supraorbital arteries.

Parietal branch
- Larger than the frontal branch, travels superficial to temporal fascia.
- Anastomoses with the posterior auricular, occipital, and contralateral arteries.

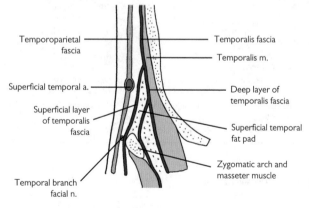

Fig. 9.32 Relationship of superficial temporal artery and facial layers, coronal section.

Reproduced courtesy of Daniel R. van Gijn.

Maxillary artery

The maxillary artery is the larger of the two terminal vessels of the ECA and supplies the areas not reached by the superficial temporal and facial branches. It courses between the neck of the mandible and sphenomandibular ligament, through the infratemporal fossa, and via the pterygomaxillary fissure, continues into the pterygopalatine fossa. Its length and respective 15 branches can be conveniently divided into thirds according to their relation to the lateral pterygoid muscle: five before, five upon, and five beyond. One branch from each part is destined for the face (Fig. 9.33):

First 'bony' part (posterior to lateral pterygoid)
Each enter a bony foramen:
• Deep auricular (external acoustic meatus).
• Anterior tympanic (petrotympanic fissure).
• Middle meningeal (foramen spinosum).
• Accessory meningeal (foramen ovale).
• Inferior alveolar (inferior alveolar canal).

Second 'muscular' part (within lateral pterygoid)
• Anterior deep temporal branches.
• Posterior deep temporal branches.
• Pterygoid branches.
• Masseteric artery.
• Buccinator artery.

Third 'pterygopalatine' part (anterior to lateral pterygoid)
See Fig. 9.34.
• Posterior superior alveolar.
• Infraorbital.
• Artery of the pterygoid canal.
• Pharyngeal artery.
• Greater palatine artery.
• Sphenopalatine artery.

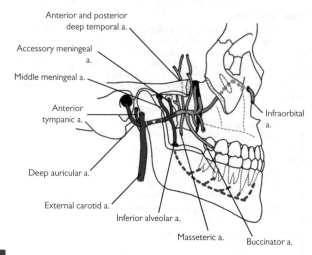

Fig. 9.33 The parts of the maxillary artery—bony part (red), muscular part (yellow), and pterygopalatine part (grey).

Reproduced courtesy of Daniel R. van Gijn.

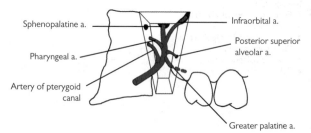

Fig. 9.34 The branches of the third part of maxillary artery within pterygopalatine fossa.

Reproduced courtesy of Daniel R. van Gijn.

Venous drainage of the face

The face is drained by the facial vein anteriorly and the retromandibular vein posteriorly. Knowledge of the venous drainage of the face is important due to the communication that exists between the facial vein and the cavernous sinus. This has implications for the retrograde spread of infection from the face to the cavernous sinus, which can result in cavernous sinus thrombosis, meningitis, and brain abscess.

Facial vein

See Fig. 9.35.
- A continuation of the *angular vein*—formed by the union of the *supratrochlear* and *supraorbital* veins.
- Follows a straight course (cf. facial artery) running obliquely inferoposteriorly across masseter towards the angle of the mandible.
- Pierces the investing layer of deep cervical fascia (passing deep to platysma) and runs superficially across the submandibular gland.
- Joined by the *anterior division of the retromandibular vein* to form the *common facial vein*.

Retromandibular vein

- Lies within the parotid gland.
- Formed by the union of the *superficial temporal* and *maxillary veins* behind the ramus of the mandible.
- Deep to facial nerve and superficial to ECA.
- Divides into an *anterior division* which joins the facial vein and a *posterior division* which joins the posterior auricular vein to form the EJV.

Communication with the cavernous sinus

The facial vein communicates with the cavernous sinus via the *superior and inferior ophthalmic veins*, the *deep facial vein*, and the *pterygoid venous plexus*.

Superior ophthalmic vein
- Begins at the inner angle of the orbit. Communicates anteriorly with the angular vein.
- Follows the ophthalmic artery.
- Passes through superior orbital fissure.

Inferior ophthalmic vein
- Begins at the floor and medial orbital wall.
- Receives contributions from vortex (meaning 'a whirlpool or eddying mass') veins and veins from inferior rectus and inferior oblique muscles, the lacrimal sac and eyelids before dividing into two branches.
- One branch continues above the inferior rectus and after passing through the inferior orbital fissure joins the pterygoid venous plexus.
- The other branch joins the cavernous sinus after passing through the superior orbital fissure

Deep facial vein and pterygoid venous plexus
- Joins the middle part of the facial vein with the pterygoid venous plexus.
- The pterygoid plexus also communicates with the maxillary vein.
- The pterygoid venous plexus in turn communicates with the cavernous sinus via emissary veins traversing the foramen ovale.

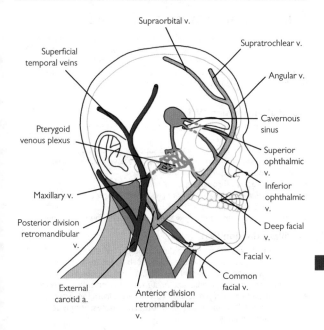

Fig. 9.35 Venous drainage of the face—facial vein (yellow) and (posterior) retromandibular vein (red).

Reproduced courtesy of Daniel R. van Gijn.

Sensory innervation of the face

The face develops from unpaired frontonasal and paired maxillary and mandibular processes, each of which is supplied by one of the three divisions
of the trigeminal nerve. The skin overlying the parotid gland and masseter
is supplied by the *greater auricular nerve* (C2). The three branches of the
trigeminal nerve are the ophthalmic, maxillary, and mandibular (Fig. 9.36
and Fig. 9.37).

Ophthalmic division (V₁)

Lies within the orbit and has five cutaneous branches—predominantly
supplying the upper eyelid.
- *Supraorbital*—from frontal nerve via superior orbital fissure.
- *Supratrochlear*—from frontal nerve. Arises above trochlea to superior
  oblique muscle.
- *Lacrimal*—passes through superior orbital fissure.
- *Infratrochlear*—from nasociliary nerve. Arises below the trochlea to
  superior oblique muscle.
- *External nasal*—emerges below the lower border the nasal bone.

Maxillary division (V₂)

Provides the cutaneous nerves to the middle part of the face.
- *Infraorbital*—passes through the inferior orbital fissure and then
  infraorbital foramen. Gives off nasal, labial, and palpebral branches (in
  addition to anterior, middle, and posterior superior alveolar nerves).
- *Zygomaticofacial* and *zygomaticotemporal*—arise from the zygomatic
  nerve and pass through foramina of the same names. Supply sensation
  to the temporal region.

Mandibular division (V₃)

- *Auriculotemporal*—from posterior division. Supplies the auricle (auricular
  branch) and temporal region (temporal branch). Supplies (external
  surface of) the tympanic membrane, external meatus, and TMJ.
- *Buccal*—sole sensory nerve from the anterior division of the mandibular
  nerve. Supplies mucosa of the inner cheek and buccal gingivae of the
  three molar teeth. It supplies a small cutaneous patch inferior to the
  zygoma.
- *Mental*—terminal branch of the inferior alveolar nerve. Branch of the
  posterior division and supplies the labial gingivae of the lower lip and
  skin of the lower lip and chin.

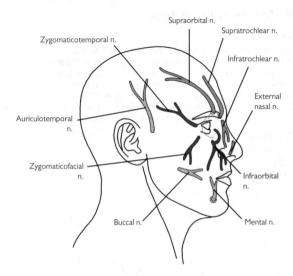

Fig. 9.36 Divisions of the trigeminal nerve. Ophthalmic division branches (grey), maxillary division branches (red), and mandibular division branches (yellow).

Reproduced courtesy of Daniel R. van Gijn.

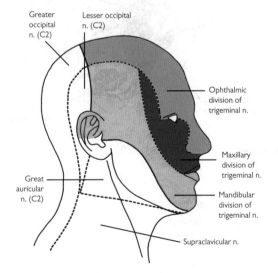

Fig. 9.37 Cutaneous innervation of the face and scalp.

Reproduced courtesy of Daniel R. van Gijn.

Motor supply to face

Overview

The main trunk of the facial nerve exits the skull via the stylomastoid for-amen. It next enters the parotid gland high up on its posteromedial surface and divides within the gland into upper *temporofacial* and lower *cervicofacial* trunks. The trunks branch further to form a parotid plexus (pes anserinus) from which five main terminal branches ultimately emerge. These branches diverge within the substance of the parotid and leave the gland via its anteromedial surface, medial to its anterior margin (Fig. 9.38).

Branches

• *Temporal*.
• *Zygomatic*.
• *Buccal*.
• *Marginal mandibular*.
• *Cervical*.

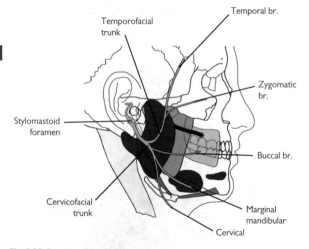

Fig. 9.38 Branches of the facial nerve.
Reproduced courtesy of Daniel R. van Gijn.

Facial nerve reconstruction

Facial nerve paralysis may be caused by congenital or acquired pathologies. In congenital disorders, it may be unclear whether it is the nerve or muscle which is defective. Acquired pathologies are usually due to trauma or malignancy, and present early. Beyond approximately 12 months of facial nerve paralysis, the motor end plates are irreversibly damaged and reconstruction of the nerve alone will not restore function.

Static reconstruction

- Tissues restored to functional position but do not produce movement.
- Brow—direct/open/endoscopic brow lift.
- Eyelid—canthopexy/canthoplasty/tarsorrhaphy.
- Mouth—direct excision and elevation, elevation with tendon or fascial sling.

Dynamic reconstruction

- Restores movement and function.
- Within 12 months—may be achieved via a nerve graft or nerve transfer (e.g. masseteric, hypoglossal, or spinal accessory nerves).
- Alternatively, transfer of innervated muscle by sliding temporalis myoplasty or free tissue transfer (gracilis, pectoralis minor)—a cross-facial nerve graft may be used as a first stage, or a donor nerve such as masseteric nerve used in a single stage.

Facial nerve identification

- *Tympanomastoid suture*—a hard ridge deep to cartilaginous portion of external auditory canal, with nerve 2–6 mm deep to its outer edge.
- *Posterior belly of digastric*—1 cm superior and parallel to the muscle near its mastoid attachment.
- *Tragal pointer (of Conley)*—nerve lies 1 cm deep and inferior to tragal cartilaginous point.
- *Styloid process*—lateral to the facial nerve.
- There is often a sentinel blood vessel situated superior to the nerve—warning of its ensuing proximity.

Fat compartments of the face

Overview

The subcutaneous fat of the face is highly partitioned (occurring in distinct anatomical compartments) and demonstrates enormous variability—both from person to person and within different regions of the face. It forms the basis of facial volume and in turn plays a key role in facial ageing. It can be considered in superficial and deep components separated by the SMAS.

Superficial fat layer

The superficial fat later consists of multiple yellow lobules interspersed between numerous fibrous septa that connect the overlying dermis to the SMAS beneath (Fig. 9.39). Named superficial compartments are:

- *Nasolabial.*
- *Medial cheek.*
- *Middle cheek.*
- *Lateral cheek.*
- *Infraorbital.*
- *Central forehead.*
- *Middle temporal.*
- *Lateral temporal forehead.*
- *Lateral temporal cheek.*
- *Jowl.*

Deep fat layer

The deep fat layer consists of paler, larger lobules with less fibrous septa between them. The deep layer of fat is found in and around adjacent musculature (Fig. 9.40)—presumably to accommodate the movement of tissue planes during muscle contraction.

Bichet's buccal fat pad

Bichet's buccal fat pad forms the mainstay of the deep fat and consists of the following five components:

- *Main body*—lies at the anterior border of masseter. Has a deep extension which lies against the posterior maxilla.
- *Buccal*—lies superficially and contributes to the contour of the cheek.
- *Pterygoid*—posterior extension into the pterygomandibular space.
- *Pterygopalatine*—extends into the pterygopalatine fossa and inferior orbital fissure.
- *Temporal*—can be subdivided into superficial and deep components. The former lies between the deep temporalis fascia and temporalis muscle while the latter lies posterior to the lateral orbital wall and extending into the infratemporal space.

Blood supply

Rich vascular supply from branches of the maxillary artery, superficial temporal, and facial arteries. Drained by tributaries of the pterygoid venous plexus.

> *Marie Francois Xavier Bichat (1771–1802)*
> French anatomist and pathologist—and largely considered the founder of general anatomy and animal histology (despite not using a microscope).

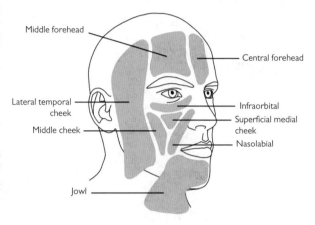

Fig. 9.39 Superficial fat compartments.
Reproduced courtesy of Daniel R. van Gijn.

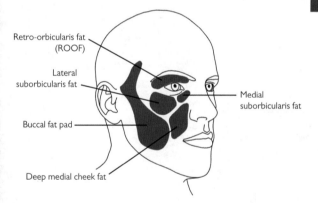

Fig. 9.40 Deep fat compartments.
Reproduced courtesy of Daniel R. van Gijn.

The orbit and its contents

Introduction

The function of the orbit is to protect and accommodate the globe in order to maximize its function. The bony orbits are paired, conical or four-sided pyramidal cavities within the skull each comprising seven bones, ranging from the paper-thin ethmoid and lacrimal plate medially to the buttress thick zygoma laterally. The conical shape consists of an apex posteriorly and a base anteriorly forming the outer margin. The medial wall and floor begin to blend towards the apex forming a posteromedial bulge as the orbit takes on a three-walled pyramidal structure. The walls are lined by peri-osteum (periorbita), which is continuous with the periosteal layer of the dura mater at the apex, the orbital septa, and the fascial sheaths of the extraocular muscles.

The margin of the orbit is formed by the junction of three bones, the zygomatic, frontal, and maxillary bones. It offers protection directly by forming a reinforced buttress to the orbit and indirectly by providing at-tachment for the fibrous orbital septum, which is suspended between the margin and tarsal plates and limits the spread of infection to and from the orbit.

The medial walls of the two orbits, interrupted only by the ethmoid sinuses and superior nasal cavity, are almost parallel to one another and the optical axis (the axes of gaze), and form an angle of approximately 23° to the orbital axis (Fig. 10.1). The difference between the two axes, combined with a natural tendency for the eye to sit in the orbital axis, accounts for the thicker medial rectus muscle and compound actions of the recti muscles (Fig. 10.1).

There are five principal openings of the orbit: three principal foramina located at the apex that transmit the neurovascular supply of the orbit and two lesser foramina (certainly lesser in size but with on par clinical implica-tions) located on the medial wall (Table 10.1).

The orbit has several clinically important relations and communications (Fig. 10.2). Superiorly, the anterior cranial fossa, containing the frontal lobe and its surrounding meninges; inferiorly, the maxillary sinus through which orbital contents may herniate in the event of fracture; medially, the nasal cavity and ethmoid and sphenoid sinuses; posterolaterally, the infratemporal and middle cranial fossae.

Protection of the eye itself is provided by the lids, acting as a shield from trauma and light while distributing the tear film across the corneal surface. The lacrimal apparatus provides a layer of protection in the form of a lubri-cant with antibacterial activity that provides a barrier to infection.

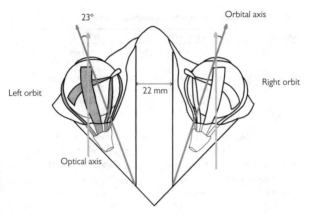

Fig. 10.1 Optical and orbital axes, superior view.
Reproduced courtesy of Daniel R. van Gijn.

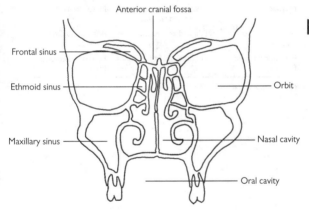

Fig. 10.2 Relationship of orbits, coronal section.
Reproduced courtesy of Daniel R. van Gijn.

Table 10.1 Summary table of orbital openings and contents

Opening	Boundaries	Structures
Optic foramen	Lesser wing of sphenoid	Optic nerve Ophthalmic artery
Superior orbital fissure	Greater and lesser wings of sphenoid	Cranial nerves III, IV, V_1, VI Ophthalmic veins Recurrent meningeal artery
Inferior orbital fissure	Greater wing of sphenoid and maxilla	Infraorbital NAV Zygomatic nerve
Supraorbital foramen	Frontal bone	Supraorbital NAV
Supratrochlear notch	Frontal bone	Supratrochlear NAV
Infraorbital groove/ foramen	Maxilla	Infraorbital NAV
Zygomatico-orbital foramen	Zygomatic bone	Zygomaticofacial NAV Zygomaticotemporal NAV
Nasolacrimal canal	Inferior nasal concha, maxilla and lacrimal bone	Nasolacrimal duct
Anterior ethmoidal foramen	Ethmoid and frontal bones	Anterior ethmoidal NAV
Posterior ethmoidal foramen	Ethmoid and frontal bones	Posterior ethmoidal NAV

NAV, nerve, artery, and vein.

Bony orbit

Roof

The roof of the orbit is thin and concave and comprised primarily of the orbital plate of the frontal bone (separating the globe from the anterior cranial fossa) and, further posteriorly towards the apex, the lesser wing of the sphenoid (Fig. 10.3).

Pertinent features

- *Frontal sinus*—may partially descend anteromedially.
- *Trochlear fovea*—found anteromedially and occasionally with a small spine for attachment of the cartilaginous pulley for the superior oblique muscle.
- *Anterior cranial fossa*—housed within the concave anterior portion.
- *Lacrimal fossa*—shallow fossa anterolaterally. Contains the orbital part of the lacrimal gland.
- *Optic canal*—bound by the roots of the lesser wing of the sphenoid.

Floor

The thin floor of the orbit is formed principally by the orbital plate of the maxilla which ascends laterally to articulate with the zygomatic bone anteriorly. Posteromedially, it articulates with the orbital process of the palatine bone. It is the only orbital wall that does not extend completely to the apex, extending from the rim to two-thirds of the depth of the orbit, where it curves and blends with the medial wall (Fig. 10.4).

Pertinent features

- *Maxillary sinus*—lies inferiorly and is separated from the orbit by a thin roof only.
- *Inferior oblique*—arises anteromedial and lateral to the nasolacrimal canal.
- *Inferior orbital fissure*—separates the floor of the orbit from the lateral wall posteriorly. It connects the orbit to the pterygopalatine fossa posteriorly and to the infratemporal fossa anteriorly.
- *Infraorbital groove*—medial edge of the floor, descending to become the infraorbital canal that ultimately opens as the infraorbital foramen. Contains the infraorbital neurovascular bundle.

Medial wall

The paper-thin lamina papyracea (orbital plate) of the ethmoid, covering the middle and posterior ethmoidal cells, forms the majority of the medial wall of the orbit. It is bound anteriorly by the orbital plate of the frontal bone and lacrimal bone and articulates posteriorly with the body of the sphenoid, which forms the remainder of the medial orbital wall.

Pertinent features

- *Nasolacrimal fossa*—contains the lacrimal sac. Bound anteriorly by the lacrimal crest of the frontal process of maxilla and posteriorly by the lacrimal crest of the lacrimal bone.
- *Anterior and posterior ethmoidal foramina*—interrupt the suture between the ethmoid bone and the orbital plate of the frontal bone.

Etymology

- *Lamina papyracea*—meaning paper-thin (papyrus being an ancient material similar to thick sheets of paper, made from the pithy stems of a water plant and used as a writing surface).

Lateral wall

The lateral wall of the orbit is the strongest, yet anteriorly it provides the least protection for the globe. Formed anteriorly by the zygomatic bone and posteriorly by the orbital surface of the greater wing of the sphenoid (Fig. 10.5).

Pertinent features

- *Zygomaticofacial and zygomaticotemporal foramina* and their respective nerves and vessels.
- *Orbital (Whitnall's) tubercle*—midpoint of lateral orbital margin. Provides attachment for three structures: check ligament of lateral rectus, lateral palpebral ligament, aponeurosis of levator palpebrae superioris (LPS).
- *Superior orbital fissure*—separates the lateral wall and roof posteriorly. Lies between the greater and lesser wings of the sphenoid inferiorly and superiorly, respectively. Communicates with the middle cranial fossa.

- *Samuel Ernest Whitnall (1876–1950)*—English doctor, anatomist, and 'Punch' columnist (For many years Whitnall authored numerous columns under the pseudonym "Tingle"—in addition to writing an 80-page spoof called *Astonishing Anatomy*).

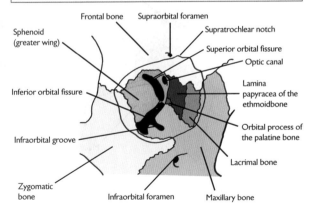

Fig. 10.3 Bones and openings of the orbit.
Reproduced courtesy of Daniel R. van Gijn.

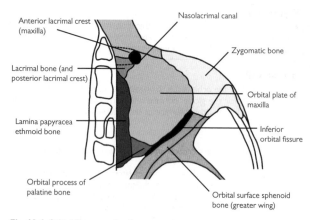

Fig. 10.4 Orbital floor, superior view.
Reproduced courtesy of Daniel R. van Gijn.

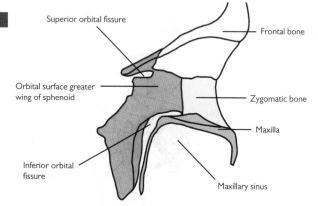

Fig. 10.5 Orbit, lateral wall.
Reproduced courtesy of Daniel R. van Gijn.

'Blow out' fracture

A 'blow out' fracture results from a fracture of a wall of the orbit with a resultant increase in orbital volume. Orbital floor fractures are the commonest cause: the floor medial to the infraorbital groove is extremely thin and vulnerable.

Clinical features

- Enophthalmos (increased orbital volume and a sunken appearance of the globe).
- Oedema/subconjunctival haemorrhage.
- Ophthalmoplegia and diplopia—downwards herniation of orbital contents including fat and muscle may limit movements and alter vision. Entrapment and the resultant strangulation of the inferior rectus muscle, in children in particular, is a surgical emergency owing to the propensity for ischaemia of this muscle and subsequent irreversible strabismus. Recognition is confounded by the presence of non-specific vagal symptoms (oculocardiac reflex) and relative absence of evidence of trauma, hence the term 'white eye' blow out fracture.
- Entrapment or neuropraxia of the infraorbital nerve causing altered sensibility of the ipsilateral midface.
- Afferent pupillary defect—Marcus Gunn pupil.

Superior orbital fissure syndrome

Superior orbital fissure syndrome (Rochon-Duvigneaud syndrome) is a clinical diagnosis supported by a sound knowledge of the involved anatomy. It occurs in 1 in 100 Le Fort II, III, or zygomatico-orbital fractures and affects structures passing through the fissure of the same name, i.e. ophthalmic vein, oculomotor, trochlear, and abducens nerves, and nasociliary, lacrimal, and frontal branches of the ophthalmic division of the trigeminal nerve (V_1).

Clinical features

- Ipsilateral ptosis.
- Proptosis.
- Ophthalmoplegia.
- Anaesthesia in the distribution of the ophthalmic branch of the trigeminal nerve.
- Dilatation and fixation of the ipsilateral pupil.
- Management is with operative reduction of the fracture with the aim of a gradual recovery of nerve function over a period of weeks.

Loss of sight coexisting with the above-listed features implies involvement of the orbital apex and therefore optic canal and optic nerve injury. This is termed the *orbital apex syndrome*.

Foramina and fissures

The globe occupies approximately one-fifth of the total volume of the orbit. The remaining space consists of orbital fat, connective tissue, and the muscles, nerves and vessels that control the functions of the eye. These neurovascular structures pass through three principal foramina and fissures at the orbital apex, namely the superior and inferior orbital fissures and the optic canal. The clinical importance of the anterior and posterior ethmoidal foramina must also be acknowledged.

Superior orbital fissure (III, IV, V₁, and VI)

The superior orbital fissure lies between the greater and lesser wings of the sphenoid. It separates the lateral wall and roof of the orbit posteriorly and connects the orbit with the middle cranial fossa (Fig. 10.6).

Structures transmitted
• Oculomotor (III), trochlear (IV), and abducent (VI) nerves.
• Branches of the ophthalmic nerve V₁ (nasociliary, frontal, lacrimal nerves).
• Ophthalmic arteries and veins.

Inferior orbital fissure

The inferior orbital fissure is bound superiorly by the greater wing of the sphenoid, inferiorly by the maxilla and orbital process of the palatine bone, and laterally by the zygomatic bone. It connects the orbit with both the pterygopalatine and infratemporal fossae (Fig. 10.6).

Structures transmitted
• Infraorbital and zygomatic branches of maxillary nerve (V₂) and associated vessels.
• Orbital rami from the pterygopalatine ganglion.
• Venous anastomosis between the inferior ophthalmic vein and the pterygoid venous plexus.

Optic canal

The optic canal is located medially at the posterior third or apex of the orbit and is enclosed by the lesser wing of the sphenoid. It connects the orbit with the middle cranial fossa. Its superior, inferior, and medial margins provide attachment for the common tendinous ring.

Structures transmitted
• Optic nerve (II) and surrounding pia, arachnoid and dura mater, and CSF.
• Ophthalmic artery.

Ethmoidal foramina

The anterior and posterior ethmoidal foramina interrupt the fronto-ethmoidal suture, indicate the level of the cribriform plate, and can be conveniently found intraoperatively at 24 mm and 36 mm respectively from the anterior lacrimal crest (Fig. 10.7). They transmit the neurovascular bundles into the ethmoid sinuses, anterior cranial fossa and lateral nasal cavity and emerge externally as the external nasal nerves and vessels.

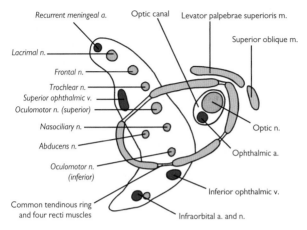

Fig. 10.6 The superior and inferior orbital fissures and optic canal (superior orbital fissure contents in italics).

Reproduced courtesy of Daniel R. van Gijn.

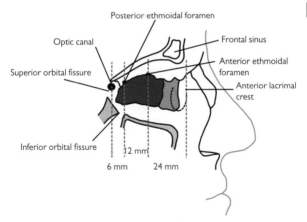

Fig. 10.7 Surface markers of the anterior and posterior ethmoidal foramen and optic canal from the anterior lacrimal crest (values in the uninjured orbit).

Reproduced courtesy of Daniel R. van Gijn.

Eyelids—lamellae

The eyelids exhibit both social and mechanical functions, ranging from the wide-eyed gaze of fright to their heavily furrowed appearance in the face of threat to the globe beneath. They act in conjunction with the lacrimal system in the distribution of tears across the corneal surface. Their intricate and delicate nature, combined with significant responsibility in the protection of sight, makes the importance of the surgical restoration of their structure and function considerable.

Structure

The eyelids can be classified clinically into three lamellae. The cross-sectional thickness at the eyelid margin is approximately 2–3 mm (two-thirds skin, one-third conjunctiva). Just anterior to the mucocutaneous junction is a surgically significant 'grey line' announcing the marginal pretarsal orbicularis oculi (more specifically the muscle of Riolan) and the point at which the lamellae may be divided in a (relatively) bloodless fashion (Fig. 10.8 and Fig. 10.9).

Anterior lamellae (from superficial to deep)
- *Skin*—the thinnest skin in the body and continuous with the conjunctiva at the margins of the palpebral fissure (where the double or triple row of eyelashes is found) and with the facial skin.
- *Orbicularis oculi*—eyelid closure and 'lacrimal pumping' towards the lacrimal canaliculi and sac. Orbital and palpebral components, the latter being divided into pretarsal (involuntary blinking) and preseptal (voluntary closure) components. Invested by SMAS.

Middle lamellae
- *Submuscular connective tissue*—continuous with the subaponeurotic layer of scalp; location of principal nerves.
- *Orbital septum*, orbital fat, and submuscular fatty tissue.

Posterior lamellae (from superficial to deep)
- *Tarsal plates*— the skeleton of the eyelids consists of concave, crescentic, thick fibrous plates (formed from the condensation of glandular tissue) that conform to and protect the anterior surface of the globe while supporting the eyelid. The superior tarsus is larger (10 mm at its midpoint) than the inferior tarsus (4 mm at its midpoint). Supported by the canthal ligaments medially and laterally and by the orbital septum.
- *Conjunctiva*—the thin, transparent lining of the inner surface of the eyelids (palpebral conjunctiva). Continues over the globe as the bulbar and limbal conjunctiva and with the skin at the free palpebral margin. Contributes to the mucinous tear film.

- *Jean Riolan (the Younger) (1580–1657)*—Royal French physician and anatomist. Also lends his name to the cremasteric muscle that covers the testis and spermatic cord. 'Cremaster' means to 'hang' or 'suspend'.

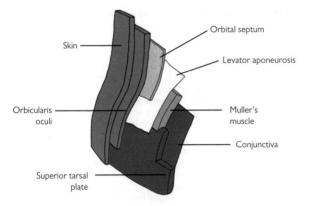

Fig. 10.8 Upper eyelid, layers and lamellae. Anterior lamellae (dark grey); middle lamellae (yellow); posterior lamellae (red).
Reproduced courtesy of Daniel R. van Gijn.

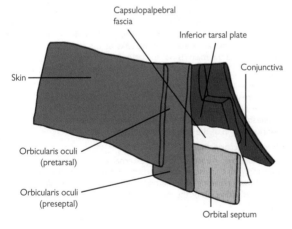

Fig. 10.9 Lower eyelid, layers and lamellae.
Reproduced courtesy of Daniel R. van Gijn.

Anatomical correlates in orbital surgery

There are several anatomical features that may be of use as landmarks in orbital surgery.

24–12–6 rule

- Distanced from anterior lacrimal crest to anterior ethmoidal foramen, anterior to middle ethmoidal foramen, and posterior ethmoidal foramen to optic canal, respectively.
- These are average values only because there may be a middle ethmoidal foramen in approximately a third of patients.
- Ethmoidal foramina may be useful guides to height of medial wall dissection.

Orbital plate of the palatine bone

- Rarely fractured in orbital blunt trauma and therefore useful as a reliable ledge on which to rest orbital reconstruction plate. Marks the posteromedial limit of the orbital floor.
- Dissection along the inferior orbital fissure should not be taken medial to the orbital plate of the palatine bone.

Approaches to the orbit

Several incisions have been described to access the orbit via the lower eyelid. Broadly speaking, they can be external (Fig. 10.10 and Fig. 10.11b) or internal/transconjunctival (Fig. 10.11c). The differences between them include the level at which the skin and orbicularis oculi muscle is incised and the layers that are dissected. The risks of the former are scar and ectropion, while the main risk of the latter is entropion.

External

- *Subciliary*—the incision is made just beneath the eyelashes and is therefore inconspicuous. Variations include a 'skin-only' flap, a 'skin-muscle' flap, or a stepped approach.
- *Subtarsal*—the incision is made at approximately the level of the inferior margin of the inferior tarsal plate.

Internal (transconjunctival)

- *Preseptal transconjunctival*—avoids external scars. Can be extended medially with a transcaruncular incision and laterally with a lateral canthotomy (splitting of the lateral canthal ligament) and inferior cantholysis (division of the inferior limb of the lateral canthal ligament).
- *Retroseptal transconjunctival*—as for preseptal transconjunctival approach, but more direct and dissection is behind the orbital septum. Theoretically, more periorbital fat is encountered. Incisions must be carefully closed to avoid an entropion (when the eyelid folds inwards).

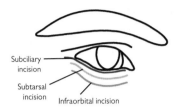

Fig. 10.10 Skin incisions for approaches to the orbit. Subciliary (red line), subtarsal (yellow line), and infraorbital (grey line).

Reproduced courtesy of Daniel R. van Gijn.

(a)

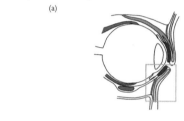

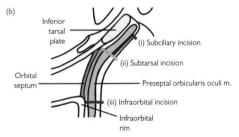

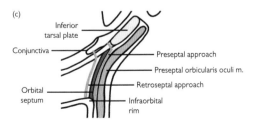

Fig. 10.11 (a) Orbit demonstrating regions magnified in subsequent images (yellow box), sagittal section. (b) Lower eyelid demonstrating skin incision approaches to the orbit: (i) subciliary (note this is a stepped incision and joins the yellow line of the subtarsal incision), (ii) subtarsal, and (iii) infraorbital. Sagittal section. (c) Lower eyelid demonstrating preseptal and retroseptal transconjunctival approaches to the orbit, sagittal section.

Reproduced courtesy of Daniel R. van Gijn.

Eyelid retractors

The eyelid retractors, orbital septum and supportive skeleton of the eyelids should be considered as a unit rather than as their individual components, with the common goal of acting upon the tarsus to protect the globe and maintain its position.

Eyelid retractors (superficial to deep)

The eyelid retractor complexes in the upper and lower eyelids consist of skeletal muscle, smooth muscle, and an aponeurosis. Collectively, they produce retraction of the tarsal plates via their attachments to the subcutaneous tissues of the eyelid. They concurrently give rise to the superior and inferior palpebral furrows which are most noticeable at the extremes of opening (Fig. 10.12, Fig. 10.13, and Table 10.2).

Skeletal muscle

- *LPS (upper lid)*—arises from the undersurface of the lesser wing of the sphenoid at the orbital apex and inserts as a wide aponeurosis into the upper edge of tarsal plate and skin. Shares common developmental and fibrous origins with superior rectus, to which it is linked by a check ligament. Supplied by the superior division of the oculomotor nerve.
- *Inferior rectus (lower lid)*—arises from the common tendinous ring inferior to the optic canal. Analogous function to LPS. Supplied by the inferior division of the oculomotor nerve.

Smooth muscle

A thin sliver of smooth muscle forms the superior and inferior tarsal muscles in the upper and lower eyelids, respectively and contributing to 1–2 mm of elevation of the eyelid on contraction. Innervated by the sympathetic nervous system and implicated in both the ptosis of Horner's syndrome (see later in topic) and the wide-eyed eye of fright.

- *Muller's muscle/superior tarsal muscle (upper lid)* —lies on the inferior surface of LPS, remaining posterior to the aponeurosis and inserting onto the upper border of the superior tarsal plate.
- *Inferior tarsal muscle (lower lid)*—less prominent and originates from the capsulopalpebral fascia of the inferior rectus, inserting onto the lower tarsus.

Aponeurosis

- *Levator aponeurosis (upper lid)*—wider continuation of the LPS, descending almost vertically posterior to the orbital septum, forming lateral and medial horns. The former divides the lacrimal gland into orbital and palpebral parts and is attached to the marginal tubercle; the latter is attached to the posterior lacrimal crest. The aponeurosis fuses with the orbital septum, skin, and pretarsal orbicularis oculi (forming upper lid crease) and superior and anterior tarsal borders.
- *Capsulopalpebral fascia (lower lid)*—anterior expansion of the fused fascial sheath of inferior rectus and inferior oblique. Fuses with the inferior border of the inferior tarsus and orbital septum.

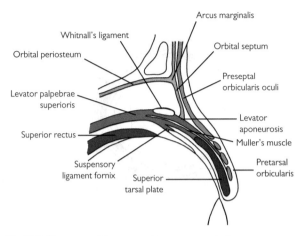

Fig. 10.12 The upper eyelid anatomy and the retractor mechanism.
Reproduced courtesy of Daniel R. van Gijn.

Horner's syndrome

A collection of (principally) ocular signs resulting from disruption of the sympathetic pathway. Signs include:

- *Ipsilateral enophthalmos*—posterior displacement of the globe in the orbit.
- *Eyelid ptosis*—interruption to the sympathetic input to Muller's smooth muscle.
- *Pupillary miosis*—constricted pupil (unopposed parasympathetic drive).
- *Anhidrosis*—lack of facial sweating.

Causes

- *Central*—hypothalamic, thalamic, or brainstem.
- *Preganglionic*—brainstem to superior cervical ganglion.
- *Postganglionic*—along internal carotid artery via cavernous sinus before joining ophthalmic division of the trigeminal nerve (V_1).

Johann Friedrich Horner (27 March 1831–20 December 1886)
Swiss ophthalmologist. Described the features of Horner's syndrome in 1869.

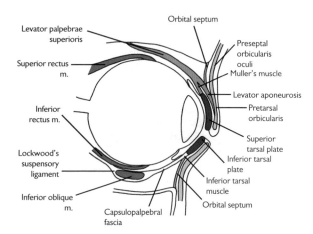

Fig. 10.13 Detail of the upper and lower eyelids, coronal section.
Reproduced courtesy of Daniel R. van Gijn.

Eyelid reconstruction

Reconstruction of the eyelid following trauma or oncological resection must consider replacement of skin, tarsus, and conjunctiva. Lid tissue is best reconstructed with lid tissue. Caution should be exercised in harvest from the upper lid due to its greater role in globe protection: a retracted upper lid causing lagophthalmos may threaten vision in the eye. A number of algorithms are described for partial- or full-thickness defects, detailing management for tissue loss of up to one-third, one-third to two-thirds, or greater than two-thirds.

Skin reconstruction

- Use a method with low risk of contraction, to reduce risk of ectropion.
- Full-thickness grafts are preferred to split-thickness skin grafts.
- Alternatively, tissue may be recruited as a local flap from opposing lid, forehead, or cheek to minimize risk of contraction.

Tarsus

- Similarly, may recruit from opposing lid, or as graft of palatal mucosa or cartilage.
- Lower lid has less retraction, and lateral canthopexy to support the lower lid may be adequate instead of tarsal reconstruction.

Conjunctiva

- From opposing lid (Hughes tarsoconjunctival flap).
- Buccal mucosal or septal mucosal graft.

Table 10.2 Equivalent upper and lower components of eyelids

Structure	Upper lid	Lower lid
Muscle (skeletal)	LPS	Inferior rectus/inferior oblique/capsulopalpebral head
Aponeurosis	LPS aponeurosis	Capsulopalpebral fascia
Muscle (smooth)	Müller's muscle (superior tarsal muscle)	Inferior tarsal muscle
Suspensory ligament	Transverse ligament of Whitnall	Lockwood's suspensory ligament

Blepharoplasty
- Dermatochalasis is an eyelid condition of skin excess.
- Blepharoplasty corrects facial ageing changes of the upper and lower eyelids: many different techniques.
- Upper lid ageing changes: typically excess skin, orbicularis oculi may be ptotic and act as lateral lid depressor, fat herniation or excess may be present.
- Lower lid ageing changes: typically minimal excess of skin, tarsoligamentous laxity, ptotic orbicularis oculi, fat herniation prominent due to fixed septum at arcus marginalis.

Upper lid blepharoplasty
- Inferior incision in supratarsal crease.
- Upper incision at upper border of a skin 'pinch test'—leave 20 mm of skin from lash margin to eyebrow.
- Skin excised together with a variable amount of orbicularis oculi.
- Some cases require conservative excision of pre- or postseptal fat: excessive resection leaves hollowed appearance.

Lower lid blepharoplasty
- Approach may be subciliary or transconjunctival (preseptal or postseptal).
- Many different techniques; current focus is on repositioning elements affected by facial ageing.
- Minimal skin and fat excision.
- Releasing insertion of septum at arcus marginalis permits redraping of fat inferiorly and treats 'puffy' lower lid appearance.

Orbital septum and support structures

Orbital septum

The orbital septum (Fig. 10.14) is continuous with the periosteum of the orbit and external skull. Lying deep to preseptal orbicularis oculi, it forms the outermost diaphragm of the orbit, maintaining the posterior position of the orbital fat pads and protecting the contents of the globe within, at the expense of forming a compartment vulnerable to both pressure and infection.

- Attached to the thickened periosteal margins of the orbit (arcus marginalis), becoming thickened at the lid margins to attach to the anterior aspect of the crescenteric tarsal plates.
- Anterior to the lateral palpebral ligament laterally and posterior to the medial palpebral ligament and nasolacrimal sac medially.
- Pierced by the lacrimal, supratrochlear, infratrochlear, and supraorbital nerves and vessels.

Supporting structures

See Fig. 10.15.

Medial palpebral ligament

The strong medial palpebral ligament is intimately related to both the orbicularis oculi and the lacrimal system. It originates by a common tendon from the anterior lacrimal crest and frontal process of the maxilla.

- It lies anterior to the orbital septum and nasolacrimal sac, providing a useful surgical landmark to the latter.
- It envelopes the lacrimal canaliculi before inserting into and anchoring down the medial ends of the upper and lower tarsi.
- The lacrimal part of the orbicularis oculi is a small thin muscle (*Horner's muscle*) arising from the posterior crest of the lacrimal bone and passing behind the lacrimal sac.

Lateral palpebral ligament

The weaker and more poorly developed lateral palpebral ligament originates from Whitnall's orbital tubercle on the zygomatic bone.

- It lies deep to the orbital septum.
- Divides into superior and inferior crura, which are inserted into the lateral angles of the upper and lower tarsi, respectively.

Whitnall's ligament

The main suspensory ligament of the upper eyelid. It is suspended from the orbital roof and spans the orbit from the trochlea of the superior oblique medially to the frontozygomatic suture laterally (approximately 1 cm above Whitnall's tubercle).

Lockwood's ligament

A condensation of the capsulopalpebral fascia and the inferior suspensory ligament of the globe. It is attached to the medial and lateral palpebral ligaments, engulfs the inferior oblique muscle, and acts as the major supportive sling of the globe.

Disruption of the medial palpebral ligament insertion secondary to naso-orbito-ethmoidal (NOE) fractures can result in 'telecanthus'— the widening of the distance between the medial canthi with a normal interpupillary distance.

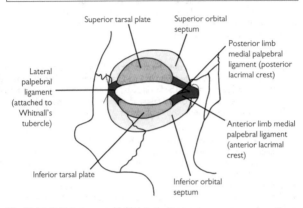

Fig. 10.14 Orbital septum, tarsi, and palpebral ligaments.
Reproduced courtesy of Daniel R. van Gijn.

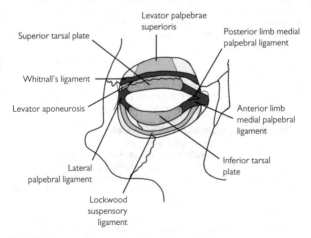

Fig. 10.15 Ligamentous support structures of the orbit.
Reproduced courtesy of Daniel R. van Gijn.

Periorbita and orbital fascia

Periorbita

The periorbita principally refers to the orbital periosteum that is loosely attached to the underling bones of the orbit. It is continuous with the external periosteum of the skull, the orbital septum of the eyelids, and the dura mater via the superior orbital fissure. It contributes to the trochlea, lacrimal fascia, and nasolacrimal sac fossa.

Orbital fascia

The fascia of the orbit includes the thin muscular fascia surrounding the muscles of the orbit associated with its important medial and lateral expansions (the check ligaments) and the fascia bulbi, or Tenon's capsule. In addition to supporting the globe, the orbital fascia allows free movement of the globe within its pocket and prevents the displacement of orbital fat (Fig. 10.16).

Muscular fascia
- Forms a sleeve surrounding each muscle of the orbit.
- Thicker anteriorly than posteriorly.
- The sleeves of the four recti muscles join to form a fascial ring that isolates the intraconal fat.
- Continuous with the fascia bulbi where the muscles pierce it.
- The sheath of superior oblique extends as far as the trochlea pulley.
- *Check ligaments*—neither 'check' nor ligaments. Rather, a strong triangular expansion of the medial and lateral recti muscle fascia, attaching to the zygomatic and lacrimal bones, respectively. Possibly limits overaction, although this checking action is questionable.
- The sheaths of inferior rectus and inferior oblique are continuous with the check ligaments and contribute to Lockwood's suspensory ligament.

Fascia bulbi (Tenon's capsule)
- Envelopes the globe from where the optic nerve enters to the corneoscleral junction (limbus).
- Forms a fibrous layer between orbital fat and the globe.
- Pierced by the ciliary nerves and vessels surrounding the optic nerve and by the tendons of the six extraocular muscles.

The orbital septum and clinical correlates

The orbital septum converts the bony orbit into a closed compartment susceptible to the accumulation of tumour, haemorrhage, and infection. The space anterior to the septum is termed the preseptal space and that posterior, the postseptal space. The latter may be divided further into intra- and extra-conal spaces, within and outside the cone of extraocular muscles, respectively (Fig. 10.17).

Infection
- *Preseptal cellulitis*—a periorbital cellulitis limited to the soft tissues anterior to the orbital septum. Commonly caused by spread of infection of the face, teeth or ocular adnexa, and treated with antibiotics.
- *Postseptal cellulitis*—infection posterior/deep to the orbital septum that may result in abscess formation requiring surgical drainage. It can be subclassified as intra- or extra-conal. May be a result of paranasal sinusitis, specifically the adjacent ethmoid sinuses. Untreated complications include cavernous sinus thrombosis, loss of vision, and intracranial abscess.

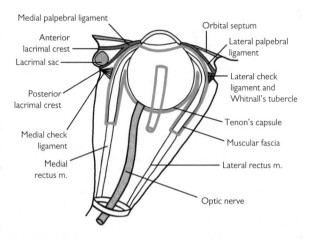

Fig. 10.16 Orbital fascia.
Reproduced courtesy of Daniel R. van Gijn.

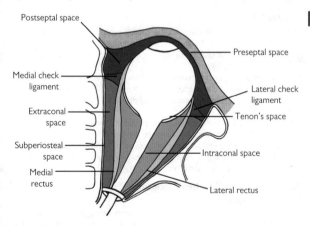

Fig. 10.17 Orbital spaces—including pre- and postseptal spaces.
Reproduced courtesy of Daniel R. van Gijn.

Periorbital fat

The fat compartments of the eye can be classified according to depth in relation to the septum and location relative to the upper and lower eyelids. Fat found deep to the orbital septum is termed the orbital fat while fat superficial to the septum and deep to the orbicularis oculi in the lower eyelid is called the *suborbicularis oculi fat* (SOOF). Between the periosteum of the supraorbital rim and orbicularis oculi in the upper eyelid is the retro-orbicularis oculi fat (ROOF).

Suborbicularis oculi fat

- Continuous with the malar fat pad of the face.
- Allows the smooth movement of muscle over periosteum.
- Consists of a medial compartment between the medial limbus and lateral canthus (adherent to the periosteum of the orbital rim) and a lateral compartment extending from the lateral canthus to the lateral orbital thickening (the lateral extension of the septum, which is continuous with the deep temporal fascia over the lateral orbital rim).

Retro-orbiculairs fat

- The 'eyebrow fat pad'.
- Found deep to orbicularis oculi and adjacent to the periosteum of the superior orbital rim.

Orbital fat

The orbital fat proper is deep to the orbital septum and preaponeurotic in nature, i.e. superficial to the levator aponeurosis. It serves as a useful surgical landmark and barometer of suspicion in soft tissue trauma in the upper eyelid (Fig. 10.18).

- *Upper eyelid*—the two fat pads that compose the upper eyelid fat are the central and the medial fat pads, separated by the trochlea for superior oblique. In the preaponeurotic space laterally is the pinker, paler lacrimal gland.
- *Lower eyelid*—the lower eyelid is comprised of medial, central, and lateral fat pads. These are posterior to the orbital septum and anterior to the lower eyelid retractors. The medial and middle fat pads are separated by the inferior oblique muscle. Prolapse of the lower fat pads is a common cosmetic concern.

Tear trough and lid–cheek junction

Tear trough (medially)

The tear trough or nasojugal groove is a depression approximately 5 mm below the orbital rim, extending inferolaterally from the medial canthus. (Fig. 10.19).

Lid–cheek junction (laterally)

A continuation from the tear trough at the midpupillary line. Lies below and parallel to the infraorbital rim. The tear trough and lid–cheek junction correlate with the cleft between the palpebral and orbital parts of orbicularis oculi. The tear trough and lid–cheek junction can be more readily seen with pressure on the globe or on upwards gaze.

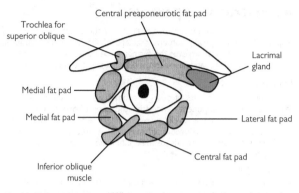

Fig. 10.18 Eyelid fat pads—posterior to the orbital septum.
Reproduced courtesy of Daniel R. van Gijn.

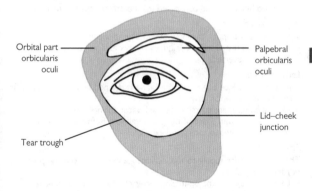

Fig. 10.19 Tear trough and lid–cheek junction.
Reproduced courtesy of Daniel R. van Gijn.

Nasolacrimal apparatus

The lacrimal system comprises four distinct structures that are collectively responsible for the production and drainage of tears. The lacrimal gland (and accessory glands) achieves the former while the superior and inferior canaliculi, lacrimal sac, and nasolacrimal duct manage the latter (Fig. 10.20).

Lacrimal gland

The lacrimal gland consists of a larger orbital (superior) and smaller palpebral (inferior) component divided by the lateral horn of the levator aponeurosis of the upper eyelid, in a similar arrangement to that of the submandibular gland and mylohyoid muscle (Fig. 10.21). Closely related small accessory glands provide residual lubrication in the event of main gland excision.

Orbital component

- Lies within the shallow lacrimal fossa formed within the orbital margin on the medial aspect of the zygomatic process of the frontal bone.
- Found superior to the LPS and lateral rectus.
- Fuses with the orbital periosteum above.
- Wedged between (and connected to) the orbital septum and orbital fat.

Palpebral component

- Lateral part of upper lid below the levator aponeurosis.
- Adherent to the superior conjunctiva fornix and may be visible when the eyelid is everted.

Lacrimal ducts

The serous produce of the lacrimal gland is drained by half a dozen main ducts into the superior fornix.

- Orbital component ducts pierce the levator aponeurosis and communicate with those of the palpebral part. Removal of the latter therefore equates to total gland excision.

Arterial supply

The neurovascular supply to the lacrimal gland enters from the posterior border (Fig. 10.22).

- Lacrimal branch of the ophthalmic artery and infraorbital branches.

Nervous supply

- Secretomotor postganglionic parasympathetic from the pterygopalatine ganglion, either directly or indirectly via the zygomatic and lacrimal branches of the maxillary nerve (V_2).
- Postganglionic sympathetic fibres from the superior cervical ganglion.

Lacrimal canaliculi

The superior and inferior lacrimal canaliculi are found posterior to the medial palpebral ligament at the puncta near the medial canthal angle of the upper and lower eyelids. They drain tears from the lacrimal lake.

- Each canaliculus is approximately 1 cm long and extends vertically approximately 2 mm before abruptly turning medially at their respective ampullae.
- Superior canaliculus is shorter and smaller.
- The superior and inferior canaliculi converge at the upper margin of the lateral wall of the lacrimal sac: the manner in which they do this is variable.

Lacrimal sac

The lacrimal sac, located in the lacrimal fossa of the anteromedial bony orbit, is the superior extent of the nasolacrimal duct and measures approximately 12 mm in length.

• *Lacrimal fascia*—an extension of orbital periosteum that envelopes the lacrimal sac between the anterior and posterior lacrimal crests.

Nasolacrimal duct

Commencing at the lacrimal sac and emptying via the inferior meatus of the nose, the 18 mm long nasolacrimal duct lies within the thin canal of the same name in the bony wall formed by the maxilla, lacrimal bone, and inferior nasal concha.

• *Ostium lacrimalis*—opening into inferior meatus.
• *Plica lacrimalis (Hasner's valve)*—fold of mucosa forming a valve.

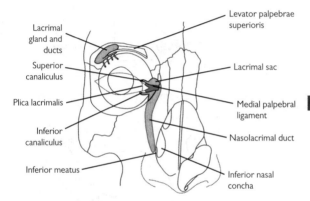

Fig. 10.20 Nasolacrimal apparatus.
Reproduced courtesy of Daniel R. van Gijn.

Nasolacrimal apparatus injury

Laceration of the nasolacrimal apparatus or excision in oncological resection prevents tear drainage, and can lead to epiphora, recurrent infections, and diplopia. Reconstruction of a canalicular injury involves insertion of a stent for a period of months. A mono-canalicular (e.g. Mini-Monoka) or bi-canalicular stent (e.g. Ritleng tube) inserted from the punctum to lacrimal sac assists reformation of the canaliculus.

Dacryocystorhinostomy

Where there is stenosis or complete destruction of the canalicular system, a dacryocystorhinostomy can directly bypass the nasolacrimal duct to assist tear drainage.

• Endonasal or external approach.
• Lacrimal bone forming lacrimal sac removed.
• Passageway is formed from the caruncle to lacrimal sac, and into nose, assisted by insertion of a stent (e.g. Lester Jones tube).

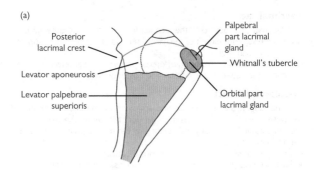

(a)

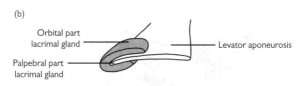

(b)

Fig. 10.21 Relationship of lacrimal gland to (a) levator palpebrae superioris and (b) its aponeurosis.

Reproduced courtesy of Daniel R. van Gijn.

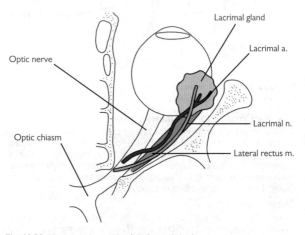

Fig. 10.22 Neurovascular supply of the lacrimal gland.

Reproduced courtesy of Daniel R. van Gijn.

- *Joseph Ritter von Artha Hasner (1819–1892)*—Austrian ophthalmologist and professor of ophthalmology in Prague. Lends his name to the mucosal fold that guards the opening of the nasolacrimal duct at the inferior meatus.

Extraocular muscles

The difference between the optical and orbital axes means that the four extraocular rectus muscles of the eye are not as straight as their name implies, and must be assisted by two oblique muscles in order to produce true upward and downward movement of the eyes. The continuous demand for torsion of the eyeball to its optical axis results in a tendency to divergence and a bulkier medial rectus muscle. The striated muscles of the globe are the four recti, two obliques, and the LPS muscle, the latter discussed previously (Fig. 10.23).

Anulus of Zinn (common tendinous ring)

The common tendinous ring is the common origin of the four rectus muscles and surrounds the optic foramen at the orbital apex, dividing the superior orbital fissure into intra- and extraconal portions.

• Connects posteriorly to the dura mater.
• Connects medially to the lesser wing of the sphenoid.
• Connects laterally to a spine on the margin of the greater wing of the sphenoid.

Rectus muscles

The four strap-shaped superior, medial, inferior, and lateral rectus muscles arise from the wonderfully named *anulus (annulus) of Zinn*, gradually widening as they pass anteriorly from the orbital apex (Fig. 10.24 and Fig. 10.25). The effect of this (in combination with intermuscular septa) is to form an anatomical cone creating intra- and extraconal compartments.

• *Blood supply*—all recti (and obliques) are supplied by the ophthalmic artery (ICA) with or without a contribution from the maxillary artery (ECA): superior rectus by the supraorbital branch of the ophthalmic artery, the inferior rectus is supplemented by the infraorbital branch of the maxillary artery, the medial rectus receives supply purely from the ophthalmic artery, and the lateral rectus by the lacrimal branch of the ophthalmic artery.
• *Nerve supply*—the oculomotor nerve supplies all but the lateral rectus, which is supplied by the abducens nerve. The inferior division of the oculomotor nerve supplies the medial and inferior rectus. The superior division supplies superior rectus.

Obliques

The superior and inferior oblique muscles lie at an angle of 51° to the optical axis and prevent the eye rotating around its long axis when the superior and inferior recti contract. See Fig. 10.24 and Fig. 10.25.

Superior oblique (works with inferior rectus)

Originates above and medial to the optic canal outside the anulus where it courses (becoming tendinous) towards the trochlea (the fibrocartilaginous pulley in the trochlear fossa of the frontal bone).

• From the trochlea, it turns laterally and posteriorly and pierces the fascial sheath between superior rectus and the globe.
• Broad fan-shaped attachment into the posterosuperior lateral quadrant of the sclera.
• *Blood supply*—ophthalmic artery and its supraorbital branch.

- *Nerve supply*—trochlear nerve.
- *Actions*—(primary) intorsion, (secondary) pure depression in the adducted position, and (tertiary) abduction.

Inferior oblique (works with superior rectus)

A thin muscle originating from the orbital surface of the maxilla, lateral to the nasolacrimal groove and close to the anterior margin.

- It courses posterolaterally between the orbital floor and inferior rectus, passing deep to lateral rectus before inserting with a broad attachment to the posteroinferior lateral quadrant of the sclera.
- *Blood supply*—ophthalmic artery and its infraorbital branch.
- *Nerve supply*—inferior division of the oculomotor nerve.
- *Actions*—(primary) extorsion, (secondary) pure elevation in the adducted position, and (tertiary) abduction.

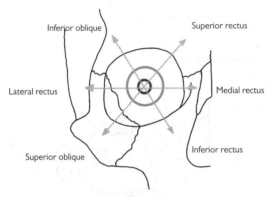

Fig. 10.23 Actions of the extraocular muscles.
Reproduced courtesy of Daniel R. van Gijn.

Johann Gottfried Zinn (1727–1759)

German anatomist, botanist, and author of *Descriptio anatomica oculi humani*. In addition to lending his name to the common tendinous ring, he described the orchid genus *Epipactis* that belongs to the orchid family.

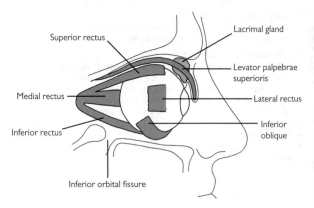

Fig. 10.24 The extraocular muscles, lateral view.
Reproduced courtesy of Daniel R. van Gijn.

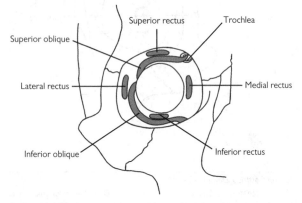

Fig. 10.25 The extraocular muscles, anterior view.
Reproduced courtesy of Daniel R. van Gijn.

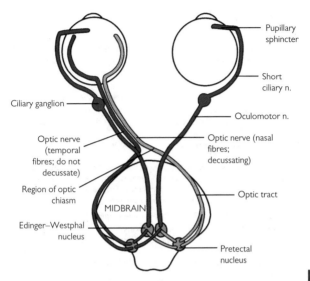

Fig. 10.26 Anatomy of the pupillary light reflex.
Reproduced courtesy of Daniel R. van Gijn.

Pupillary light reflex and relative afferent pupillary defect (RAPD)

The pupillary light reflex allows the size of the pupil(s) to respond appropriately to changing light conditions, both directly and consensually. It is entirely dependent on functioning *afferent* and *efferent* subcortical pathways (Fig. 10.26).

Afferent pathway

Consists of the optic nerve, optic chiasma, optic tract, pretectal nucleus, and Edinger–Westphal nucleus.

Efferent pathway

Consists of the oculomotor nerve and its preganglionic parasympathetic fibres from the Edinger–Westphal nucleus to the ciliary ganglion. Postganglionic fibres thereafter innervate the ciliary and constrictor muscles of the iris.

Relative afferent pupillary defect test (RAPD test)

The swinging light test is a useful test to detect unilateral lesions of the optic nerve or disease of the retina. A positive RAPD therefore implies that there is a difference in the afferent pathways of the two eyes and there will be less pupillary constriction in the eye with an optic nerve lesion. Both pupils will constrict further when the light is shone in the normal eye and when the light is shone back into the abnormal eye both pupils will dilate once more. This is known as a *Marcus Gunn pupil*.

Nerve supply

Motor

The orbit and its associated structures receive contributions from the second to sixth cranial nerves inclusive and from two autonomic ganglia (Fig. 10.27).

Oculomotor (III)

The oculomotor nerve divides into superior and inferior divisions which enter the orbit via the superior orbital fissure through the common tendinous ring, remaining intraconal to supply their respective muscles (Fig. 10.28).

- *Superior division*—passes above the optic nerve and supplies the superior rectus and LPS.
- *Inferior division*—lateral, central, and medial branches. The lateral branch supplies inferior oblique and communicates with the ciliary ganglion. The central branch supplies inferior rectus. The medial branch passes beneath the optic nerve to supply medial rectus.

Trochlear (IV) ('SO4'— superior oblique muscle supplied by IV)

- Traverses the lateral wall of the cavernous sinus.
- Enters the orbit through the superior orbital fissure above the common tendinous ring.
- Passes above the oculomotor nerve and LPS before innervating superior oblique.

Abducens (VI) ('LR6'— lateral rectus muscle supplied by VI)

Travels within the substance of the cavernous sinus, lateral to the ICA after passing through Dorello's canal (bound superiorly by the petroclinoid ligament of Gruber).

- Enters orbit through superior orbital fissure, passing through common tendinous ring.
- Passes between superior and inferior divisions of oculomotor nerve.
- Enters and supplies lateral rectus via its medial surface.

Robert Marcus Gunn (1850–1909)

Scottish ophthalmologist. Lends his name to the *Marcus Gunn pupil* seen in RAPDs and the 'jaw winking (congenital) ptosis' associated with synkinetic movements of the upper eyelid with mastication, due to aberrant connections between the motor contributions of the trigeminal nerve controlling the muscles of mastication and the superior division of the oculomotor nerve supplying LPS. This may explain the phenomenon of the reflex opening of the mouth when applying mascara or eye drops.

Oculomotor nerve palsy

Caused by damage to the third cranial nerve, resulting in a classic 'down and out' appearance of the globe due to the unopposed actions of lateral rectus and superior oblique, respectively (unopposed by superior rectus, inferior rectus and inferior oblique). Associated with ptosis resulting from paralysis of LPS. Third nerve palsies may crudely be classified as 'surgical' and 'medical'. The former involves pupillary dilation (mydriasis) due to interruption of the parasympathetic supply that accompanies the third nerve. The pupil is spared in a 'medical' third nerve palsy.

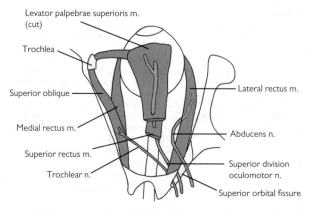

Fig. 10.27 The motor nerves of the right orbit, superior view.
Reproduced courtesy of Daniel R. van Gijn.

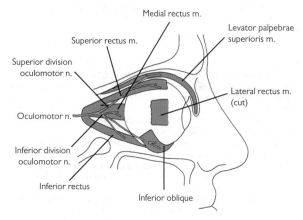

Fig. 10.28 Superior and inferior divisions of oculomotor nerve, lateral view.
Reproduced courtesy of Daniel R. van Gijn.

Sensory

The sensory nerves of the orbit are the second cranial nerve and the first two divisions of the fifth. While the former remains loyal to the confines of the orbit, the latter merely considers the orbit a convenient channel *en route* to supply the face and jaws (Fig. 10.29).

Optic nerve (II)

The optic nerve is an outpouching of the diencephalon rather than a true peripheral nerve and is ensheathed in dura, arachnoid, CSF, and pia. It can be divided into four segments:

- *Intraocular*—lies within the retina before it emerges through the mesh-like lamina cribrosa, a defect in the sclera medial to the posterior pole.
- *Intraorbital*—approximately 20 mm and gently tortuous within the orbit allowing for movements of the globe. It is surrounded by CSF and dura and is in continuity with the subarachnoid space, which allows for the clinical detection of papilloedema with increased intracranial pressure.
- *Intracanalicular*—where the optic nerve exits through the anulus of Zinn and optic canal (inferior to the ophthalmic artery). At the optic foramen, the dural sheath of the nerve blends with the periorbita.
- *Intracranial*—approximately 10 mm in length before joining its contralateral fellow at the chiasma.

Ophthalmic nerve (V₁) ('NFL'—from medial to lateral, nasociliary, frontal, lacrimal)

Arises from the trigeminal ganglion within Meckel's cave and passes along the lateral wall of the cavernous sinus, Divides into its three branches before breaching the superior orbital fissure. The nasociliary branch passes through the anulus while the frontal and lacrimal branches pass above and are therefore extraconal.

Nasociliary (through anulus of Zinn)

See Fig. 10.30.

- Enters the orbit through the common tendinous ring.
- Crosses the optic nerve obliquely (with the ophthalmic artery) to reach the medial orbit. It divides into anterior and posterior ethmoidal nerves and the infratrochlear nerve.
- *Infratrochlear nerve*—passes inferior to the trochlea before piercing the orbital septum and orbicularis oculi to supply the medial upper and lower eyelids, lacrimal sac, and superolateral external nose.
- *Anterior ethmoidal nerve*—exits the orbit via the foramen of the same name to enter the cranial cavity, where it courses along the cribriform plate towards an opening into the nasal cavity lateral to the crista galli; grooves the internal surface of the nasal bone and divides further into internal and external nasal branches.
- *Posterior ethmoidal nerve*—leaves the orbit via the posterior ethmoidal foramen and supplies the ethmoid and sphenoidal sinuses.
- *Long ciliary nerves*—two or three in number running between sclera and choroid to supply the ciliary body, iris, and cornea. Contain postganglionic sympathetic fibres (from the superior cervical ganglion) to dilator pupillae.

Frontal

The largest branch of the ophthalmic nerve, enters the orbit through the superior orbital fissure and passes above the common tendinous ring between to the trochlear and lacrimal nerves.

- It rides LPS to the orbital rim, dividing halfway into the supraorbital and supratrochlear nerves that supply the skin and conjunctiva of the upper eyelid, the skin of the forehead and scalp, and mucous membrane of the frontal sinus.

Lacrimal

Enters the orbit through the superior orbital fissure, passing above the common tendinous ring.

- Remains lateral and runs along lateral rectus towards and through the lacrimal gland and orbital septum to supply the conjunctiva and skin of the lateral upper eyelid.
- May carry postganglionic parasympathetics (from pterygopalatine ganglion via the zygomatic branch of V_2) to the lacrimal gland.

Maxillary nerve (V_2)

After leaving the skull through the foramen rotundum it divides within the pterygopalatine fossa into its zygomatic and infraorbital branches, which enter the orbit via the inferior orbital fissure. The former divides further after entering the orbit into the zygomaticotemporal and zygomaticofacial nerves, destined for the face via the one or two foramina of the same name through the lateral orbital wall.

Infraorbital

Grooves the floor of the orbit before entering a canal of the same name near the orbital rim, emerging onto the face at the infraorbital foramen to supply the skin of the lower eyelid, nose, and upper lip.

Johann Friedrick Meckel, the Elder (1724–1774)

Professor of anatomy and the 'head' of a dynasty of anatomists—most notably his grandson Johann Friedrich Meckel, 'the Younger' who lends his name to *Meckel's cartilage* (the cartilaginous bar of the mandibular arch) and *Meckel's diverticulum* among others.

'The Elder' Meckel described *Meckel's cave*, the CSF-containing dural pouch that houses the trigeminal ganglion. It is found in the posteromedial part of the middle cranial fossa closely associated with the cavernous sinus and the ICA. Meckel the Elder discovered the submandibular ganglion and lends his name to the pterygopalatine (sphenopalatine) ganglion.

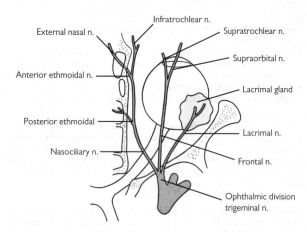

Fig. 10.29 Sensory innervation right orbit, superior view (cutaneous and upper eyelid branches of lacrimal nerve not shown).
Reproduced courtesy of Daniel R. van Gijn.

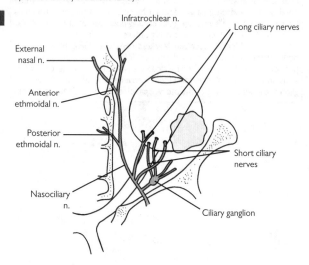

Fig. 10.30 The nasociliary nerve, right orbit.
Reproduced courtesy of Daniel R. van Gijn.

Blood supply

Ophthalmic artery

The principal artery of the orbit is the ophthalmic artery, arising from the internal carotid artery as it emerges from the roof of the cavernous sinus. Entering the orbit through the optic canal, initially inferior and lateral to the optic nerve, it turns medially to pass superior to it. On reaching the medial orbital wall, it courses forward, beneath superior oblique before dividing into its two terminal branches, the frontal (supratrochlear) and dorsal nasal arteries. It is responsible for supplying the extraocular muscles, the lacrimal gland, and the globe. Its numerous branches show considerable variation and may be classified into orbital and ocular groups (Fig. 10.31 and Fig. 10.32):

Orbital branches

The branches of the orbital group mimic those of the frontal and lacrimal branches of the ophthalmic nerve, supplying the ethmoid sinus, nasal cavity, external nose, eyelids, and forehead.

Lacrimal artery

Large lateral branch of the ophthalmic artery arising near (or before) the optic canal. Travels with the nerve of the same name atop lateral rectus. Supplies and crosses the lacrimal gland, destined ultimately for the eyelids. Its branches include:

- *Lateral palpebral*—branches run medially in the upper and lower eyelids and anastomose with the medial palpebral arteries.
- *Zygomatic*—one to two in number: one to the cheek (via the zygomaticofacial foramen) anastomosing with the transverse facial artery, and the other to the temporal fossa (via the zygomaticotemporal foramen) to anastomose with the deep temporal arteries.
- *Recurrent meningeal*—exits the orbit through the lateral aspect of the superior orbital fissure and anastomoses with the middle meningeal artery. Occasionally replaces lacrimal artery.

Supraorbital artery

Accompanies the supraorbital nerve medial to superior rectus and LPS (which it supplies), having left the ophthalmic artery where it crosses the optic nerve. After passing through the supraorbital foramen, it divides into superior and inferior branches.

- Supplies skin, muscle, periosteum and diploe of frontal bone.
- Supplies the mucoperiosteum of the frontal sinus.
- Anastomoses with the supratrochlear and frontal branches of the superficial temporal artery.

Anterior and posterior ethmoidal arteries

- Follow the nerves of the same name and pass through the anterior and posterior ethmoidal foramina, respectively of the medial orbital wall.
- After supplying the ethmoid and frontal sinuses, they both provide meningeal branches to the dura and nasal branches that descend into the nasal cavity via the cribriform plate to supply the lateral wall, septum, and dorsum of the nose.

Medial palpebral artery
- Superior and inferior branches arise directly from the ophthalmic artery opposite the trochlea of the superior oblique.
- Form superior and inferior arches, respectively, passing between the tarsi and orbicularis oculi and anastomose with lateral palpebral branches of the lacrimal artery (among the other arteries mentioned previously).

Frontal artery (supratrochlear)
- A terminal branch of the ophthalmic that exits the orbit along with the supratrochlear nerve at its medial angle.
- Anastomoses with the supraorbital branch and contributes to its aforementioned supply of the layers of the forehead and brow.

Dorsal nasal artery
- A terminal branch of the ophthalmic artery.
- Exits the orbit between medial palpebral ligament and the trochlea.
- Supplies upper part of the nasolacrimal sac and dorsum of nose.
- Anastomoses with the facial artery, its contralateral fellow, and the lateral nasal branch of the facial artery.

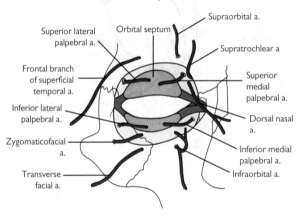

Fig. 10.31 The arterial supply to the eyelids and periorbital region.
Reproduced courtesy of Daniel R. van Gijn.

Ocular branches (ophthalmic artery)
While the orbital branches of the ophthalmic remain largely peripheral, the ocular branches stay central (Fig. 10.32).

Central artery of retina
The first branch to arise from the ophthalmic artery within the dural sheath. It runs inferior to the optic nerve before piercing the subarachnoid space, entering the nerve, and passing to the retina.
- Supplies the meninges of the optic nerve and the retina.

Short and long posterior ciliary artery
Numerous ciliary arteries (15–20 short posterior ciliary arteries, 1–2 long posterior ciliary arteries) pierce the sclera near the optic nerve and are destined for the major arterial circle of the iris and the choroid. They anastomose with branches of the central retinal artery at the optic disc.

Muscular arteries
- Form superior and inferior branches, generally accompanying the branches of the oculomotor nerve.
- The inferior branch provides the anterior ciliary vessels that ride the tendons of the recti and are bound for the eyeball, ultimately piercing the sclera and contributing to the major arterial circle of the iris.

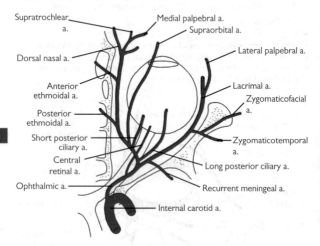

Supratrochlear a.
Medial palpebral a.
Supraorbital a.
Dorsal nasal a.
Lateral palpebral a.
Anterior ethmoidal a.
Lacrimal a.
Zygomaticofacial a.
Posterior ethmoidal a.
Short posterior ciliary a.
Zygomaticotemporal a.
Central retinal a.
Long posterior ciliary a.
Ophthalmic a.
Recurrent meningeal a.
Internal carotid a.

Fig. 10.32 The ophthalmic artery.
Reproduced courtesy of Daniel R. van Gijn.

Retrobulbar haemorrhage and orbital compartment syndrome

Introduction

Blunt trauma to the orbit can result in orbital fractures with subsequent bleeding from either shearing of the vessels within the periorbital fat or from the infraorbital, anterior, or posterior ethmoidal arteries. The orbital soft tissues are contained within the rigid walls of the orbit and anteriorly by the orbital septum, medial and lateral canthal tendons, and the globe itself. A rise in orbital volume and pressure gives rise to an orbital compartment syndrome and causes a reduction in the blood flow to the optic nerve and retina. If the orbit is not decompressed, loss of vision may ensue (Fig. 10.33).

Symptoms

- Asymptomatic if small.
- Nausea and vomiting.
- Proptosis (abnormal forward displacement of the globe).
- Pain.
- Raised intraocular pressures.
- Periorbital bruising (ecchymosis).
- Ophthalmoplegia (reduced/absent eye movements).
- RAPD.
- Loss of vision.

Treatment

The definitive management is urgent surgical decompression in the form of a lateral canthotomy and inferior cantholysis under local anaesthesia (Fig. 10.34). Medical management including steroids, mannitol, and acetazolamide should not delay surgical intervention.

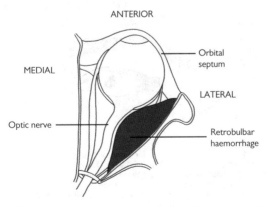

Fig. 10.33 Axial section demonstrating schematic of retrobulbar haematoma right orbit causing optic nerve compression.
Reproduced courtesy of Daniel R. van Gijn.

(a)

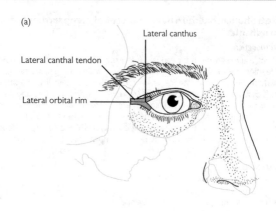

Lateral canthus

Lateral canthal tendon

Lateral orbital rim

(b)

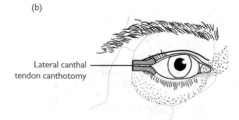

Lateral canthal tendon canthotomy

(c)

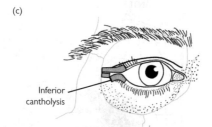

Inferior cantholysis

Fig. 10.34 (a) Position of skin incision for lateral canthotomy. Note distance between lateral canthus and orbital rim 0.5–1.0 cm. Dotted line demonstrates line of incision. (b) Illustration demonstrating lateral canthotomy—splitting of the lateral canthal tendon. (c) Illustration demonstrating inferior cantholysis—division of the inferior limb of lateral canthal tendon to free lower eyelid attachment from orbit.

Reproduced courtesy of Daniel R. van Gijn.

Venous drainage

The venous channels of the orbit allow for direct valve-devoid communication between the veins of the face and intracranial veins, with the potential for significant clinical ramifications. The three principal vessels involved are the superior and inferior ophthalmic veins and the infraorbital vein (Fig. 10.35).

Superior ophthalmic vein

The superior ophthalmic vein commences above the medial palpebral ligament, having received tributaries from the frontal, supraorbital, and angular veins from the forehead region and face, respectively.

- Travels between the optic nerve and superior rectus with the ophthalmic artery.
- From anterior to posterior, it receives tributaries from the superior vortex veins of the globe, the central vein of the retina (which may drain directly into the cavernous sinus), and the inferior ophthalmic vein.
- Drains into the cavernous sinus after crossing the superior orbital fissure above the anulus of Zinn.

Inferior ophthalmic vein

The inferior ophthalmic vein commences medially at the anterior orbital floor, communicating at the inferior margin with the facial vein.

- Travels above the inferior rectus muscle, receiving contributions from tributaries draining inferior rectus and inferior oblique before passing through the inferior orbital fissure to drain into the pterygoid venous plexus.
- From anterior to posterior it receives tributaries from the nasolacrimal sac, the eyelids, and the inferior vortex veins.
- An alternative drainage route intracranially is either directly, or indirectly via the superior ophthalmic vein, through the superior orbital fissure to the cavernous sinus.

Infraorbital vein

Follows the nerve and artery of the same name through the infraorbital foramen.

- Drains structures of the orbital floor.
- From anterior to posterior it communicates with the facial vein and inferior ophthalmic vein, ultimately draining into the pterygoid venous plexus via the inferior orbital fissure.

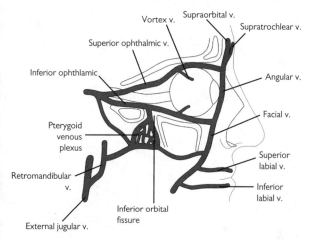

Fig. 10.35 Venous drainage of orbit.
Reproduced courtesy of Daniel R. van Gijn.

The mouth

Introduction

The mouth is the common aperture to the aerodigestive tract allowing for the convenient passage of food and airway adjuncts in the event of emergency. With the coordinated assistance of the tongue and lips, it contributes to the formation of meaningful sound, while the presence of intact dental arches allows for effective mastication. See Fig. 11.1.

The red, capillary-rich lips, in addition to providing a prominent visual impact upon the face, are involved in the fine tuning of the production of sound and in the process of oral intake. The numerous additional roles of the lips become ever more apparent in the loss of tissue in the presence of disease and surgery.

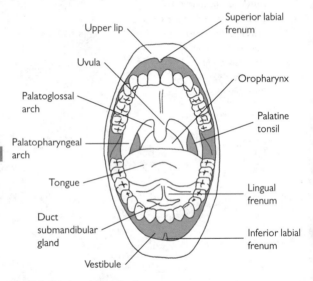

Fig. 11.1 Overview of the oral cavity.
Reproduced courtesy of Daniel R. van Gijn.

Oral cavity

Introduction

The oral cavity proper represents the atrium beyond the lips, reaching to the palatoglossal arches posteriorly, where the oropharynx begins beyond the oropharyngeal isthmus (→ Fig. 11.4, p. 403). It is the area located internal to the teeth and is restricted by the cheeks laterally, the hard and soft palate superiorly (separating the mouth from the nasal cavity), and the mobile tongue resting on the mylohyoid muscle inferiorly. The paired major salivary glands (parotid, submandibular, and sublingual) drain into the oral cavity together with numerous minor salivary glands.

Oral mucosa

The oral mucosa is continuous with the skin at the vermilion border and with the oropharynx at the oropharyngeal isthmus. It is classically divided into lining, masticatory, and specialized mucosa. The specialized mucosa of the anterior two-thirds of the tongue will be discussed later in this chapter (→ Tongue, p. 408).

Lining mucosa

- Covers the majority of the oral cavity, ie the soft palate, ventral tongue, floor of mouth, internal lips and cheeks, and the alveolar processes up to the mucogingival junction, where the gingival masticatory mucosa take over.

Masticatory mucosa

- Firmly bound to bone or the neck (cervical) region of the teeth.
- Keratinized over the palate, gingivae, and dorsal tongue.
- Gingivae are further subdivided into free (around cervical margin) and attached (to periosteum and teeth, stippled).
- Gingivae and midline palatine raphe have no submucosa.

Maxillary blood supply

The maxillary arch gingivae are supplied by branches of the maxillary artery.
- *Buccal gingivae*—perforating and gingival branches (posterior superior alveolar artery), buccal artery.
- *Anterior labial gingivae*—labial branches of the infraorbital artery and perforating branches from the anterior superior alveolar artery.
- *Palatal gingivae*—greater palatine artery (descending palatine artery from the maxillary artery).

Mandibular blood supply

The mandibular arch gingivae are supplied by branches of the maxillary and lingual arteries:
- Buccal gingivae—buccal branch and perforating branches from the inferior alveolar artery (maxillary artery).
- Anterior labial gingivae—mental artery and perforating branches of the incisive artery (inferior alveolar branch of maxillary artery).
- Lingual gingivae—perforating and lingual branches of the inferior alveolar artery and the lingual artery proper (external carotid artery).

Nerve supply
See Fig. 11.2.
- Maxillary arch—supplied by the maxillary division of the trigeminal nerve (V₃) via its greater palatine, nasopalatine, and anterior, middle and posterior superior alveolar branches.
- The mandibular arch is supplied by the mandibular division of the trigeminal nerve via its inferior alveolar, lingual, and buccal branches.

Lymphatic drainage
The lingual and palatal gingivae drain into the jugulodigastric lymph nodes. The buccal and labial gingivae of both arches drain into the submandibular lymph nodes, but note that the labial gingivae of the mandibular incisors may drain submentally.

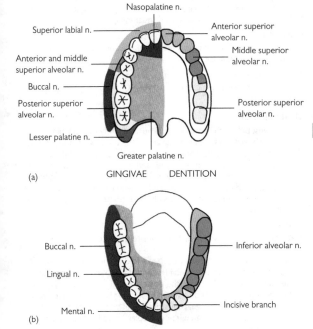

Fig. 11.2 Sensory innervation to the maxillary (a) and mandibular (b) arches: gingival/mucosal innervation on left and dental innervation on right.
Reproduced courtesy of Daniel R. van Gijn.

Cheek and oral vestibule

Cheek

The cheek is the part of the face extending from the nasolabial fold anteriorly to the anterior border of masseter posteriorly, and bound superiorly and inferiorly by the alveolar processes of the maxilla and mandible, respectively. It consists of skin externally and a mucosal lining internally, the latter tightly adherent to buccinator. From superficial to deep are the following layers and structures (Fig. 11.3 and Fig. 11.4):

• *Skin*.
• *Superficial fascia*—containing zygomaticus major and risorius, buccal branches of the mandibular and facial nerves (sensory and motor respectively), parotid duct, and buccal fat bad of Bichat.
• *Buccinator muscle*—covered by the buccopharyngeal fascia.
• *Submucosal layer*—containing mucus-secreting 'molar' glands.
• *Mucosa*—non-keratinized stratified squamous.

Blood supply

• Buccal branch of the maxillary artery supplies buccinator, buccal fat pad, and the buccal mucosa.

Nerve supply

• Zygomaticofacial and infraorbital nerves (V_2).
• Buccal (V_3).

Oral vestibule

The oral vestibule is the narrow yet almost infinitely expandable space between the cheeks and the buccal surface of the teeth. With the teeth in occlusion, there is a communication between the vestibule and the oral cavity via a gap between the last molar tooth and the ramus of mandible, and, to a lesser extent, between the interdental spaces. The cheek is limited superiorly and inferiorly by the maxillary and mandibular vestibuli, anteriorly by the labial commissure, and posteriorly by the intermaxillary commissure and retromolar trigone.

Features

• *Parotid duct (of Stensen)*—opens opposite the second upper molar tooth.
• *Pterygomandibular raphe*—enclosed in a fold of mucosa between maxillary and mandibular alveoli (extends from pterygoid hamulus of the medial pterygoid plate to the posterior end of the mylohyoid line). It forms a tendinous band to which buccinator is attached anteriorly and the superior pharyngeal constrictor is attached posteriorly. An important landmark for an inferior alveolar nerve block in dental anaesthesia.
• *Frenula*—maxillary and mandibular midline mucosal folds, bridging the vestibule and connecting the gingivae to the lips.

Frenulum injuries

A torn labial frenum in a child is often considered to be pathognomonic of non-accidental injury and should be investigated appropriately. Mechanisms include force feeding, twisting, shaking, and a direct blow.

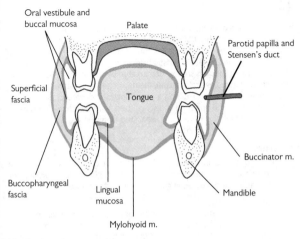

Fig. 11.3 Oral cavity, coronal section.
Reproduced courtesy of Daniel R. van Gijn.

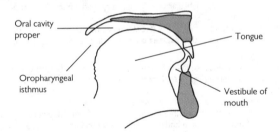

Fig. 11.4 Oral cavity, sagittal section.
Reproduced courtesy of Daniel R. van Gijn.

Lips

The lips are paired, highly mobile musculofibrous folds that act as tactile sensory organs throughout life: they occupy a disproportionate area of the cortical sensory homunculus. The lips consist of the hair-bearing skin of the face and cheek and the characteristic hairless red or vermilion zone of the lip proper; the transition is sharply demarcated by the vermilion border and further characterized by the philtrum, the depressed area between the base of the columella of the nose, and a pronounced midline concavity of the vermilion border. The upper lip is distinguished from the cheek laterally by the nasolabial folds; the lower lip is separated from the chin by way of the labiomental groove (Fig. 11.5).

Structure

The lips are based upon a muscular foundation of orbicularis oris and the various elevators and depressors that act upon the upper lip, modiolus, or lower lip. These are discussed in greater detail in ⟁ Chapter 9.

Blood supply

The blood supply to the lips comes from branches of the facial and maxillary arteries (external carotid artery). Buccinator receives its supply principally from the buccal artery (second part of the maxillary artery), which travels between the medial pterygoid and temporalis muscles *en route* to the outer surface of buccinator (Fig. 11.6).

- *Upper lip*—superior labial artery (facial artery) and infraorbital artery (maxillary artery).
- *Lower lip*—inferior labial artery (facial artery), mental artery (inferior alveolar artery from the first part of the maxillary artery) (Fig. 11.7).

Nerve supply

Sensation to the lips is supplied by the maxillary and mandibular divisions of the trigeminal nerve (Fig. 11.6). Motor supply is from the facial nerve and is discussed elsewhere.

- *Upper lip*—superior labial nerve (infraorbital nerve V₂).
- *Lower lip*—mental nerve (inferior alveolar nerve from V₃). Exits the mental foramen of the mandible below the second premolar tooth. Supplies the lower lip, chin, and buccal gingivae.
- *Buccal nerve (long buccal nerve, V₃)*.

Lymphatic drainage

- *Upper lip*—to ipsilateral submandibular lymph nodes (and then to jugulodigastric nodes). Occasionally to periparotid/preauricular groups.
- *Lower lip*—ipsilateral submandibular nodes from the lateral lip and bilateral submental nodes from the central lip.

Etymology

- *Cupid's bow*—the shape of the upper lip contour resembles the double-curved bow belonging to Cupid, the Roman god of love.
- *Philtrum*—meaning 'love potion' or 'love charm'. In Jewish mythology, thought to be the remnant of being tapped on the lip by an Angel to hush an infant from telling secrets learned *in utero*.

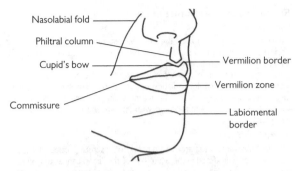

Fig. 11.5 Surface markings of the lips.
Reproduced courtesy of Daniel R. van Gijn.

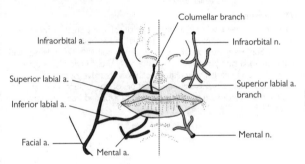

Fig. 11.6 Arterial and nerve supply of the lips.
Reproduced courtesy of Daniel R. van Gijn.

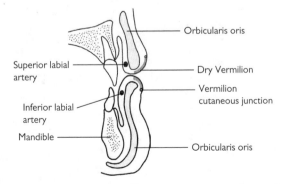

Fig. 11.7 The relationship of the labial arteries to orbicularis oris and position of the vermilion cutaneous junction.
Reproduced courtesy of Daniel R. van Gijn.

Squamous cell carcinoma of the lip

Overview

Cancer of the lip is one of the commonest cancers of the head and neck region, the commonest type being squamous cell carcinoma (SCC). Clinical presentation is normally either an exophytic or ulcerated firm lesion. The lower lip is more commonly affected than the upper. Risk factors include ultraviolet radiation exposure, pipe smoking, thermal injury, immunosuppression, and chronic infection (interestingly, alcohol and tobacco use have less association with lip cancer than other oral SCC subtypes).

Anatomical subtypes

The lip represents an anatomical junction of discrete groups of cancer: cutaneous cancer affecting the white skin of the lip; lip cancer beginning at the vermilion border and including only that part of the vermilion component of the lip that comes into contact with the upper lip; oral/mucosal cancer affecting the labial mucosa.

Management

Treatment is generally by surgical excision of the primary cancer with local reconstruction of the defect to restore aesthetics and function of the lip. Surgery to remove the draining lymph nodes (submandibular and submental) is rarely required given the early presentation of most cancers of the visible lip. A multitude of reconstructive options are available, depending on the size and location of the defect, ranging from simple primary closure to multi-staged local flaps and free tissue transfer (Figs. 11.8–11.10).

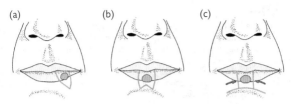

Fig. 11.8 Lip reconstruction by primary closure. (a) Simple wedge excision. (b) W-wedge. (c) Bilateral advancement flaps.

Reproduced courtesy of Daniel R. van Gijn.

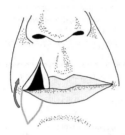

Fig. 11.9 Abbe–Estlander 'lip-switch' flap for commissure defects. Based on the inferior labial artery.

Reproduced courtesy of Daniel R. van Gijn.

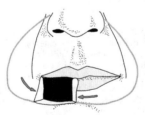

Fig. 11.10 Karapandzic bilateral advancement-type flap for larger defects. Based on the superior and inferior labial arteries.

Reproduced courtesy of Daniel R. van Gijn.

Tongue

The tongue is a thick, mucosa-covered muscular structure concerned with taste, mastication, swallowing and talking. A convenient landmark of the dorsal tongue is the sulcus terminalis, dividing the tongue into a presulcal, mobile oral two-thirds and a fixed postsulcal pharyngeal third. The V-shaped sulcus terminalis extends from the lateral palatoglossal arches to a median pit, the foramen caecum, which marks the site of the superior end of the thyroglossal duct (Fig. 11.11).

Oral part

Dorsal surface

Characterized by four types of papillae:

- *Circumvallate*—arranged in a V shape anterior to the sulcus terminalis. Each is surrounded by a sulcus scattered with taste buds and serous glands of von Ebner; 8–12 in number.
- *Fungiform*—situated along the side, apex, and dorsum of the tongue; contain taste buds.
- *Filiform*—minute conical projections over the entire dorsal surface. Thought to increase friction between tongue and food.
- *Foliate*—mucosal folds found at the lateral borders of the tongue near the sulcus terminalis; contain taste buds.

Ventral surface

The inferior surface is covered with mucosa that is continuous with the floor of the mouth and lingual and labial gingivae. The lingual frenum connects the ventral tongue to the floor of the mouth and is flanked bilaterally by the deep lingual veins, the sublingual papillae, and the plica fimbriata (folds) most laterally.

Pharyngeal part

Posterior to the palatoglossal arch, the pharyngeal (post-sulcal) tongue forms the base of the tongue and the anterior wall of the oropharynx. The covering mucosa is continuous laterally with that covering the palatine tonsils and pharynx and posteriorly with the epiglottis via the median and paired lateral glossoepiglottic folds. The valleculae lie between these folds (Fig. 11.12). The post-sulcal tongue is devoid of papillae. It contains lymphoid nodules that collectively constitute the lingual tonsil which is a component of *Waldeyer's ring*.

Etymology

- *Tongue*—from the old English word *tunge* meaning the organ of phonation. Associations with the Latin *lingua* meaning tongue or language.
- *Victor von Ebner (1842–1925)*—Austrian anatomist and histologist. Lines of von Ebner are the incremental lines seen in the dentine and cementum of a tooth which represent daily dentine deposition.

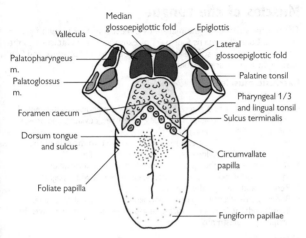

Fig. 11.11 The dorsum of tongue, superior view.
Reproduced courtesy of Daniel R. van Gijn.

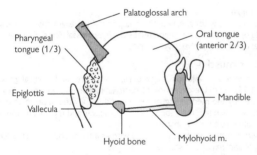

Fig. 11.12 The tongue, lateral overview.
Reproduced courtesy of Daniel R. van Gijn.

Muscles of the tongue

The tongue is divided in the midline by a median fibrous septum fixed to the hyoid bone. It contains four pairs of extrinsic muscles attached to the mandible, hyoid bone, soft palate, styloid processes, and pharynx, and four pairs of intrinsic muscles that alter its shape.

Extrinsic muscles

See Fig. 11.13.

* *Genioglossus*—from the genial tubercles of the mandible to the ventral tongue from root to apex. Protrudes, depresses, deviates, and prevents the tongue falling backwards.
* *Hyoglossus*—from the greater cornu of the hyoid to the side of the tongue, medial to styloglossus. Depresses the tongue.
* *Styloglossus*—from the tip of the styloid process/stylomandibular ligament to the side of the tongue, where it blends with hyoglossus. Retracts and elevates the tongue.
* *Palatoglossus*—from the palatine aponeurosis to the lateral tongue. Blends with the intrinsic muscles. Elevates the tongue and narrows the oropharyngeal isthmus.

Blood supply

Sublingual branch of the lingual artery and submental branch of the facial artery.

Nerve supply

All muscles of the tongue, with the exception of palatoglossus (essentially a muscle of the palate) are innervated by the hypoglossal nerve. Palatoglossus is innervated via the pharyngeal plexus.

Intrinsic muscles

The superior and inferior longitudinal, transverse, and vertical muscles (Fig. 11.14). With the exception of decussating fibres at the apex, they are separated by the median lingual septum and occupy the upper part of the tongue lying beneath the submucous fibrous layer and mucous membrane. Their role is to alter the shape of the tongue.

* *Superior longitudinal muscle*—works with its inferior counterpart (*inferior longitudinal muscle*) to shorten the tongue.
* *Transverse fibres*—cause narrowing and elongation.
* *Vertical fibres*—at the lateral borders of the anterior tongue. Flatten and broaden the tongue.

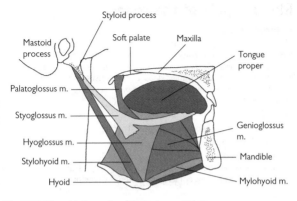

Fig. 11.13 The extrinsic muscles of the tongue, sagittal view.
Reproduced courtesy of Daniel R. van Gijn.

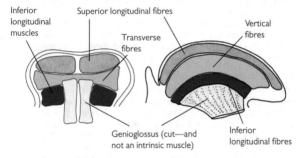

Fig. 11.14 The intrinsic muscles of the tongue, coronal and sagittal views.
Reproduced courtesy of Daniel R. van Gijn.

Blood supply of the tongue

Arterial supply

The e tongue is supplied by the lingual artery, which arises anteriorly from the ECA, immediately posterior to the hyoid bone and beneath the posterior belly of digastric. After giving off a tonsillar branch, it exits the submandibular triangle and courses deep to hyoglossus *en route* to the floor of mouth. It can be considered in three parts according to its relation to hyoglossus (Fig. 11.15):

Posterior to hyoglossus

- Crossed superficially by the hypoglossal nerve.
- Gives off suprahyoid branch.

Deep to hyoglossus

- Travels anteriorly between hyoglossus and genioglossus.
- Gives off two or three dorsal lingual arteries to the posterior third of the tongue.

Anterior to hyoglossus

- The lingual artery gives off the sublingual artery, which passes between genioglossus and mylohyoid to supply the sublingual gland and surrounding area.
- The lingual artery proper continues anteriorly towards the ventral surface, becoming the deep lingual artery where it anastomoses with its contralateral fellow and is accompanied by branches from the lingual nerve (V_3).

Venous drainage

The paired lingual veins join the facial vein and anterior retromandibular vein (forming the common facial vein) before ultimately emptying into the IJV near the greater cornu of the hyoid bone. They are formed from the union of two systems: the dorsal lingual veins that accompany the lingual artery and travel deep to hyoglossus and the deep lingual and vena comitans superficial to hyoglossus that accompany the hypoglossal nerve (Fig. 11.16):

- *Dorsal lingual*—drains the dorsum and sides of tongue. Accompanies the lingual artery.
- *Deep lingual*—travels from the tip of the tongue just deep to the mucous membrane of the inferior surface of the tongue, joined by the *sublingual* vein.
- *Vena comitans*—a vein of considerable size that accompanies the hypoglossal nerve.

Lymphatic drainage

The principal lymphoid tissue in the tongue is the lingual tonsil of the pharyngeal part. The anterior tongue drains into the marginal and central vessels and the posterior tongue into the dorsal vessels. More central regions may drain bilaterally, which is of clinical significance in the context of malignant disease and spread (Fig. 11.17 and Fig. 11.18).

- *Marginal vessels*—drain the apex, lateral margins, and sublingual region to submental, submandibular, jugulo-omohyoid, or jugulodigastric nodes. They may cross under the frenulum to the contralateral nodes.

- *Central vessels*—ascend between the genioglossi. They drain into jugulo-omohyoid and jugulodigastric nodes or pierce mylohyoid to access the submandibular nodes.
- *Dorsal vessels*—drain the postsulcal region and join the marginal vessels towards the jugulo-omohyoid and jugulodigastric nodes after piercing the pharyngeal wall.

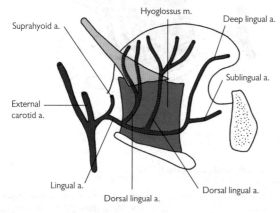

Fig. 11.15 Arterial supply to the tongue.
Reproduced courtesy of Daniel R. van Gijn.

Pirogov's triangle
The space bound by the intermediate tendon of digastric inferiorly, the posterior border of the mylohyoid muscle anteriorly, and the hypo-glossal nerve superiorly. The lingual artery can be found within, deep to hyoglossus.

Nikolay Pirogov (1810–1881)
Russian scientist, surgeon, and founder of 'field surgery': he used anaes-thesia in the field while working as an army surgeon in the Crimean War.

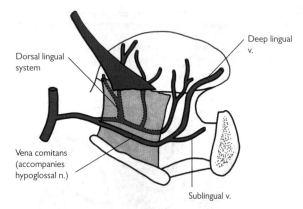

Deep lingual v.

Dorsal lingual system

Vena comitans (accompanies hypoglossal n.)

Sublingual v.

Fig. 11.16 Venous drainage of the tongue.
Reproduced courtesy of Daniel R. van Gijn.

Oral squamous cell carcinoma

Overview
The oral tongue is the most common location for intraoral SCC, typically presenting as a non-healing, painless, indurated ulcer or a mass in the neck representing metastatic cervical disease. The most common causative factors are alcohol and tobacco abuse. There is often invasion of the intrinsic muscles of the tongue at presentation given the absence of anatomical barriers.

Investigations
Following a histological diagnosis by incisional/punch biopsy, the patient should undergo local regional and staging imaging in the form of magnetic resonance imaging and CT, respectively, prior to discussion at a multidisciplinary team meeting consisting of head and neck surgeons, oncologists, radiologists, pathologists, dieticians, and speech and language therapists. Further preoperative considerations include an assessment of medical comorbidities and general fitness to undergo extensive surgery.

Management
Surgery remains the mainstay of tongue tumours with a margin of 1 cm. Neck dissection (cervical lymphadenectomy) should be offered electively for small cancers and performed therapeutically for those tumours thicker than 4 mm. The former offers overall survival benefits. Reconstruction of the primary defect may be achieved by local or regional pedicled flaps or microvascular free tissue transfer, most commonly in the form of a radial forearm free flap, anterolateral thigh flap, or medial sural artery perforator flap with the aim of restoring aesthetics and function.

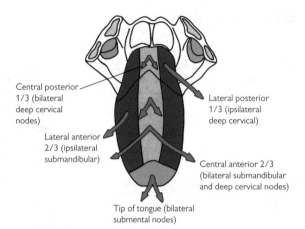

Central posterior 1/3 (bilateral deep cervical nodes)

Lateral posterior 1/3 (ipsilateral deep cervical)

Lateral anterior 2/3 (ipsilateral submandibular)

Central anterior 2/3 (bilateral submandibular and deep cervical nodes)

Tip of tongue (bilateral submental nodes)

Fig. 11.17 Lymphatic drainage of the tongue.
Reproduced courtesy of Daniel R. van Gijn.

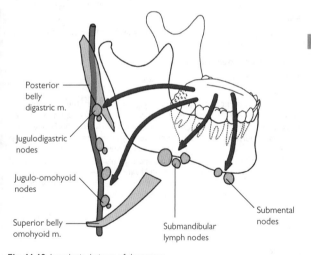

Posterior belly digastric m.

Jugulodigastric nodes

Jugulo-omohyoid nodes

Superior belly omohyoid m.

Submandibular lymph nodes

Submental nodes

Fig. 11.18 Lymphatic drainage of the tongue.
Reproduced courtesy of Daniel R. van Gijn.

Nerves of the tongue

See Fig. 11.19, Table 11.1, and Table 11.2.

Lingual nerve

The lingual nerve arises from the posterior trunk of the mandibular division of the trigeminal nerve. It leaves the infratemporal fossa and is joined, at an acute angle, by the chorda tympani of the facial nerve before passing between the mandible and medial pterygoid muscle *en route* to the lateral tongue (Fig. 11.20). It has the following important relationships:

- Passes beneath the pterygomandibular raphe and superior pharyngeal constrictor muscle.
- Intimately related to the periosteum of the medial mandible and distolingual root of the last third molar, where it is covered only by mucoperiosteum.
- Progresses anteromedially resting upon the deep part of the submandibular gland and the lingual surface of mylohyoid.
- It is crossed (from medial to lateral) by the submandibular duct before heading superiorly and medially to enter the tongue.
- Within the tongue it travels laterally to hyoglossus and genioglossus and supplies the lingual mucosa via its terminal branches.
- Several additional branches connect the lingual nerve to the submandibular ganglion, hypoglossal nerve, and inferior alveolar nerve.

Function

Sensory to the floor of the mouth, mandibular lingual gingivae, and anterior two-thirds of the tongue.

Glossopharyngeal nerve

See Fig. 11.21.

Structure

Shortly after leaving the anteromedial jugular foramen, the glossopharyngeal nerve travels deep to the styloid process and associated structures, piercing the superior pharyngeal constrictor muscle from superficial to deep (or passing between it and the middle pharyngeal constrictor) to supply the posterior third of the tongue (including the sulcus terminalis and vallate papillae), tonsils, oral mucous glands, and pharyngeal mucosa. Branches of note (distal to the tympanic and carotid branches) are:

- *Pharyngeal*—unite with branches of the vagus to form the pharyngeal plexus lying on the middle pharyngeal constrictor.
- *Muscular*—supplies stylopharyngeus.
- *Tonsillar*—forms a plexus around the palatine tonsil. Communicates with palatine nerves.
- *Lingual*—supplies the vallate papillae, tongue base and mucosa covering posterior tongue. Communicates with the lingual nerve.

Hypoglossal nerve

The hypoglossal nerve is the motor supply to all the muscles of the tongue except palatoglossus. After exiting the hypoglossal canal, it is intimately related to the IJV, ICA, and IX and X. At first medial and then lateral to these structures, it next descends vertically between the vessels and anterior to

X (Fig. 11.21). It appears in the carotid triangle at approximately the level of the angle of the mandible and proceeds anteriorly, with the following important relationships:

- Passes above or below the occipital artery (covered by skin, superficial fascia, and platysma and crossed by the common facial vein).
- Passes deep to posterior belly of digastric and stylohyoid muscles.
- Appears in the digastric triangle and travels anteriorly between the hyoglossus and mylohyoid muscles.
- While between hyoglossus and mylohyoid, it travels inferior to the deep part of the submandibular gland, submandibular duct, and the lingual nerve before piercing genioglossus.

Table 11.1 Summary of tongue innervation. Note: palatoglossus is innervated by the pharyngeal plexus

	General sensation	Taste	Motor
Anterior 2/3	Lingual nerve (V₃)	Chorda tympani (VII)	Hypoglossal (except palatoglossus)
Posterior 1/3	Glossopharyngeal (IX)	Glossopharyngeal (IX)	Hypoglossal (except palatoglossus)
Valleculae	Glossopharyngeal (IX)	Internal branch superior laryngeal nerve (X)	

Referred otalgia

Overview

Earache or 'otalgia' can be either primary, arising from problems of the ear itself, or secondary referred otalgia, in which the source of the pain arises at a site distant from the ear. The ear receives its sensory innervation from cranial nerves V, VII, IX, and X and upper cervical nerves. Pathology in the distribution of any these nerves may give rise to otalgia.

Glossopharyngeal nerve-related otalgia

The glossopharyngeal nerve supplies the posterior one-third of the tongue, tonsillar fossa, pharynx, and para/retropharyngeal spaces. Pathology in any of these areas may refer pain to the ear via the tympanic branch of the glossopharyngeal nerve (Jacobsen's nerve).

Trigeminal nerve related otalgia—mandibular division V₃

The lingual, buccal, and inferior alveolar branches of V₃ supply the cheek, floor of mouth, and anterior tongue. Pathology in any of these areas may result in referred otalgia via the auriculotemporal branch of V₃.

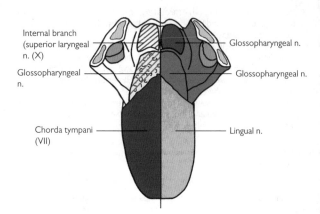

Fig. 11.19 Sensory innervation of the tongue, schematic summary.
Reproduced courtesy of Daniel R. van Gijn.

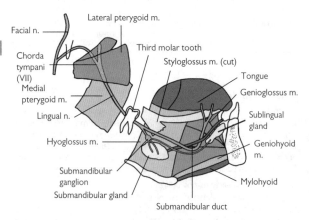

Fig. 11.20 Schematic anatomy of the lingual nerve.
Reproduced courtesy of Daniel R. van Gijn.

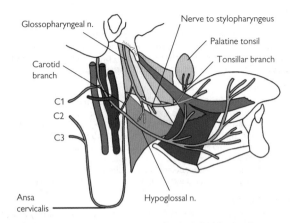

Fig. 11.21 Schematic anatomy of the glossopharyngeal and hypoglossal nerves.
Reproduced courtesy of Daniel R. van Gijn.

Table 11.2 Development of tongue innervation involves all pharyngeal arches

	Pharyngeal arch	Nerve supply
Touch sensation		
Anterior 2/3 tongue	1st pharyngeal arch	Lingual nerve (V_3)
Posterior 1/3 tongue	3rd pharyngeal arch	Glossopharyngeal nerve
Tongue base	4th pharyngeal arch	Vagus nerve
Taste sensation		
Anterior 2/3 tongue	2nd pharyngeal arch	Chorda tympani (VII)
Posterior 1/3 tongue	3rd pharyngeal arch	Glossopharyngeal nerve
	4th pharyngeal arch	Vagus nerve
Motor		
All muscles of tongue (except palatoglossus)	6th pharyngeal arch	Hypoglossal nerve

Floor of the mouth

The floor of the oral mouth is an important anatomical area with significant surgical and pathological correlates. It represents an aggregation of structures that declare themselves superficially on the ventral surface of the tongue and is intimately related to the sublingual space.

Structure

The floor of the mouth is formed by the mylohyoid muscles. Its horseshoe shape is bound laterally by the lingual surface of the mandibular teeth and it is loosely divided into two halves by the midline lingual frenulum, which extends onto the inferior surface of the tongue. Structures lateral to the frenulum (from medial to lateral) are the sublingual papillae and sublingual folds (Fig. 11.22).

- *Sublingual papillae*—the openings of the submandibular ducts.
- *Sublingual folds*—cover the submandibular ducts and sublingual glands.

Blood supply

The blood supply of the floor of the mouth is via the lingual artery and its sublingual and deep lingual branches.

Muscles of the floor of the mouth

Mylohyoid

A flat, triangular muscle superior to the anterior belly of the digastric muscle which forms a diaphragm with its contralateral counterpart. Posteriorly, its free edge cleaves the submandibular gland, dividing it into a deep and superficial lobe. Inferior to mylohyoid lie the anterior bellies of digastric (covered superficially by platysma), the superficial lobe of the submandibular gland, the facial vessels, and the mylohyoid neurovascular bundle. Superior to mylohyoid are the geniohyoid, hyoglossus, and styloglossus muscles, the hypoglossal and lingual nerves and submandibular ganglion, the sublingual and deep part of the submandibular gland and duct, and the sublingual and lingual vessels (Fig. 11.23 and Fig. 11.24).

- *Origin*—the whole length of the mylohyoid line of the mandible; the two muscles unite at a midline raphe (occasionally absent, thus the mylohyoid forms a continuous sheet).
- *Insertion*—body of hyoid bone.
- *Blood supply*—mylohyoid branch of the inferior alveolar artery (from the first part of maxillary artery).
- *Nerve supply*—mylohyoid nerve (from the inferior alveolar nerve, V_3).
- *Action*—elevates the floor of the mouth, hyoid bone, and tongue. Depresses mandible.

> **Etymology**
> - *Frenum/frenulum*—from Latin, meaning 'little bridle'.
> - *Papilla*—from Latin, meaning 'nipple' (the diminutive of *papula* meaning 'swelling').
> - *Mylohyoid*—from the Greek *myle/mylo* meaning 'mill'. The word was given to the posterior/molar teeth owing to their ability to 'grind'. Myle became *mola* in Latin and subsequently *molar*. *Mylohyoid* therefore relates to the posterior part of the jaw and the hyoid bone.

Geniohyoid

A narrow muscle found superior to the mylohyoid near the midline. It lies shoulder to shoulder with its contralateral fellow (occasionally fusing with it or genioglossus) and is one of the four suprahyoid muscles. Laterally lie the sublingual gland and submandibular duct, the deep part of the submandibular gland, and the hypoglossal nerve (Fig. 11.25). Superiorly lies the lingual neurovascular bundle.

- *Origin*—inferior mental spine of mandible.
- *Insertion*—anterior surface of the body of the hyoid bone.
- *Blood supply*—branches of the lingual artery.
- *Nerve supply*—C1 via hypoglossal nerve (from the ansa cervicalis).
- *Action*—brings the hyoid bone up and forward during deglutition. Depresses mandible when the hyoid is fixed.

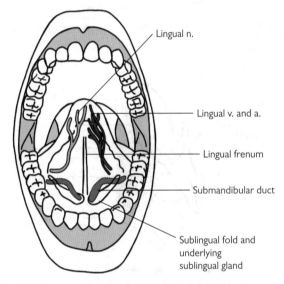

Lingual n.

Lingual v. and a.

Lingual frenum

Submandibular duct

Sublingual fold and underlying sublingual gland

Fig. 11.22 Structures of ventral tongue and floor of mouth, open mouth view.
Reproduced courtesy of Daniel R. van Gijn.

Mylohyoid boutonniere

From boutonniere meaning buttonhole. A variation of normal in which there is a focal discontinuity or hiatus of the mylohyoid muscle which may allow the sublingual gland (the 'bouton'), in combination with fat and/or vessels, to herniate from the sublingual space into the submandibular space.

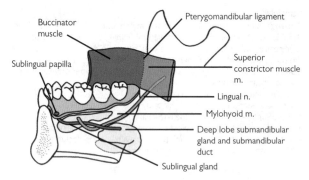

Fig. 11.23 Relationship of structures of the floor of mouth, internal view of right hemimandible.
Reproduced courtesy of Daniel R. van Gijn.

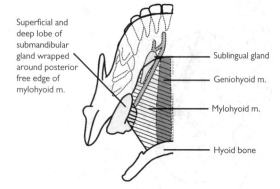

Fig. 11.24 The mylohyoid and geniohyoid muscles and relationship of the submandibular gland to the mylohyoid muscle, inferior view.
Reproduced courtesy of Daniel R. van Gijn.

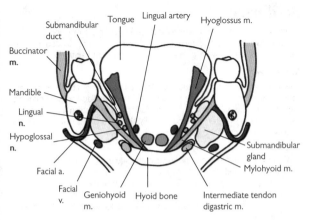

Fig. 11.25 The structures of the floor of the mouth, coronal section.
Reproduced courtesy of Daniel R. van Gijn.

Hard palate

The palate forms the roof of the mouth, separating the oral and nasal cavities and participating in speech and swallowing. It can be divided into two parts: an anterior bony hard palate and posterior soft palate (Fig. 11.26).

Structure

The hard palate forms three-quarters of the entire length of the palate and consists of the paired palatine processes of the maxillae and the horizontal processes of the palatine bones (articulating at the median and transverse palatine sutures). Anteriorly and laterally the hard palate is bound by the alveolar processes of the maxilla (Fig. 11.27).

Features

- *Mucous membrane*—keratinized stratified squamous epithelium bound tightly to the underlying periosteum. This in turn is bound to the bone by multiple Sharpey's fibres. The mucous membrane and periosteum over the horizontal plates of the palatine bones are separated by minor mucous-type salivary glands that may eventually coalesce at the paired palatine fovea.
- *Palatine raphe*—a narrow midline ridge devoid of submucosa.
- *Incisive papilla*—oval prominence at the anterior extremity of the palatine raphe marking the site of the incisive fossa.
- *Incisive fossae*— marks the junction of the premaxilla and maxilla.

The oral opening of the incisive canals carrying the (ascending) greater palatine neurovascular bundle and the (descending) nasopalatine nerve.

- *Greater palatine foramen*—adjacent to the secondary maxillary molar between the palatine bone and maxilla. Transmits the greater palatine nerve (V_2) and artery (third part of the maxillary artery) via the canal of the same name.
- *Lesser palatine foramen*—an inferior opening of the greater palatine canal that perforates the pyramidal process of the palatine bone, posterior to the greater palatine foramen. Transmits the lesser palatine nerve and arteries.

Neurovascular supply

⮑ See Fig. 11.28 and 11.29, p. 427.

- *Greater palatine artery and nerve*—emerge from the greater palatine foramen and pass anteriorly in a groove near the alveolus of the maxilla towards the incisive canal through which they ascend and anastomose with septal branches of the nasopalatine (sphenopalatine) artery and nerve. They supply the gingivae, palatine glands, and mucous membrane.
- *Lesser palatine arteries and nerves*—also pass through the greater palatine foramen but emerge through the more posterior lesser palatine foramina to supply the uvula, tonsil, and soft palate.

William Sharpey (1802–1880)
Scottish anatomist and physiologist, described as the father of British physiology. Lends his name to those fibres that join the lamellae of bone together and anchor bone to tendon.

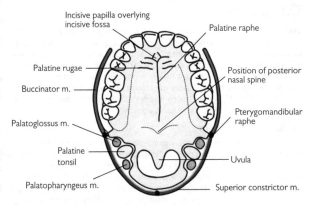

Fig. 11.26 Palate and associated structures, inferior view.
Reproduced courtesy of Daniel R. van Gijn.

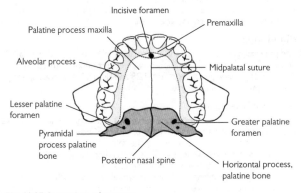

Fig. 11.27 Bony palate, inferior view.
Reproduced courtesy of Daniel R. van Gijn.

Soft palate

The soft palate arises as a fibromuscular shelf hanging from the posterior border of the bony hard palate. It consists of a fibrous aponeurosis to which five pairs of muscle are attached, and numerous nerves and vessels, lymphoid tissue, and mucous tissue, the latter constituting almost half of its substance. Its posterior edge makes contact with the posterior pharyngeal wall during swallowing, effectively closing off the nasopharynx from the oropharynx (Fig. 11.30). Although it is technically part of the oropharynx the soft palate is described here for continuity.

Surfaces and borders

Curving posteroinferiorly as the *velum palatinum*, the soft palate has a posterior free edge interrupted only by the midline uvula. Laterally, it extends to the sides of the posterior tongue as the palatoglossal arches (anterior pillar of the fauces), and to the lateral wall of the pharynx as the palatopharyngeal arches (posterior pillar of the fauces). The anterior and posterior pillars of the fauces contain the palatoglossus and palatopharyngeus muscles, respectively; the palatine tonsil lies between the arches in the tonsillar fossa.

- *Inferior (oral) surface*—concave, with a median raphe. Covered by stratified squamous epithelium.
- *Posterior (nasal) surface*—convex, continuous with the nasal floor, and covered with ciliated columnar epithelium.

Blood supply of the palate

The principal blood supply of the soft palate is from the ascending palatine branch of the facial artery, occasionally with contributions from a branch of the ascending pharyngeal artery (Fig. 11.28 and Fig. 11.31). Venous drainage is via the pterygoid venous plexus.

Nerves of the palate

- *General sensation*—lesser palatine nerve (V_2), pharyngeal branches of glossopharyngeal nerve, and tonsillar branches of both nerves.
- *Taste*—taste buds on oral surface of the soft palate, via the lesser palatine nerve which passes through the pterygopalatine ganglion and joins the greater petrosal branch of the facial nerve.
- *Secretomotor*—postganglionic parasympathetic fibres usually travel via the lesser palatine nerve from the pterygopalatine ganglion but some may travel via branches from the otic ganglion.

Le Fort I osteotomy blood supply

During a Le Fort I level osteotomy, performed electively as part of orthognathic surgery, both the nasopalatine and descending/greater palatine vessels may be compromised or even sacrificed. The maxilla maintains its blood supply via the soft palate and the ascending palatine artery (from the facial artery) and ascending pharyngeal arteries (from ECA) (Fig. 11.28). Despite this, there are rare reports of the maxilla or parts of the maxilla, becoming non-viable during Le Fort I osteotomy.

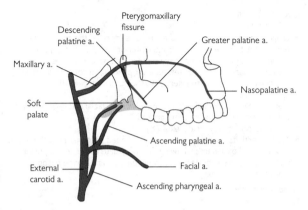

Fig. 11.28 Blood supply to the palate.
Reproduced courtesy of Daniel R. van Gijn.

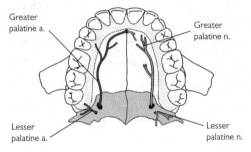

Fig. 11.29 Neurovascular contributions to the hard palate.
Reproduced courtesy of Daniel R. van Gijn.

Muscles of the soft palate

The muscles of the soft palate are attached to a thin, fibrous palatine aponeurosis, which is composed of the expanded tendons of the tensor veli palatini muscles: all the muscles act to alter the shape and position of the soft palate. There are five paired muscles, only two of which are purely palatal, the others are muscles associated with the tongue and pharynx (Fig. 11.32). All are supplied by the pharyngeal plexus (X) with the exception of tensor veli palatini, which is supplied by the nerve to medial pterygoid (V_3).

Levator veli palatini
See Fig. 11.33.
- *Origin*—quadrilateral area on the inferior surface of the apex of the petrous part of the temporal bone (anterior to carotid canal) and the cartilaginous part of the pharyngotympanic (Eustachian) tube.
- *Insertion*—passes medial to the superior pharyngeal constrictor (through the sinus of Morgagni) to insert onto the nasal surface of the palatine aponeurosis.
- *Blood supply*—ascending palatine branch of the facial artery and greater palatine branch of the maxillary artery.
- *Nerve supply*—pharyngeal plexus (X).
- *Action*—with its counterpart, forms a V-shaped sling that pulls the palate upwards and backwards, allowing the soft palate to touch the posterior wall of the pharynx during swallowing, thus separating the nasopharynx from the oropharynx.

Tensor veli palatini
See Fig. 11.33.
- *Origin*—medial pterygoid plate, medial aspect of the spine of the sphenoid, and the pharyngotympanic (Eustachian) tube.
- *Insertion*—fibres converge as a thin tendon that turns medially around the pterygoid hamulus to pass through the attachment of buccinator and insert onto the palatine aponeurosis and horizontal process of the palatine bone.
- *Blood supply*—ascending palatine branch of the facial artery and greater palatine branch of the maxillary artery.
- *Nerve supply*—nerve to medial pterygoid (V_3). (Remember 'Tensor – Trigeminal')
- *Action*—tightens and flattens the arch of the soft palate. Helps to open the pharyngotympanic tube, equalizing air pressure between the middle ear and nasopharynx (and the reason why opening your mouth and swallowing on flights helps to unblock ears).

Palatoglossus
See Fig. 11.33.
Forms the palatoglossal arch (with its overlying mucosa).
- *Origin*—oral surface of the palatine aponeurosis, continuous with its contralateral fellow.
- *Insertion*—side of tongue, anterior to the palatine tonsil. Fibres may interdigitate within the dorsum of tongue with the intrinsic transverse muscles.
- *Blood supply*—ascending palatine branch of the facial artery, ascending pharyngeal artery.
- *Nerve supply*—pharyngeal plexus (X).
- *Action*—closes the oral cavity from the oropharynx, elevating the tongue and bringing the left and right arches together.

Palatopharyngeus
See Fig. 11.33.
Consists of two heads or fasciculi. Forms the palatopharyngeal arch (posterior pillar of the fauces) with its overlying mucosa.

- *Origin*—the anterior head arises from the posterior border of the hard palate and pharyngeal surface of the palatine aponeurosis. The posterior head arises further posteriorly on the pharyngeal surface.
- *Insertion*—the two heads combine to insert into the lateral wall of the pharynx posterior to the tonsil. A slip continues inferiorly, blending with stylopharyngeus and salpingopharyngeus to insert into the thyroid lamina.
- *Blood supply*—the ascending palatine branch of the facial artery, the pharyngeal branch of the ascending pharyngeal artery, and the greater palatine branch of the maxillary artery.
- *Nerve supply*—pharyngeal plexus (X).
- *Action*—narrows the oropharyngeal isthmus, lowers the soft palate, and elevates the larynx and pharynx.

Musculus uvulae
See Fig. 11.33.
- *Origin*—posterior nasal spine of the palatine bone and pharyngeal surface of the palatine aponeurosis.
- *Insertion*—runs above the sling formed by levator veli palatini and inserts into the mucosa of the uvula.
- *Blood supply*—ascending palatine branch of the facial artery, descending palatine branch of the maxillary artery.
- *Nerve supply*—pharyngeal plexus (X).
- *Action*—increases midline bulk of the soft palate, aiding levator palatine, which in turn, assists velopharyngeal closure.

Bartolomeo Eustachi (approx. 1500–1574)

Italian anatomist and contemporary of Andreas Vesalius. Considered to be one of the founders of human anatomy. In addition to describing the pharyngotympanic tube that bears his name, he described the muscles of the malleus and the stapedius muscle, the cochlea, the presence of deciduous and secondary teeth, and the adrenal glands.

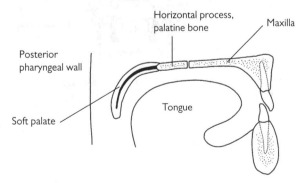

Fig. 11.30 The hard and soft palate, sagittal view.
Reproduced courtesy of Daniel R. van Gijn.

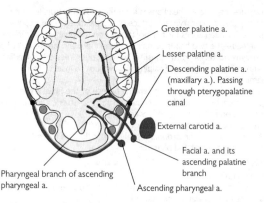

Fig. 11.31 Arterial supply of the hard and soft palate, inferior view.
Reproduced courtesy of Daniel R. van Gijn.

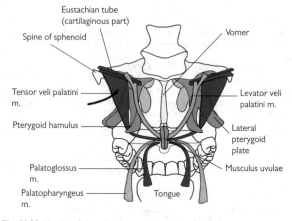

Fig. 11.32 Muscles of the soft palate, posterior view of nasopharynx.
Reproduced courtesy of Daniel R. van Gijn.

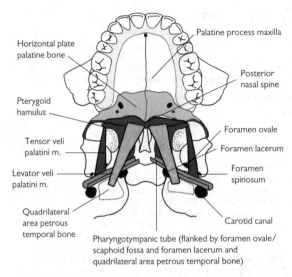

Palatine process maxilla

Horizontal plate palatine bone

Posterior nasal spine

Pterygoid hamulus

Tensor veli palatini m.

Levator veli palatini m.

Foramen ovale

Foramen lacerum

Foramen spinosum

Quadrilateral area petrous temporal bone

Carotid canal

Pharyngotympanic tube (flanked by foramen ovale/ scaphoid fossa and foramen lacerum and quadrilateral area petrous temporal bone)

Fig. 11.33 The palate and skull base demonstrating the relationships of levator veli palatini and tensor veli palatini, inferior view.
Reproduced courtesy of Daniel R. van Gijn.

Palatine tonsils

The palatine tonsils are located in the tonsillar fossa, created by the palatoglossal and palatopharyngeal arches. They represent the largest collection of lymphoid tissue in Waldeyer's ring. The palatine tonsil has a thin capsule (which differentiates it from the lingual and pharyngeal tonsils) consisting of pharyngobasilar fascia covering its deep (lateral) surface.

Waldeyer's ring

The gatekeeper loop of uninterrupted lymphoid tissue found at the upper end of the pharynx, circumscribing the naso- and oropharynx. It consists of the palatine, lingual, pharyngeal (adenoid), and tubal tonsils, along with aggregates of intervening lymphoid tissue throughout the pharynx (Fig. 11.34).

Surfaces

- *Medial (free) surface*—multiple surface pits or crypts containing lymphoid tissue which may extend superiorly into the soft palate as the *pars palatina* and anteroinferiorly to the tongue as a mucosal fold called the *plica semilunaris*. Both tend to involute with age.
- *Lateral (deep) surface*—the superior pharyngeal constrictor muscle (and fibres from palatopharyngeus) covered by the fascial tonsillar hemicapsule, adherent to the tongue, palatoglossus, and palatopharyngeus (Fig. 11.35). Lateral to the muscular wall, and occasionally piercing it, are the neurovascular supply to the tonsil (Fig. 11.34). The styloid process and its attachments are closely related. The ICA lurks approximately 25 mm behind and lateral.

Neurovascular supply

Arteries

Three arteries supply the tonsil at its lower pole (after piercing the superior pharyngeal constrictor) and two reach the tonsil via its superior pole (Fig. 11.36):

- *Tonsillar artery* (branch of facial or ascending palatine arteries).
- *Dorsal lingual* artery (branches of lingual artery).
- *Ascending palatine artery* (branch of facial artery).
- *Ascending pharyngeal arteries* (enter superior pole).
- *Greater and lesser palatine arteries*— from the descending palatine artery (third part of the maxillary artery); enter superior pole.

Veins

A tonsillar venous plexus forms around the capsule before piercing the superior pharyngeal constrictor and draining into the pharyngeal plexus. It consists of:

- *Venae comitantes* of the tonsillar artery.
- *Paratonsillar (or external palatine) vein*—receives tributaries from the tonsillar bed prior to piercing superior pharyngeal constrictor. May be a source of post-tonsillectomy bleeding.
- *Tonsillar branch of the lingual vein*—drains into the lingual vein.
- *Accessory tonsillar veins*—drains to pharyngeal plexus.

Nerves

The mucous membranes of the tonsil are supplied by tonsillar branches of the maxillary nerve (via the lesser palatine nerve) and tonsillar branches of the glossopharyngeal nerve, which combine to form a *circulus tonsillaris* around the tonsil. The soft palate and oropharyngeal isthmus receive contributions from this plexus.

Lymphatic drainage

Lymphatic vessels pierce the hemicapsule and superior pharyngeal constrictor to drain either directly into the deep cervical lymph nodes or indirectly via the retropharyngeal group. The jugulodigastric (level 2, or tonsillar) node immediately behind the angle of the mandible and anterior to SCM is most predominantly affected in inflammatory processes of the tonsil.

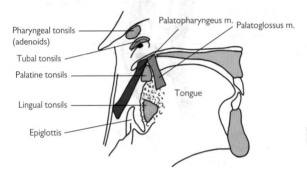

Fig. 11.34 Components of Waldeyer's ring, sagittal view.
Reproduced courtesy of Daniel R. van Gijn.

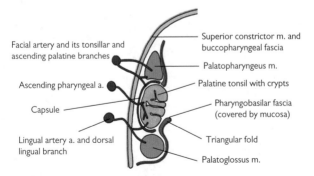

Fig. 11.35 The right tonsil demonstrating the relationship of the superior constrictor muscle and anterior and posterior pillars, transverse view.
Reproduced courtesy of Daniel R. van Gijn.

Etymology
- *Heinrich Wilhelm Gottfried von Waldeyer-Hartz (1836–1921)*—German anatomist after whom Waldeyer's lymphoid ring is named. Perhaps better known for coining the terms 'chromosome' and 'neuron' among others.

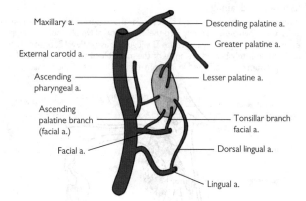

Fig. 11.36 The blood supply of the palatine tonsil.
Reproduced courtesy of Daniel R. van Gijn.

Chapter 12

The salivary glands

Introduction

There are three paired major salivary glands of the head and neck, all named according to their location. They all contribute to the production of saliva and salivary enzymes, and empty into the oral cavity via their respective ducts to assist with mastication and digestion (Fig. 12.1). At rest, the lion's share (60%) of saliva production is by the submandibular glands. On stimulation, the parotid contribution increases from 20% to 50%. Up to 1000 minor salivary glands are found within the submucosa of the oral cavity; they are 1–2mm in size and predominantly mucous in nature.

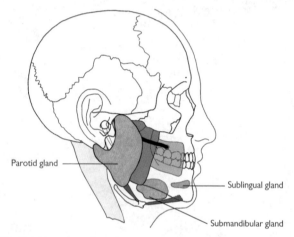

Fig. 12.1 Major salivary glands, overview.
Reproduced courtesy of Daniel R. van Gijn.

Etymology
- *Parotid*—from 'para-' (besides/next to) and 'ot-' (pertaining to the ear) and therefore literally meaning 'besides the ear', which is a surprisingly little-known etymological fact.

Parotid gland

The parotid glands are irregular shaped masses of lobulated glandular tissue (loosely triangular when viewed side-on) situated on the side of the face, extending from the zygomatic arch superiorly to the upper part of the neck inferiorly, where they overlie the posterior belly of digastric and upper part of SCM (Fig. 12.2). Anteriorly, the gland lies between the posterior border of the mandibular ramus (where it spills over the masseter muscle) before continuing inferior to the external acoustic meatus towards the mastoid process posteriorly (Fig. 12.3). This 'wedging' around the posterior ramus forms arbitrary superficial and deep 'lobes', connected by a broad isthmus, providing a theoretical plane for the plexiform passage of the main branches of the facial nerve and a surgically convenient division point of the gland. All gland lateral to the nerve is deemed to be in the superficial portion, while that medial to the nerve is termed the deep portion. This plane is theoretical because the two lobes of the parotid intimately fuse around and between the branches of the facial nerve (Fig. 12.4 and Fig. 12.5).

Borders, ends, and surfaces—and associated structures

As a pyramidal wedge, the parotid gland can be described as having two ends (superior and inferior), two borders (anterior and posterior), and three surfaces (superficial, anteromedial, and posteromedial) (Fig. 12.3).

- *Superficial/lateral*—covered by skin, SMAS, and the outer leaf of the parotidomasseteric fascia (destined for the zygomatic arch).
- *Anteromedial*—grooved by the ramus of the mandible and its attached muscles (masseter and medial pterygoid). A pterygoid process may extend between ramus and medial pterygoid; the parotid duct and branches of the facial nerve emerge through this surface.
- *Posteromedial*—grooved by the ECA and in contact with the mastoid process and the attached SCM and posterior belly of digastric. Separated from the carotid sheath by the styloid process and its associated muscles (stylohyoid, stylopharyngeus, styloglossus).
- The junction (medial margin) of the anteromedial and posteromedial surfaces may project deeply, bulging into the superior pharyngeal constrictor muscle and highlighting the importance of intraoral examination in the assessment of deep lobe involvement.
- *Superior end/surface*—concave and related to the posterior aspect of the TMJ and the cartilaginous part of the external acoustic meatus. Closely associated structures are the auriculotemporal nerve, superficial temporal vessels and the temporal branch of the facial nerve (Fig. 12.2).
- *Inferior end/apex*—overlies the posterior belly of digastric and the carotid triangle. Associated structures are the anterior and posterior divisions of the retromandibular vein and the cervical branch of the facial nerve.

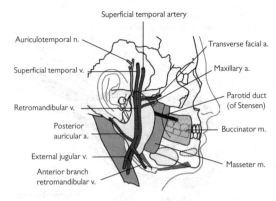

Fig. 12.2 Structures related to the parotid gland and its superior pole.
Reproduced courtesy of Daniel R. van Gijn.

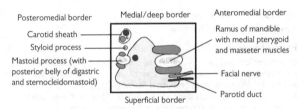

Fig. 12.3 Borders of the parotid gland and associated features.
Reproduced courtesy of Daniel R. van Gijn.

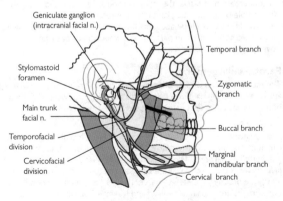

Fig. 12.4 Structures related to the anterior border of the parotid gland and facial nerve anatomy.
Reproduced courtesy of Daniel R. van Gijn.

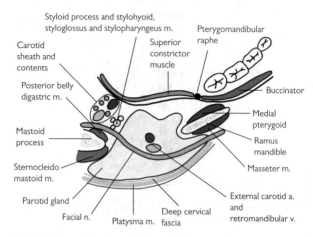

Fig. 12.5 Relationships of the parotid gland, axial view.
Reproduced courtesy of Daniel R. van Gijn.

Parotid capsule

Both superficial and deep 'lobes' of the parotid are tightly bound by a split superior extension of the investing layer of deep cervical fascia, that forms a parotidomasseteric fascia or parotid capsule (Fig. 12.6).

- The superficial lamina is thick and fibrous, blending intimately with the masseter and attaching superiorly to the zygomatic arch.
- The deep, thinner lamina is attached to the tympanic plate and styloid process of the temporal bone.
- A condensation of fascia, the stylomandibular ligament, separates the lower pole of the parotid gland from the submandibular gland.
- Its tight, fibrous envelope accounts for the significant pain experienced in pathological swelling, in part due to stimulation of branches of the overlying great auricular nerve.

Parotid enlargement

The multiple causes of a swollen parotid gland range from inflammatory, autoimmune, drug reactions, and neoplastic. An acute swelling of the parotid gland within its tight capsule causes pain.

Inflammatory

Inflammatory causes of parotid enlargement include acute viral infections (mumps, an RNA paramyxovirus, most commonly) and acute bacterial (suppurative) parotitis. The latter is most frequently seen in elderly, infirm, dehydrated, and debilitated patients where reduced salivary flow and poor oral hygiene result in ascending (usually staphylococcal) infection with unilateral painful swelling and leaking of pus from the duct.

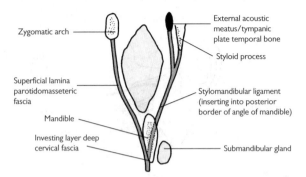

Fig. 12.6 The parotid and submandibular glands and their associated fascia, coronal view.

Reproduced courtesy of Daniel R. van Gijn.

Parotid duct

The parotid (Stensen's) duct carries saliva from the serous secretory units of the parotid glands to the oral cavity. It is approximately 5 cm long with a maximum diameter of a little over 2 mm.

• After leaving the anteromedial surface of the superior gland, the duct crosses masseter before heading medially to pierce buccinator and the buccal fat pad and enter the oral cavity opposite the second upper molar tooth.
• A change of angle combined with a short submucosal passage provides a valve effect and prevents the retrograde passage of air and subsequent inflation of the gland when oral cavity pressure increases.
• The middle third of a line drawn from tragus to philtrum marks the surface marking of the duct and must be borne in mind when assessing sharp injuries in the vicinity (Fig. 12.8).
• The transverse facial artery and accessory parotid gland accompany the duct superiorly.
• The buccal branch of the facial nerve passes inferior to the gland: on occasion the duct is crossed by branches passing between the buccal and zygomatic divisions of VII (Fig. 12.7).

Parotid duct injury

Injuries to the parotid gland and duct can result in leakage of saliva into the soft tissues and collections of saliva (sialocele). Injuries of the parotid duct should ideally be repaired in the operating theatre with good lighting and under general anaesthesia, so as to provide the best environment for proper wound exploration and repair. Management depends on the location of the injury:

• *Proximal (intraglandular) duct*—closure of parotid capsule and pressure dressing.
• *Mid-duct or terminal duct*—repair of the duct over a silicone catheter/cannula is performed and left in place for 10–14 days. More distal injuries should be drained directly into the mouth.

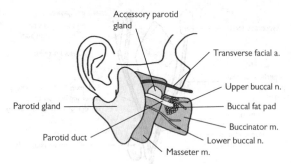

Fig. 12.7 Relationships of the parotid duct.
Reproduced courtesy of Daniel R. van Gijn.

Surface anatomy of the parotid gland

See Fig. 12.8.

- *Anterior border*—from the upper border of the mandibular condyle to a point on the central masseter, then to a point 2 cm below and behind the angle of the mandible.
- *Posterior border*—from the tip of the mastoid process to a point 2 cm below and behind the angle of the mandible.
- *Upper border*—from the upper border of the mandibular condyle to the mastoid process.

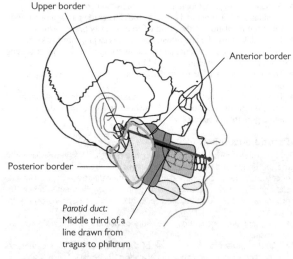

Fig. 12.8 Surface anatomy of the parotid gland and parotid duct.
Reproduced courtesy of Daniel R. van Gijn.

- *Niels Stensen* (also known as Nicolas Steno) *(1638–1688)*—Danish anatomist, geologist, and Catholic bishop who first described the parotid duct in a sheep. Stensen also made significant contributions to the neurosciences, with early pathophysiological investigations on hydrocephalus. He lends his name to stenonite, a mineral containing aluminum, barium, carbon , fluorine, oxygen, sodium and strontium.

Neurovascular supply to parotid

Blood supply

The blood supply to the parotid is derived from the numerous vessels that traverse its substance:

- *Arteries within the gland*—ECA directly and via its maxillary, superficial temporal and transverse facial branches (Fig. 12.9).
- *Retromandibular vein*—formed from the union of the superficial temporal and maxillary veins. Lies superficial to the ECA, drains via anterior and posterior branches, the former joining the facial vein and the latter joining the posterior auricular/external jugular vein.

Nerve supply

Carried by the auriculotemporal nerve, which arises from the posterior division of V_3 via two roots that encircle the middle meningeal artery, before uniting as a single nerve that passes between the neck of the mandibular condyle and sphenomandibular ligament and then runs laterally behind the TMJ related to the upper part of the parotid gland.

- *Somatosensory innervation*—directly via the auriculotemporal nerve (Fig. 12.9).
- *Parasympathetic*—postganglionic secretomotor fibres from the otic ganglion hitchhike with the auriculotemporal nerve to reach the gland. (Preganglionic fibres arise from cells in the inferior salivatory nucleus and travel via the tympanic branch of IX to the tympanic plexus and the lesser petrosal nerve to the otic ganglion (Fig. 12.10).
- *Sympathetic*—postganglionic vasomotor fibres reach the gland from the superior cervical ganglion via external carotid and middle meningeal artery plexuses.

Frey's syndrome (gustatory sweating)

Minor starch-iodine testing identifies 80% of patients affected following superficial parotidectomy, but only 20% report symptoms.

Aetiology

- Parasympathetic secretomotor nerves supplying the parotid gland and travelling with the auriculotemporal nerve are divided.
- Cholinergic sympathetic fibres to sweat glands in the overlying skin are also transected.
- Aberrant innervation of sweat glands on the face by regenerating parasympathetic secretomotor axons that would previously have innervated the parotid gland produces abnormal communications that result in gustatory sweating.
- Injection of botulinum toxin A is an effective treatment.

Lucja Frey (1889–1942)
Polish physician and neurologist who died in the Lwów ghetto during the
Holocaust. While others described the syndrome before Frey (including
Brown-Sequard and Henle), she was thought to be the first to describe
the anatomical and pathological bases of gustatory sweating, and the
auriculotemporal nerve syndrome.

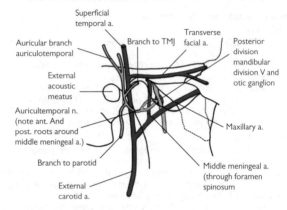

Fig. 12.9 Neurovascular supply to the parotid gland, right lateral view.
Reproduced courtesy of Daniel R. van Gijn.

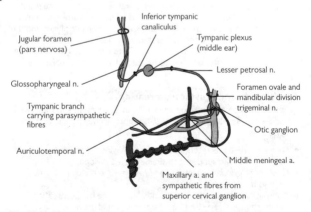

Fig. 12.10 Parasympathetic and sympathetic supply to the parotid gland.
Reproduced courtesy of Daniel R. van Gijn.

Parotid gland tumours

The majority (80%) of parotid gland tumours are benign. The main benign tumours are pleomorphic adenomas and Warthin tumours (cystadenolymphoma, generally in older male smokers, may be bilateral).

Malignant parotid tumours include mucoepidermoid, adenoid cystic, acinic cell carcinoma, and SCC. Presentation is often with a painless, slowly enlarging preauricular mass. Deep lobe tumours may present with an intraoral mass. Facial nerve involvement at presentation is a concerning feature and suggests malignant rather than benign disease. Acinic cell carcinoma has the greatest tendency for perineural invasion and therefore facial nerve involvement. Surgical treatment options depend on pathology and broadly include extracapsular dissection, superficial parotidectomy, and total parotidectomy with or without nerve sacrifice. With more aggressive tumours the surgeon needs to balance the risks of higher local recurrence with nerve preservation yet improved quality of life.

Facial nerve identification

A nerve stimulator may be used to guide identification, but the nerve should be identified at a number of points during the procedure:

- Stylomastoid foramen.
- Tragal pointer—1 cm deep and anteroinferior to the tragal cartilage.
- Deep to medial insertion of posterior belly of digastric.
- 6–8 mm inferior to tympanomastoid suture.
- Lateral to styloid process.

Facial nerve landmarks

Retrograde dissection of the nerve may be required.

- *Frontal branch*—Pitanguy's line, drawn from 0.5 cm inferior to the tragus to 1.5 cm superior to the lateral brow.
- *Buccal branch*—1 cm below a line drawn from the tragus to the nasal ala, along the parotid duct.
- *Inferior trunk*—travels with the retromandibular vein at the inferior margin of the parotid gland.
- *Marginal mandibular branch*—inferior to the lower border of the body of the mandible, but with a variable course; crosses the facial vein.

Intraparotid lymph nodes

The parotid glands (in comparison with the other major salivary glands) encapsulate late during development and have their own lymph nodes (Fig. 12.11). Intraparotid lymph nodes are frequently the first echelon nodes from cutaneous malignancy, most commonly SCC affecting the ear, cheek, temple, forehead, and (anterior) scalp. The majority of intraparotid lymph nodes are found within the superficial lobe, along the retromandibular vein.

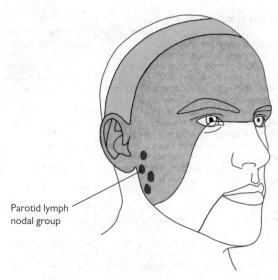

Parotid lymph
nodal group

Fig. 12.11 Lymphatic drainage of frontotemporal region, ear, and scalp (yellow shaded area) to parotid lymph node group.

Reproduced courtesy of Daniel R. van Gijn.

Submandibular gland

The submandibular gland is substantially smaller than the parotid (often compared to the size and shape of walnut). Situated within the digastric triangle, it is horseshoe shaped, consisting of a large superficial lobe and smaller deep lobe, wrapped around the posterior free edge of the mylohyoid muscle.

Deep part

Lies predominantly against the mylohyoid muscle except posteriorly, where it rests against hyoglossus, related closely to the lingual and hypoglossal nerves on their routes to the tongue (Fig. 12.12).

Superficial part

In the digastric or submandibular triangle, reaching as far anteriorly as the anterior belly of digastric and posteriorly separated from the tail of the parotid gland by the stylomandibular ligament. It is wedged between the mandible and the mylohyoid muscle, leaving an impression on the former (below the mylohyoid line) as the submandibular fossa (Fig. 12.12).

Relations of the submandibular gland

- *Superficially*—covered by skin, platysma, and the investing layer of deep cervical fascia. The latter divides into a superficial slip (from the greater cornu of the hyoid bone to the inferior border of the body of the mandible) and a deep layer (attached superiorly to the mylohyoid line of the mandible, covering the medial surface of the gland) (Fig. 12.13).
- *Inferiorly*—crossed by the facial vein and cervical branch of the facial nerve.
- *Laterally*—submandibular fossa of the mandible. The posterosuperior aspect of the gland is grooved by the facial artery *en route* to the face, as it crosses the lower border of the mandible (also indented) at the anterior border of masseter.
- *Medially*—mylohyoid nerve and artery (intervening between gland and mylohyoid muscle). Between the gland and hyoglossus lie, from superior to inferior, styloglossus, lingual nerve and submandibular ganglion, hypoglossal nerve, and the deep lingual vein.

Blood supply

Branches of the facial and lingual artery supply the gland.

Nerve supply

- *Secretomotor*—from the small fusiform submandibular ganglion, which is suspended from the lingual nerve by anterior and posterior roots. Lies superior to the deep part of the gland on the surface of hyoglossus. Preganglionic parasympathetic fibres from cell bodies in the superior salivatory nucleus travel in the chorda tympani (VII) to the ganglion. Postganglionic fibres from the ganglion are secretomotor to both the submandibular and sublingual glands.
- *Sympathetic*—postganglionic fibres from the plexus associated with the facial artery are vasomotor to vessels supplying submandibular and sublingual glands.
- *Sensory*—lingual nerve.

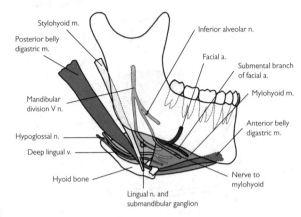

Fig. 12.12 Deep relations of the superficial lobe of the submandibular gland.
Reproduced courtesy of Daniel R. van Gijn.

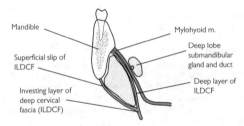

Fig. 12.13 Schematic relationship of deep cervical fascia to submandibular gland, coronal view.
Reproduced courtesy of Daniel R. van Gijn.

Submandibular (Wharton's) duct

- Emerges from the medial surface of the superficial part of the submandibular gland, posterior to the free edge of mylohyoid, where it makes an acute bend (genu).
- Runs anteriorly beneath the mucosa of the floor of the mouth, initially between hyoglossus and mylohyoid, and later between the sublingual gland and genioglossus, before opening at the summit of the sublingual papilla, which is closely adjacent to the lingual frenum.
- Is double-crossed by the lingual nerve, which runs lateral, inferior, and then medial to the nerve (Fig. 12.14).

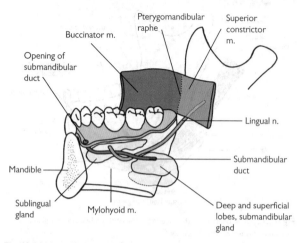

Fig. 12.14 View of right hemimandible demonstrating the relationship of the submandibular duct, lingual nerve, and opening of duct.

Reproduced courtesy of Daniel R. van Gijn.

Sialolithiasis

Salivary calculi are the commonest pathology of the salivary glands, most frequently affecting the submandibular gland and located in Wharton's duct. History delineates the pathology, usually unilateral, commoner in men, with onset of pain and inflammation on salivary stimulation. Obstruction of a salivary duct causes constant pain and inflammation, predisposing to the risk of infection.

Submandibular salivary calculi are more frequently located in the distal third of the duct, enabling their surgical removal, whereas parotid calculi are more commonly located in the gland itself. Minor salivary gland calculi may present in the buccal mucosa or upper lip, mimicking a tumour.

Digastric triangle

Boundaries

The digastric (submandibular) triangle is a subdivision of the anterior triangle of the neck, bounded by the anterior and posterior bellies of digastric and the inferior border of the mandible. It is in broad communication with the sublingual space via the gap between the mylohyoid and hyoglossus muscles (Fig. 12.15).

• *Roof*—covered superficially by skin, superficial fascia, and platysma and the investing layer of deep cervical fascia.
• *Floor*—mylohyoid anteriorly and hyoglossus and middle pharyngeal constrictor muscle posteriorly.

Contents

- *Submandibular gland*—superficial part almost fills triangle; submandibular duct.
- *Submandibular lymph nodes*—three to five in number; may be missed during neck dissection and superior retraction of facial vessels to protect marginal mandibular nerve (Hayes Martin manoeuvre).
- *Anterior and posterior (retromandibular) facial veins*—cross superficial to the gland and enter the carotid triangle where they unite to form the common facial vein.
- *Facial artery*—lies deep to gland with its submental branch.
- *Mylohyoid nerve*—deep to gland. A branch of the inferior alveolar nerve which supplies the anterior belly of digastric and mylohyoid.
- *Hypoglossal nerve*—runs posterior and deep to the junction of the anterior and posterior bellies of digastric. Runs in a plane deep to the submandibular gland.

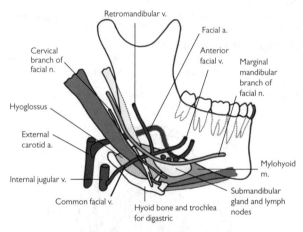

Fig. 12.15 Digastric triangle and the superficial relations of the submandibular gland.
Reproduced courtesy of Daniel R. van Gijn.

Sublingual gland

The sublingual gland is narrow, flat, and the smallest of the three pairs of major salivary glands (almond-sized, if loyal to the culinary comparisons). It is situated between mylohyoid and the mucosa of the floor of the mouth (which it raises to form the sublingual folds), and immediately anterior to the deep part of the submandibular gland. It rests against the sublingual fossa of the mandible laterally and is related to the submandibular duct and lingual nerve medially, which separate the gland from the genioglossus muscles. Anteriorly, it almost meets its contralateral fellow (Fig. 12.16).

Blood supply

See Fig. 12.16 and Fig. 12.17.
- *Sublingual branch of the lingual artery.*
- *Submental branch of the facial artery.*

Nerve supply

Postganglionic parasympathetic secretomotor fibres via the lingual nerve, originating from the submandibular ganglion (Fig. 12.17).

Sublingual (Bartholin's) duct

- The gland is predominantly mucous, secreting via up to 20 ducts, which open either onto the sublingual fold or directly into the submandibular duct.
- Occasionally, a major sublingual (Bartholin's) duct is formed, opening with or near to the submandibular duct.

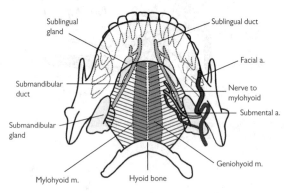

Fig. 12.16 Inferior view. Relationship of submandibular and sublingual glands and ducts.

Reproduced courtesy of Daniel R. van Gijn.

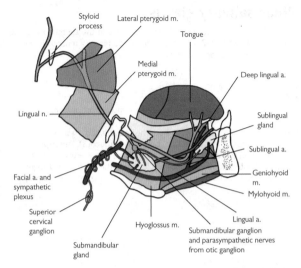

Fig. 12.17 Blood and nerve (sensory and autonomic) supply to the submandibular and sublingual glands.

Reproduced courtesy of Daniel R. van Gijn.

Malignant tumours of the salivary glands

Malignant tumours of the major salivary glands become increasingly common with decreasing size of the gland:

• 15% of parotid tumours are malignant.
• 35% of submandibular gland tumours are malignant.
• 85% of sublingual gland tumours are malignant.

Minor salivary glands

Up to 1000 minor salivary glands are found within the submucosa of the oral cavity. They are 1–2 mm in size and predominantly mucous in nature, with either individual or shared excretory ducts.

Locations
- *Labial*—mucous and serous glands.
- *Buccal*—mucous and serous glands.
- *Palatoglossal*—mucous glands, located around the oropharyngeal isthmus.
- *Palatal*—mucous glands within both the soft and hard palates.
- *Lingual*—anterior and posterior (both mainly mucous). Anterior glands are found on the ventral tongue and open via ducts near the lingual frenum. Posterior lingual glands are found on the root of the tongue. Serous glands of von Ebner occur around the (circum)vallate papillae.

Chapter 13

The nose and paranasal sinuses

Introduction

The external nose is a marked proboscis occupying a central position on the face. Its aesthetic and anatomical variations are multiple, its prominence is perhaps best exemplified by its absence (Bibi Aisha by Jodi Bieber, Time Magazine, August 2010). The subtle and not so subtle deflections, flicks, and variations in angle, bulbosity, and form of the nose may be assessed for clues regarding the owner's heritage and sporting prowess among other factors. A link between attractiveness and symmetry is clear. In addition to being the subject of much aesthetic scrutiny, the central position and protrusion of the nose, coupled with a lack of support from the underlying facial skeleton, makes it vulnerable to trauma and external forces. The external nose is the most proximal component of the respiratory tract, leading into the nasal cavity, which is the principal site for humidification and warming of inspired air and for olfaction, and also contributes in no small measure to the sense of taste and to the character of the voice (as a supraglottic resonator).

Surface markings

Anatomical landmarks

For reconstructive, cephalometric, and cosmetic purposes, the nose may be described in terms of topographic landmarks. These are independent of the aesthetic subunits of the nose described later (Fig. 13.1 and Fig. 13.2).

- *Glabella*—the most anterior midpoint on the fronto-orbital soft tissue contour. Situated between the brows superficially and underlying bony superciliary ridges.
- *Nasion*—most anterior point on frontonasal suture.
- *Radix (subnasion)*—deepest concavity and junction of frontal bone and dorsum of nose. Root of the nose.
- *Rhinion*—osseocartilaginous junction.
- *Supratip break*—area just above the tip of the nose; depression where the nasal dorsum joins the lobule.
- *Tip-defining point*—may be localized clinically by light reflex on nasal tip. Represents the highest point of the intermediate crus of the lower lateral cartilages.
- *Pronasale*—the most anterior point of the nasal tip in lateral view. Confusingly used interchangeably with the tip-defining point.
- *Infratip lobule*—part of the tip lobule between the tip-defining point and the columella–lobule angle.
- *Subnasale*—junction between the columella and philtrum.
- *Columella*—links tip to nasal base; separates the nares and is the inferior part of the nasal septum.
- *Pogonion*—most anterior point of the mandibular symphysis.

Nasal reconstruction

The earliest recordings of nasal reconstruction are from ancient Egypt, and subsequently from India. Nasal amputation as a means of punishment and humiliation has continued with time: 'To pay through the nose' is a term suggested to originate from a time when Danes amputated the noses of Irish people who would not pay taxes. In the eighteenth century, it is said that a king ordered the nasal amputation of all male inhabitants in Kitipoor, Nepal, before changing its name to Naskatapoor—the city without noses.

With the prevalence of such trauma, nasal reconstruction has evolved.

- Sushruta Samhita reported in detail a cheek flap in 700 BCE.
- Vaghbat described protecting the pedicle of a cheek flap in the fourth century.
- In Europe, the Italian surgeon Branca de Branca reported waltzing an arm flap to the nose in six stages in the fourteenth century.
- Benedetti described a two-stage arm flap and detailed its vasculature in the fifteenth century.
- The 'Indian' forehead flap has become the cornerstone of nasal reconstruction. Utilized for several hundred years in India prior to awareness of the procedure in Europe, which began in a letter to Gentleman's Magazine in 1794, with a report of the case of a bullock driver for the British army in India, whose nose was amputated and subsequently reconstructed with a forehead flap.

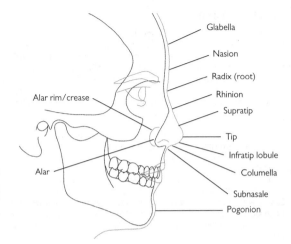

Fig. 13.1 Anatomic landmarks of the nose, lateral view.
Reproduced courtesy of Daniel R. van Gijn.

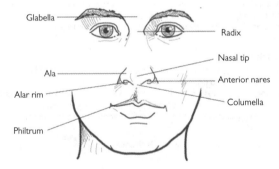

Fig. 13.2 Anatomic landmarks of the nose, frontal view.
Reproduced courtesy of Daniel R. van Gijn.

Etymology
- *Glabella*—from the diminutive of *glaber* meaning smooth or bald.
- *Columella*—from the diminutive of columna, a small column or pillar.

External nose

The external nose is pyramidal in shape. It has an osseocartilaginous framework. The root, or radix, of the nose is continuous with the forehead. Inferiorly, the nose ends as the apex or nasal tip. At this most anterior point, the nose turns acutely inwards to become the midline soft tissue columella, anterior to the nasal septum and separating the paired elliptical nares, which open into the nasal cavities. The dorsum of the nose is the prominent ridge that is formed by the midline convergence of the sloping lateral surfaces.

Skin

The skin of the nose forms a mobile layer overlying the nasal muscles. It can be divided into vertical thirds. The skin is of varying thickness, and how it drapes over its underlying support will indirectly influence the result of rhinoplasty.
- *Upper third*—fairly thick, tapering towards the middle third.
- *Middle third*—thinnest over the osseocartilaginous junction.
- *Lower third*—equal thickness to upper third and with a greater number of sebaceous glands at the tip, particularly in men. This is conveniently demonstrated in the condition rhinophyma, where there is progressive hypertrophy of the sebaceous glands.

Aesthetic subunits

The soft tissue of the external nose can be discussed in terms of aesthetic subunits, in order to divide the surgical anatomy of the nose into reconstructive segments. Where 50% or greater of a subunit is lost, consider replacing the entire subunit using local, regional, or free flaps and grafts (Fig. 13.3).

Muscles

The muscles acting on the nose are found deep to skin in the nasal SMAS. They consist of two principal opposing groups: the elevators and depressor and the dilators and compressor (Fig. 13.4). These work synergistically and are involved in respiration and facial expressions. In conjunction with orbicularis oris, they contribute to the formation of certain sounds.

Elevators
Procerus and levator labii superioris alaeque nasi.

Depressor
Depressor septi.

Dilators
Dilator naris anterior and dilator naris posterior (alar part of nasalis).

Compressor
Compressor naris (transverse part of nasalis).

When resecting a skin cancer, if greater than 50% of a subunit is involved, resecting all of the subunit may be considered in order to improve homogeneity and cosmesis of the reconstruction.

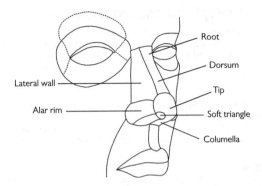

Fig. 13.3 Aesthetic subunits of the external nose.
Reproduced courtesy of Daniel R. van Gijn.

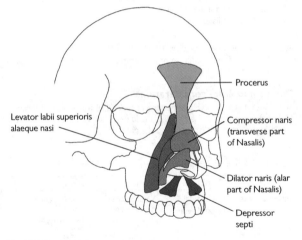

Fig. 13.4 Muscles of the external nose.
Reproduced courtesy of Daniel R. van Gijn.

Blood supply to the external nose

The rich blood supply to the subdermal vascular plexus of the nose is derived from three main vessels: predominantly from the facial artery and its branches (ECA) but also from branches of the anterior ethmoidal artery (ophthalmic artery) and the infraorbital artery (maxillary artery) (Table 13.1 and Fig. 13.5).

Facial artery
* *Alar*—a branch of the superior labial branch of the facial artery, supplying the ala of the nose.
* *Lateral nasal*—a branch from the angular artery, a continuation of the facial artery running deep to the nasolabial fold as it approaches the medial eye.

Ophthalmic artery
* *Dorsal nasal*—one of the two terminal branches of the ophthalmic artery. Pierces the orbital septum above the medial palpebral ligament and gives off two branches.
* *External nasal*—terminal branch of the anterior ethmoidal artery. Travels onto the dorsum of the nose between the nasal bones and upper lateral cartilages.

Maxillary artery
Gives off multiple branches after entering the pterygopalatine fossa.
* *Nasal branch of infraorbital*—a branch from the maxillary artery. Supplies the lateral nose.

Open rhinoplasty considerations
The bilateral lateral nasal arteries travel superficial to the alar cartilages. They are not compromised during a columellar approach in rhinoplasty, alleviating concerns of ischaemia to the nasal tip.

Table 13.1 Arterial contributions to the nose

	Ophthalmic	Maxillary	Facial
External nose	Dorsal nasal External nasal	Nasal branch of infraorbital	Alar (superior labial) Lateral nasal
Nasal septum	Anterior ethmoidal Posterior ethmoidal	Sphenopalatine Greater palatine	Septal branch of superior labial
Nasal cavity	Anterior ethmoidal Posterior ethmoidal	Sphenopalatine Greater palatine	Septal branch of superior labial

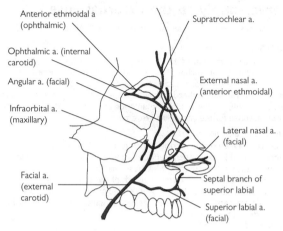

Fig. 13.5 Arterial supply to the external nose.
Reproduced courtesy of Daniel R. van Gijn.

Nerve supply to the external nose

General sensation to the external nose is supplied by V$_1$ and V$_2$ (Fig. 13.6).

Ophthalmic division (V$_1$)

The ophthalmic division of the trigeminal nerve divides into nasociliary, frontal, and lacrimal branches ('NFL' is used as a mnemonic) before entering the orbit via the superior orbital fissure. The frontal and lacrimal branches are destined for the forehead and globe respectively, while the nasociliary nerve gives off, among others, the anterior ethmoidal and infratrochlear nerves destined for the internal and external nose.

Anterior ethmoidal nerve

A terminal branch of the nasociliary nerve, it travels from the orbit to the anterior cranial fossa via the anterior ethmoidal foramen in the medial orbital wall. It leaves the anterior cranial fossa via the nasal slit.

- *External nasal branch*—a terminal branch of the anterior ethmoidal nerve. It leaves the nasal cavity between the nasal bone and upper lateral nasal cartilage and supplies general sensation to the lower half of the external nose and nasal tip.

Infratrochlear nerve

The infratrochlear nerve is given off from the nasociliary nerve in the orbit. It runs superiorly to the medial rectus muscle before exiting the orbit beneath the pulley of the superior oblique. It supplies the skin of the eyelids and the side of the nose above the medial canthus, the conjunctiva, lacrimal sac and the lacrimal caruncle.

Maxillary division (V$_2$)

Infraorbital nerve

The infraorbital nerve emerges onto the face at the infraorbital foramen, where it lies between levator labii superioris and levator anguli oris. It gives off palpebral, nasal and superior labial branches. The nasal branches supply the skin of the side of the nose and the movable part of the nasal septum and join the external nasal branch of the anterior ethmoidal nerve.

Nerve blocks to anaesthetize the external nose

Excision of skin malignancies and reconstruction of traumatic defects of the nose is frequently performed under local anaesthesia, and injections directly to the nose can be painful. A knowledge of sensory innervation and nasal nerve block techniques are important, and should precede direct infiltration to utilize the effects of adrenaline.

Infraorbital nerve
- Supplies lateral nasal sidewall, ala, and columella.
- Emerges from the infraorbital foramen, approximately 7 mm below infraorbital rim in a line inferior to medial limbus of the iris in neutral gaze.

Can anaesthetize at its exit from the foramen
- With direct infiltration perpendicular to the skin.
- From nasolabial fold, a few millimetres lateral to alar groove.
- Via an intraoral approach, directed towards the infraorbital foramen (less painful).

Dorsal nasal nerve
- Innervates cartilaginous dorsum and tip.
- Anaesthetized at caudal border of nasal bones, 5–10 mm lateral to midline.

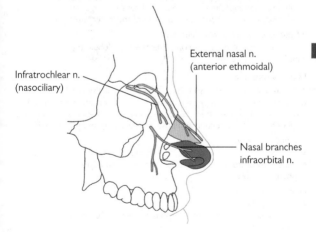

Fig. 13.6 Sensory nerve supply to the external nose, right lateral view.
Reproduced courtesy of Daniel R. van Gijn.

Osteocartilaginous skeleton

The skeleton of the nose is formed from bone, cartilage, and fibro-fatty elements. Its components articulate with the piriform aperture and can be conveniently classified into upper, middle, and lower thirds, each with key structures and relationships (Fig. 13.7).

Piriform aperture

The piriform aperture forms the bony foundation and footprint of the external nose, the sharp-edged anterior limit of the nasal skeleton. The aperture is formed by the paired nasal bones superiorly and the maxilla inferolaterally. The most inferior horizontal border is bound by the alveolar processes of the maxillae, which converge to form the anterior nasal spine (anterior insertion of the septal cartilage) in the midline.

Vault

See Fig. 13.8.

Superior third—upper bony vault

The upper third is bony, consisting of the paired nasal bones which articulate with the nasal processes of the frontal bones superiorly and the frontal processes of the maxillae laterally. The nasal bones are thick superiorly and become progressively thinner as they join the upper lateral cartilage.

Middle third—upper cartilaginous vault

The middle third is occupied by the osseocartilaginous junction and the important relationships between the upper lateral cartilages and septum (the nasal valve, see below) and the upper lateral and lower lateral cartilages.

Inferior third—lower cartilaginous vault

The lower third of the nose comprises the nasal lobule (tip, supratip, and infratip) and nasal base (columella, alar rim, and nasal sill).

Nasal valve area

The anterior part of the nose forms the region of the nasal valve, which is responsible for airflow resistance. It can be divided into external and internal nasal valves; the latter must be recognized and preserved during nasal surgery to avoid obstruction and postoperative asymmetry (Fig. 13.9).

External nasal valve

- Formed by the columella, nasal floor, and nasal rim.
- Dilated by dilator naris anterior and posterior during inspiration, preventing collapse.

Internal nasal valve

- 'True' nasal valve.
- Narrowest part of the nose, forming an angle of 10–15° between the nasal septum and upper lateral cartilages.
- Formed by the nasal septum, caudal border of the upper lateral cartilages, inferior turbinate, and piriform aperture.

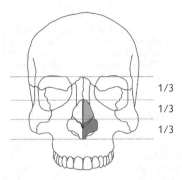

Fig. 13.7 Division of osteocartilaginous skeleton into thirds.
Reproduced courtesy of Daniel R. van Gijn.

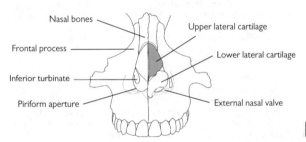

Fig. 13.8 Osteocartilaginous skeleton of the nose.
Reproduced courtesy of Daniel R. van Gijn.

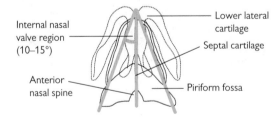

Fig. 13.9 Internal nasal valve region, inferior view.
Reproduced courtesy of Daniel R. van Gijn.

Nasal obstruction

Nasal obstruction may contribute to difficulty in breathing, and require correction of the septum, inferior turbinates, or nasal valves. Rhinoplasty can address the pathology through reshaping, excision, or reconstruction. Access to the nasal framework can be through an open approach, with a columellar incision, or a closed approach, with a mucosal incision.

Septal deviation

- Septoplasty to reshape the cartilaginous septum.
- Posterior septal deviation may need submucous resection.

Inferior turbinate hypertrophy

- Where the septum is deviated, the contralateral turbinate will hypertrophy to equalize nasal resistance.
- Lateral outfracture of inferior turbinate for reduction, or alternatively submucosal electrocautery.

External nasal valve

- Comprised of alar rim, nasal sill, and membranous septum.
- Opening valve usually requires cartilage grafts from the nasal septum or concha.
- Columellar strut grafts give more projection; alar batten grafts prevent collapse of the alar rim.

Internal nasal valve

- Acute angle of 10–15° formed by the cartilaginous septum and the caudal upper lateral cartilages.
- Cottle's manoeuvre places lateral traction on the cheek, opening the internal nasal valve and improving airflow where it is narrowed.
- Open rhinoplasty approach with cartilaginous spreader grafts to open the angle, most commonly harvested from nasal septum.

Cartilaginous vault

The cartilaginous structure of the nose proper, forming the dorsum and apex of the nose, is mobile, demonstrates significant variation from person to person, and has the unfortunate tendency to lie in the path of all manner of traumatic objects. It is formed by paired upper (lateral) cartilages, which underlie the nasal bones and contribute to the internal nasal valve, and lower lateral (major) cartilages, combined with additional minor nasal cartilages that surround the ala (Fig. 13.10). The paired cartilages of the nose contribute to the outward appearance of the nose and are therefore of interest to the aesthetic surgeon.

Upper lateral nasal cartilages

See Fig. 13.11 and Fig. 13.12.
- Also referred to as the triangular cartilages.
- Overlapped superiorly by the nasal bones, to which they are attached along with the frontal process of the maxilla.
- Inferiorly, they overlap the superior margins of the lower lateral cartilages, connected by fibrous tissue.
- The paired upper lateral cartilages meet one another in the midline and superiorly are supported by and connected to the nasal septum, forming the internal nasal valves.
- More inferiorly, the upper lateral cartilages do not directly unite with the septal cartilage and have a free edge just lateral to the midline of the nose. At this point, the septum alone contributes to the anterior projection of the nose.

Lower lateral (major) cartilages

See Fig. 13.10.
- Paired, thin curved plates of cartilage that contribute to the nasal lobule, base of nose, and nostril patency.
- The relationship between the upper lateral and lower lateral cartilages is called the scroll area, which is an anatomically significant region for tip support.
- Each is composed of a medial, intermediate, and lateral crus:
  - *Medial crus*—reaches its contralateral counterpart in the midline; connected to it and the septal cartilage by fibrous tissue, forming the midline columella that separates the nares.
  - *Intermediate (or middle) crus*—analogous to the infratip region of the nose, anterior and cephalad to the columella. The junction point of the intermediate and lateral crus of the lower lateral cartilages form the nasal domes, the apex or hinge point of each alar cartilage and the tip-defining point.
  - *Lateral crus*—continues posterolaterally from the nasal dome passing obliquely above the alar crease to attach to the free margin of the piriform aperture via a fibrous membrane containing the minor alar cartilages.

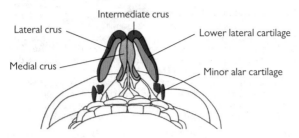

Fig. 13.10 Lower lateral and minor cartilages, inferior view.
Reproduced courtesy of Daniel R. van Gijn.

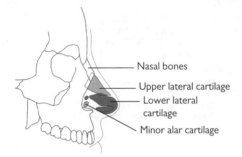

Fig. 13.11 Nasal cartilages, lateral view.
Reproduced courtesy of Daniel R. van Gijn.

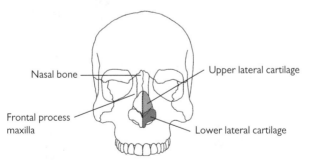

Fig. 13.12 Nasal cartilages, frontal view.
Reproduced courtesy of Daniel R. van Gijn.

Full-thickness nasal reconstruction

The nose is composed of skin, an osseocartilaginous framework, and mucosa. Assessment of a defect must consider these three elements individually, and reconstruction should aim to replace like with like. The workhorse flap currently used for replacement of skin in large nasal defects is the paramedian forehead flap.

Reconstruction may be with grafts or flaps, with the osseocartilaginous framework usually replaced with a graft. Two grafts cannot be placed adjacent to each other; defects requiring replacement of mucosa when a cartilage graft has been used require a vascularized surface as a flap.

Reconstructive options for skin

- Full-thickness skin graft.
- Wide range of local flaps. For large defects use free tissue transfer (e.g. radial forearm free flap).

Reconstructive options for osseocartilaginous framework

- Cartilage graft (harvested from septum, concha, rib).
- Bone graft (harvested from rib, split calvaria).

Reconstructive options for mucosa

- Buccal mucosal graft/flap.
- Split-thickness skin graft.
- Local turnover skin flaps.
- Intranasal mucosal flaps.
- Free tissue transfer.

Nasal cavity

The nasal cavity, perhaps best appreciated in coronal section where it forms an approximately triangular shape, forms the central space of the skull, sandwiched between the anterior and middle skull base superiorly and the roof of the mouth inferiorly (Fig. 13.13). It extends from the nares anteriorly to the choanae posteriorly, where it communicates with the nasopharynx. It is divided into two symmetrical halves by the midsagittal osseocartilaginous nasal septum and is flanked by the maxillary and ethmoidal sinuses, situated intimately adjacent to allow for their drainage into the nasal cavity. Each half of the nasal cavity consists of medial and lateral walls, a roof, and a floor (Fig. 13.14).

Medial wall

The bony cartilaginous nasal septum forms the medial wall of each nasal cavity.

Floor

- The anterior three-quarters of the floor are formed by the paired palatine processes of the maxillary bone.
- Horizontal processes of the palatine bones form the posterior third.
- A mucosal depression found anteriorly by the nasal septum marks the position of the incisive canals which transmit the greater palatine artery and the nasopalatine nerves into the oral cavity.

Roof

- From anterior to posterior, the roof of the nasal cavity first inclines upwards along the nasal spine of the frontal and nasal bones.
- It then flattens out along the undersurface of the cribriform plate of the ethmoid bone, which separates the nasal cavity from the anterior cranial fossa and transmits the olfactory nerves, associated meninges and CSF (and the anterior ethmoidal neurovascular bundle via a separate foramen).
- Posteriorly, the roof slopes downwards along the anterior aspect of the body of the sphenoid.

Lateral wall

The lateral wall of the nose is complicated and is formed of six bones that articulate with the medial aspect of the maxilla. Four act more specifically to reduce the size of the impressive maxillary hiatus that leads to the maxillary sinus.

- *Lacrimal*—forms part of the medial bony wall of the nasolacrimal duct with the inferior turbinate.
- *Ethmoid*—composed of the superior and inferior turbinates.
- *Inferior nasal turbinate*—individual bone superimposed on the lateral wall.
- *Perpendicular plate of the palatine bone*—covers the posterior part of the maxillary hiatus.
- *Nasal bone.*
- *Medial pterygoid plate of sphenoid*—most posterior aspect of lateral wall.

The terms nasal 'turbinates' and 'conchae' are generally used interchange-ably, although the latter is technically used if the bones contain an air sac. Pneumatization of the middle turbinate is not uncommon and is known as a concha bullosa.

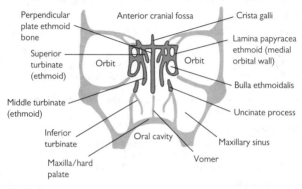

Fig. 13.13 Relationships of the nasal cavity, coronal section.
Reproduced courtesy of Daniel R. van Gijn.

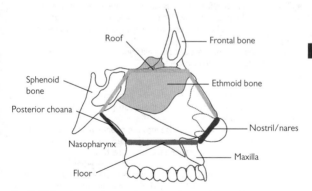

Fig. 13.14 Boundaries and anterior/posterior relations of the nasal cavity.
Reproduced courtesy of Daniel R. van Gijn.

Lateral wall of the nose

Superimposed upon the lateral wall are the superior and middle turbinates (medial protrusions of the ethmoid), the solitary inferior turbinate, and their respective meati. The turbinates are delicate, mucosa-covered bony scrolls that converge towards one another posteriorly (Fig. 13.15).

Inferior turbinate

A separate bone that closes off the inferior portion of the maxillary hiatus and articulates with the following:

- The nasal surface of the maxilla anteriorly.
- The perpendicular plate of the palatine bone posteriorly.
- The inferior portion of the lacrimal bone anterosuperiorly via its lacrimal process.
- The posterior aspect of the uncinate process of the ethmoid bone via its ethmoidal process.

Inferior meatus

- The inferior meatus is the largest of the meati, occupying most of the anteroposterior distance of the lateral wall.
- The nasal opening of the nasolacrimal duct is found anteriorly.

Middle turbinate

A projection from the medial process of the ethmoidal labyrinth.

- Articulates with the perpendicular plate of the palatine bone.
- The sphenopalatine foramen is posterior to the middle turbinate, connecting the nasal cavity with the pterygopalatine fossa and transmitting the sphenopalatine artery and nasociliary and superior nasal nerves.
- *Ager nasi cell*—a prominence at the anterior end of the middle turbinate. Overlies the lacrimal sac.

Middle meatus

Found beneath the middle turbinate, the anatomy of the middle meatus is perhaps the most complicated of the meati (Fig. 13.16). It presents the following principal features:

- *Ethmoidal bulla*—a rounded bulge into the middle meatus produced by a group of the largest and least variable anterior ethmoidal air cells. A variable number of ostia may be found on the bulla.
- *Hiatus semilunaris*—deep gutter lying between the ethmoid bulla superiorly and the hook-shaped uncinate process inferiorly. Contains ostia of anterior ethmoidal cells and the larger maxillary ostium posteriorly.
- *Uncinate process of ethmoid*.
- *Infundibulum*—represents the anterior end of the hiatus semilunaris. Leads to the maxillary ostium.
- *Frontal recess*—the region of the middle meatus superior and anterior to the infundibulum. Receives secretions of the frontal sinus via the frontonasal duct.

Superior turbinate

- The shortest of the three turbinates (about half the length of the middle turbinate). It forms a roof above the superior meatus.
- The *sphenoethmoidal* recess is an area between the posterior aspect of the superior turbinate and the anterior surface of the body of the sphenoid.

Superior meatus

Receives the posterior ethmoidal sinuses into its anterior aspect.

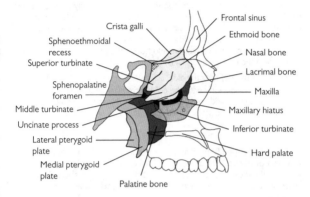

Fig. 13.15 Lateral wall of the nose.
Reproduced courtesy of Daniel R. van Gijn.

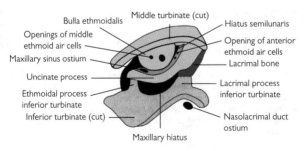

Fig. 13.16 Amplified detail of middle meatus anatomy.
Reproduced courtesy of Daniel R. van Gijn.

Nasal septum

The nasal septum acts as the main sagittal midline support structure of the nose, and represents the medial walls of the paired nasal cavities. It is fundamental in dorsal and tip support to the nose and is involved in maintaining the patency of the nasal airways and in providing a foundation for the overlying nasal mucosa. It consists of bone posteriorly, hyaline cartilage anteriorly, and a small exclusively membranous contribution (Fig. 13.17).

Bony components

The bony components of the septum consist principally of the perpendicular process of the ethmoid bone and the vomer. The broad articular surface of the nasal bones, the nasal spine of the frontal bones, and the rostrum and crest of the sphenoid contribute to the superior boundary while the crests formed by the maxillae and horizontal processes of the palatine bones form the inferior boundary.

Perpendicular plate of the ethmoid
- Continuous superiorly with the cribriform plate (which has potential clinical sequelae) and constitutes the upper third of the septum.
- Anterior spine articulates with the frontal spine and crest of the nasal bones.

Vomer
- Triangular-shaped bone. The upper border approximates to the inferior aspect of the body of the sphenoid, where it expands into an ala on each side. It extends anteroinferiorly, becoming progressively broader where it articulates with a groove on the superior aspect of the hard palate.
- Forms the posterior border of the septum.
- Indented bilaterally by the nasopalatine nerves.

Cartilaginous and soft tissue components

Quadrangular cartilage
- Extends from the internasal suture between the nasal bones superiorly, almost as if an inferior unossified continuation of the perpendicular plate of the ethmoid bone.
- Posteriorly, a narrow segment extends between the perpendicular plate of the ethmoid and the vomer.
- Terminates anteriorly in the supratip area.
- Continuous with the upper lateral cartilages anterosuperiorly.
- Anteriorly, it is connected to the lower lateral cartilages by fibrous tissue.
- Its inferior border articulates with the vomer posteriorly and anteriorly sits in a groove formed by the nasal crest and anterior nasal spine.

Vomeronasal cartilage
- A small strip of cartilage situated between the vomer and the inferior border of the septal cartilage.
- It encompasses the vomeronasal organ, an auxiliary sense organ of olfaction integral to the flehmen response and detection of pheromones.
- The vomeronasal organ allegedly regresses after birth, persisting as a simple epithelium-lined sac that opens into the base of the nasal cavity.

Membranous septum
- Represents the mobile most anterior element of the septum.
- Lies between the anterior border of the septal cartilage and columella, accounting for the mobility in this area.
- Is formed by the union of the septal mucous membranes (which blend with the skin of the columella). Supported by the medial crura of the lower lateral cartilages.

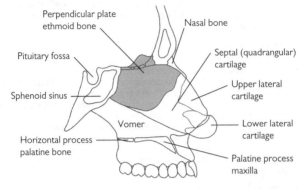

Fig. 13.17 Components of the nasal septum.
Reproduced courtesy of Daniel R. van Gijn.

Vomeronasal organ and the flehmen response

The vomeronasal or Jacobson's organ (Ludwig Jacobson, 1813) is an accessory olfactory organ situated at the base of the nasal septum thought to be involved in the detection of chemical stimuli—in particular, pheromones. It is considered responsible for the *flehmen response*.

Flehmen response
From the German 'flehmen' meaning to 'bear the upper teeth'. It involves inhalation and the curling upwards of the upper lip—presumably to aid in the transfer of pheromones and other chemical stimuli to the vomeronasal organ. Stallions are particularly known for their impressive flehmen response in their attempts at detection of pheromones in the urine of mares in oestrus.

Blood supply to the nasal cavity

The nasal septum relies upon variable anastomoses from five vessels: two branches from the ophthalmic artery, two from the maxillary artery, and one from the facial artery. Collectively, they form the troublesome *Kiesselbach's* plexus or *Little's* area (Fig. 13.18). This high-flow confluence of vessels carries with it the burden of dramatic and occasionally life-threatening epistaxis, from the inadvertent pass of the surgeon's instrument or secondary to an aggressive ulcer. A working knowledge of the vascular anatomy is required in order to successfully expose and ligate the proximal arterial contributions of the offending vessel(s).

Ophthalmic artery
See Fig. 13.19.
- *Anterior ethmoidal artery (lateral and septal branches)*—pierces the medial orbital wall to enter the anterior cranial fossa, giving off nasal branches into the nasal cavity through the nasal slits adjacent to the crista galli. Supplies the anterior third of the septum and corresponding lateral wall of the nose via septal and lateral branches, respectively.
- *Posterior ethmoidal artery (lateral and septal branches)*—leaves the orbit through the posterior ethmoidal foramen where it passes into the anterior cranial fossa in the region of the cribriform plate. Gives off septal and lateral nasal branches to supply the posterosuperior septum and superior nasal turbinate, respectively.

Maxillary artery
See Fig. 13.19.
- *Sphenopalatine artery (lateral and septal branches)*—passes into the anterior nasal cavity via the sphenopalatine foramen (immediately behind the posterior end of the middle nasal turbinate) and divides into lateral (essentially conchal) and septal posterior nasal arteries.
  - The *lateral posterior nasal* artery is the larger of the two, usually dividing to pass alongside the middle and inferior turbinates before anastomosing with branches of the anterior ethmoidal artery.
  - The *septal posterior nasal* branch of the sphenopalatine, as its name suggests, heads toward the septum and courses anteroinferiorly to the incisive foramen where it anastomoses with the greater palatine artery.
- *Greater palatine artery*—continuation of the descending palatine artery (a terminal branch of the maxillary artery that passes through the pterygopalatine canal). Exits the pterygopalatine fossa by descending through the greater palatine foramen and travels anteriorly along the hard palate to resurface into the nasal cavity via the midline incisive foramen. Anastomoses with the septal posterior nasal branch of the sphenopalatine artery.

Facial artery
See Fig. 13.19.
- *Septal artery*—branch of the superior labial artery which courses along the upper lip (between mucous membrane and orbicularis oris) before giving off the septal (or coronary) artery that anastomoses with the septal posterior nasal branch of the sphenopalatine artery to supply the vestibule of the nose and septum.

- *James Lawrence Little (1836–1885)*—American surgeon. First described the area in 1879.
- *Wilhelm Kiesselbach (1839–1902)*—German otolaryngologist.

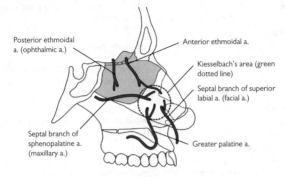

Fig. 13.18 Blood supply of the nasal septum.
Reproduced courtesy of Daniel R. van Gijn.

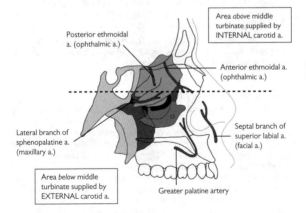

Fig. 13.19 Blood supply of the lateral wall of the nose.
Reproduced courtesy of Daniel R. van Gijn.

Epistaxis

Bleeding from the nose is usually minor, but in some cases can be life-threatening. Causes of epistaxis are local or systemic and can be classified as anterior or posterior; the majority are anterior, originating from Little's area. Posterior bleeding is more likely to be arterial in origin and may cause airway compromise, aspiration, and difficulty in control.

Anterior bleeding

- Can usually be managed by pressure to the nasal alae with the patient sitting up.
- Adjunctive measures include silver nitrate sticks or diathermy.
- Nasal packing or a nasal tampon may be required if simple measures are unsuccessful.

Posterior bleeding

Can be more challenging as it is difficult to identify a source. Posterior packing or a balloon catheter can act as a tamponade.

Intractable bleeding

- May require interventional radiology or surgery.
- The sphenopalatine artery is accessed endoscopically at the rear of the middle turbinate. The anterior and posterior ethmoidal arteries are accessed via a medial orbital skin incision.
- Ligation of the maxillary artery may be achieved with a Caldwell–Luc incision in the upper buccal sulcus to access the pterygopalatine fossa.
- As a final measure, the ECA can be ligated.

Septal haematomas present as cherry-red swellings of the mucoperichondrium of the nasal septum; incision and drainage are imperative to prevent necrosis of the cartilage.

Sphenopalatine artery ligation

The sphenopalatine artery is one of the vessels supplying the nasal cavity responsible for significant epistaxis, and has (not unreasonably) been labelled as the 'artery of epistaxis'. A terminal branch of the maxillary artery (ECA), it traverses the sphenopalatine foramen from the pterygopalatine fossa and divides into medial and lateral posterior nasal arteries, ultimately contributing to Kiesselbach's plexus.

If epistaxis persists despite conservative measures (anterior and posterior nasal packing, vasoconstrictor agents, reversal of haematological causes, oxidized cellulose, etc.), proximal embolization or ligation of the offending vessel can be considered. The sphenopalatine artery enters the nasal cavity adjacent to the posterior attachment of the medial concha, where it can be endoscopically ligated.

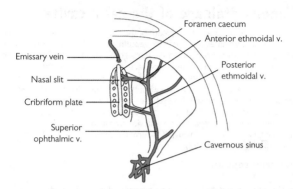

Fig. 13.20 Venous drainage of nose—schematic demonstrating intracranial communication.

Reproduced courtesy of Daniel R. van Gijn.

Venous drainage of the nasal cavity

The dense submucosal venous plexus of the nose, particularly of the middle and inferior turbinates and posterior septum, resemble that of the erectile tissues. This warm pool of blood, although beneficial in the warming of inspired air, is less welcome in the face of engorgement and resultant nasal obstruction. The veins accurately accompany the arteries (principally the sphenopalatine, facial, and ophthalmic vessels) and are perhaps best considered according to which part of the septum they drain and the deep veins to which they drain. Occasionally, the foramen caecum (at the frontoethmoidal suture within the anterior cranial fossa) may be patent and an emissary vein passes through it to form the origin of the superior sagittal sinus (➲ Fig. 13.20, p. 483).

Anterior septum

See Fig. 13.21.

- Drainage principally by veins accompanying the anterior and posterior ethmoidal arteries, into the superior ophthalmic vein and cavernous sinus.
- Some veins may drain into facial veins.
- Some veins enter the anterior cranial fossa, via either the cribriform plate or a patent foramen caecum, and drain into the superior sagittal sinus.

Posterior septum

See Fig. 13.21.

- Drainage via the sphenopalatine vein (accompanying the artery of the same name) into the pterygoid venous plexus, and thence into the cavernous sinus.

An external nasal plexus overlying the alar cartilages drains towards the external nasal opening and is thereafter destined for the facial vein. The communication between external nasal veins and the septal venous system with the intracranial venous sinuses represents a potential pathway for the spread of infection.

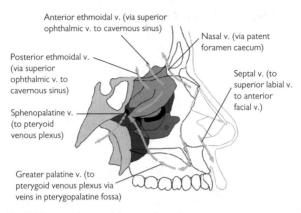

Anterior ethmoidal v. (via superior ophthalmic v. to cavernous sinus)

Nasal v. (via patent foramen caecum)

Posterior ethmoidal v. (via superior ophthalmic v. to cavernous sinus)

Septal v. (to superior labial v. to anterior facial v.)

Sphenopalatine v. (to pteryoid venous plexus)

Greater palatine v. (to pterygoid venous plexus via veins in pterygopalatine fossa)

Fig. 13.21 Venous drainage of the nose, schematic.
Reproduced courtesy of Daniel R. van Gijn.

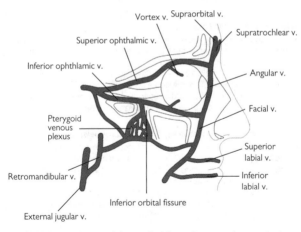

Vortex v. Supraorbital v.

Superior ophthalmic v.

Supratrochlear v.

Inferior ophthlamic v.

Angular v.

Facial v.

Pterygoid venous plexus

Superior labial v.

Retromandibular v.

Inferior labial v.

Inferior orbital fissure

External jugular v.

Fig. 13.22 Venous drainage of the superficial face and intracranial communication.
Reproduced courtesy of Daniel R. van Gijn.

Nerve supply to the nasal cavity

General sensation to the internal nose is carried by branches of the ophthalmic and maxillary divisions of the trigeminal nerve. Branches from the latter reach the nose either directly or via the pterygopalatine ganglion (Fig. 13.23 and Fig. 13.24).

Ophthalmic division (V₁)

Anterior ethmoidal nerve

The anterior ethmoidal nerve is a branch of the nasociliary nerve. It enters and supplies the roof of the nasal cavity, grooving the inner surface of the nasal bone before continuing as the external nasal nerve. It provides the following branches to the internal nose:

- *Lateral internal nasal nerve*—supplies anterolateral nasal wall.
- *Medial internal nasal nerve*—supplies anterosuperior septum.

Maxillary division (V₂)

The maxillary division of the trigeminal nerve supplies the mucosa of the nasal cavity, both directly via branches of the maxillary nerve proper as it traverses the orbit and indirectly via branches of the pterygopalatine ganglion which pass through the sphenopalatine foramen to enter the nasal cavity.

Direct branches to the nasal cavity

- *Infraorbital nerve*—the maxillary nerve enters the infraorbital canal and passes through the infraorbital foramen to become the infraorbital nerve. Supplies the nasal vestibule.
- *Anterior superior alveolar nerve*—a branch given off within the infraorbital canal before the maxillary division exits the infraorbital foramen. Communicates with the middle superior alveolar nerve and gives off a nasal branch to supply the inferior turbinate and the floor of the nasal cavity.

Indirect branches to the nasal cavity from the pterygopalatine ganglion

- *Greater palatine nerve*—enters the pterygopalatine canal to emerge into the hard palate via the greater palatine foramen. Before emerging, the greater palatine nerve gives off lateral posterior inferior nasal nerves to supply the inferior meatus and turbinate.
- *Posterior superior nasal nerve*—passes through the sphenopalatine foramen; divides into medial and lateral branches to supply the posterior septum and the region of superior and middle turbinates, respectively.
- *Nasopalatine nerve*—travels alongside the septal branch of the sphenopalatine artery, entering the nasal cavity via the sphenopalatine foramen and coursing anteroinferiorly across the septum (which it supplies) towards the incisive canal. Supplies the mucosa of the gingivae and hard palate immediately posterior to the upper central incisors.

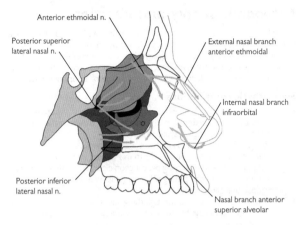

Fig. 13.23 Nerve supply of the lateral nasal wall.
Reproduced courtesy of Daniel R. van Gijn.

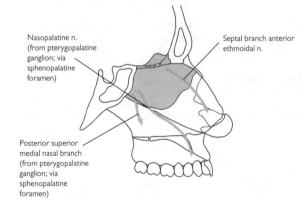

Fig. 13.24 Nerve supply of the nasal septum.
Reproduced courtesy of Daniel R. van Gijn.

Autonomic supply and olfaction

As well as relaying general sensory information and pain and temperature, the maxillary nerve (more specifically, the nasal branches from the pterygopalatine ganglion) carries the sympathetic contributions to the nasal blood vessels and the parasympathetic secretomotor fibres that drive the nasal mucous glands. Olfaction is conveyed by the olfactory nerve (I).

Sympathetic contributions

- Preganglionic input from neurons in T1-T3 segments of the spinal cord. Fibres ascend bilaterally in the sympathetic trunks to the superior cervical ganglia, where they synapse.
- Postganglionic fibres travel as a plexus around the ICA.
- The deep petrosal nerve, derived from this plexus, unites with the greater petrosal nerve (carrying preganglionic parasympathetic fibres), to form the nerve of the pterygoid canal (vidian nerve) which enters the pterygopalatine ganglion posteriorly
- The sympathetic fibres pass through the ganglion without synapsing and are distributed along the blood vessels of the nasal mucosa, mediating vasoconstriction.

Parasympathetic contributions

- Derived from the greater petrosal nerve (a branch from the geniculate ganglion, VII).
- Preganglionic parasympathetic fibres travelling in the nerve of the pterygoid canal (see above) synapse in the ganglion.
- Postganglionic secretomotor parasympathetic fibres travel within nasal palatine and nasal branches to the nasal mucosa.

Olfactory nerve

- The olfactory nerve arises within the olfactory epithelium covering the superior aspects of the nasal septum and lateral nasal cavity.
- On each side, the olfactory nerve proper, up to 20 bundles of minute axons and their supporting glia, surrounded by CSF and a meningeal sheath, travels through the cribriform plate into the anterior cranial fossa and enters the olfactory bulb lying on the plate.
- The olfactory bulb represents the rostral expansion of the olfactory tract.
- Olfactory nerves can regenerate, a quality apparently bestowed upon them by their ensheathing cells. Manipulation of these cells remains of interest in the continuing search for ways to encourage effective regeneration of damaged CNS tissue.

Etymology
- *Vidian*—from Vidus Vidius, a sixteenth-century Italian surgeon and anatomist.

Paranasal sinuses

The frontal, sphenoidal, ethmoidal and maxillary sinuses are air-filled cavities located in the bones of the same name and known collectively as the paranasal sinuses (Fig. 13.25). They are lined with mucosa continuous with that covering the nasal meatus into which they drain, facilitating clearance of mucus into the nose by way of the mucociliary escalator. Their function remains unclear, both vocal resonance and facilitating craniofacial enlargement have been postulated.

Frontal sinus

The frontal sinuses are paired structures lying between the outer and inner tables of the frontal bone. They are typically asymmetrical; the septum between them usually deviates from the median plane and the parts extending into the frontal bone and medial orbital roof vary in size.

Structure
- Underlies a triangular area formed by the nasion, a point 3 cm superior to the nasion, and the junction between the medial one-third and lateral two-thirds of the supraorbital margin.
- Extends superiorly above the medial brow.
- Extends posteriorly to the medial orbital roof, and occasionally to the lesser wing of the sphenoid.
- Aperture opens into the middle meatus via the ethmoidal infundibulum or an elongated frontonasal duct (Fig. 13.26).

Neurovascular supply
- Arterial supply by supraorbital and anterior ethmoidal arteries.
- Venous drainage into an anastomotic vein connecting the supraorbital and superior ophthalmic veins.
- Lymphatic drainage to the submandibular nodes.
- Innervation from the supraorbital branches of the ophthalmic nerve (V_1).

Frontal sinus fractures
Overview
Frontal sinus fractures result from blunt trauma, either in isolation or alongside additional facial fractures and intracranial injury. They may be complicated by cosmetic deficit, CSF leak, and intracranial infection including sinusitis, mucocele, mucopyocele, osteomyelitis, and cerebral abscess.

Classification
Fractures involving the frontal sinus may be classified as those involving the anterior wall only, posterior wall, floor (is the frontonasal duct involved?), or combinations of these.

Management
Management is broadly directed at addressing any contour/cosmetic defects and making the sinus 'safe', i.e. reducing the risk of lifetime ascending infection if there is direct communication between the outside world and the intracranial cavity via the frontonasal duct. Procedures include obliteration of the frontal sinus with sealing of the frontonasal duct and cranialization.

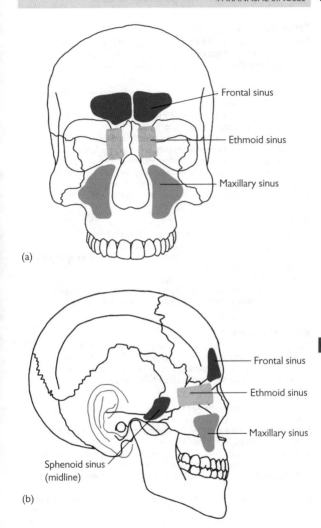

(a)

(b)

Fig. 13.25 The approximate positions of the paranasal sinuses, (a) anteroposterior and (b) lateral views.

Reproduced courtesy of Daniel R. van Gijn.

Sphenoid sinus

Two large irregular cavities within the body of the sphenoid, located posterior to the upper nasal cavity. They are in close proximity to the optic canals, occasionally encircling them reflecting variable pneumatization.

Structure

- The optic canals, ICAs, and cavernous sinus lie adjacent to the lateral wall of each sinus.
- Related to the optic chiasm and hypophysis cerebri superiorly.
- The pterygoid canal lies at the floor of each sinus.
- A lateral recess may extend into the greater and lesser wings of the sphenoid or the pterygoid processes, and may invade the basilar part of the occipital bone almost to the foramen magnum.
- Anterior midline septum often deviated to one side posteriorly; identification is important in trans-sphenoidal surgery.
- The aperture for the sinus is high on the anterior wall in the sphenoethmoidal recess (Fig. 13.26).

Neurovascular supply

- Arterial supply from the posterior ethmoidal branch of the ophthalmic artery and nasal branch of the sphenopalatine artery.
- Venous drainage is via the posterior ethmoidal vein draining into the superior ophthalmic vein.
- Lymphatic drainage is to retropharyngeal nodes.
- General sensation is mediated by the posterior ethmoidal nerves. Parasympathetic secretomotor fibres run in orbital branches of the pterygopalatine ganglion.

Ethmoidal sinus

Multiple small, thin-walled sinuses between the upper nasal cavity and orbit on each side, within the ethmoidal labyrinth. The openings into the nasal cavity can be highly variable and are divided into anterior and posterior groups separated by the basal lamella of the middle concha.

Structure

- Boundary formed by the frontal, maxillary, lacrimal, sphenoid, and palatine bones.
- Separated from the orbit by the paper-thin lamina papyracea (which is a poor barrier to infection and force).
- *Anterior group*—composed of anterior and middle ethmoidal air cells. Anterior air cells open into ethmoidal infundibulum or frontonasal duct. Middle air cells open into middle meatus by the ethmoidal bulla (Fig. 13.26).
- *Posterior group*—lies close to optic nerve and canal. Open into superior meatus and occasionally sphenoid sinus. *Onodi cells* refer to extension of this group into the anterior clinoid process and involving the optic canal, resulting in catastrophe to the misguided ENT surgeon or in the face of infection.

Neurovascular supply

- Arterial supply from nasal branches of the sphenopalatine artery and anterior and posterior ethmoidal branches of the ophthalmic artery.
- Venous drainage to corresponding veins.

- Lymphatic drainage is to submandibular nodes (from anterior group) and to retropharyngeal nodes (posterior group).
- General sensation is mediated by the anterior and posterior ethmoidal branches of the ophthalmic nerve.
- Parasympathetic secretomotor fibres run in orbital branches of the pterygopalatine ganglion.

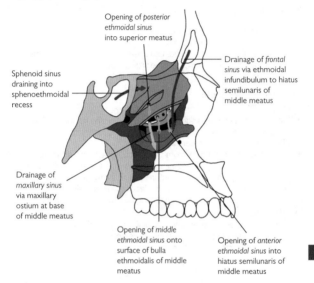

Opening of *posterior ethmoidal sinus* into superior meatus

Drainage of *frontal sinus* via ethmoidal infundibulum to hiatus semilunaris of middle meatus

Sphenoid sinus draining into sphenoethmoidal recess

Drainage of *maxillary sinus* via maxillary ostium at base of middle meatus

Opening of *middle ethmoidal sinus* onto surface of bulla ethmoidalis of middle meatus

Opening of *anterior ethmoidal sinus* into hiatus semilunaris of middle meatus

Fig. 13.26 Overview of the drainage of the paranasal sinuses.
Reproduced courtesy of Daniel R. van Gijn.

Maxillary sinus (antrum of Highmore)

The paired maxillary sinuses are the largest paranasal sinuses. Each is pyramidal in shape, located within the body of the maxilla and drains into the middle meatus via the hiatus semilunaris. Tumours or infection may pass through the thin walls of the sinus, leading to pathology in the orbit, nose, infratemporal fossa or mouth.

Structure
- Base is medial and forms most of the lateral wall of the nasal cavity.
- Floor is the alveolar process and part of the palatine process of the maxilla and is related to the roots of the maxillary teeth.
- Roof forms a major part of the floor of the orbit and is ridged by the infraorbital canal.
- Lateral wall extends as an apex into the zygomatic process.
- Medial wall is deficient posterosuperiorly at the maxillary hiatus.
- Anterior wall is the facial part of the maxilla.

- Posterior wall is the infratemporal aspect of the maxilla. It transmits the posterior superior alveolar nerves and vessels to the molar teeth.
- The ostium of the maxillary sinus is located at the junction of the roof and medial wall of the sinus

Neurovascular supply
- Arterial supply from maxillary, infraorbital, and greater palatine arteries.
- Corresponding veins drain to the facial vein or the pterygoid venous plexus.
- Lymphatic drainage is to submandibular nodes.
- General sensation is mediated by the maxillary nerve via the infraorbital nerves and the anterior, middle, and posterior superior alveolar nerves.
- Parasympathetic secretomotor fibres run in nasal branches of the pterygopalatine ganglion.

Ostiomeatal complex
See Fig. 13.27.
- Area bounded by the middle turbinate medially, the lamina papyracea laterally, and the basal lamellae superiorly and posteriorly.
- Inferior and anterior borders are open.
- The final drainage pathway from the frontal, sphenoidal, ethmoidal, and maxillary sinuses into the middle meatus. It is composed of the ostium of the maxillary sinus, ethmoid infundibulum, hiatus semilunaris and frontal recess. Persistent obstruction leads to chronic sinusitis.

> **Etymology**
> - *Sinus*—Latin for curve or hollow in land or bay/gulf.
> - *Antrum*—meaning a cave or cavity of the body.

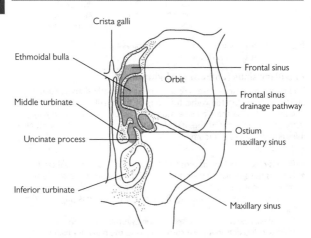

Fig. 13.27 Ostiomeatal complex (area shaded yellow).
Reproduced courtesy of Daniel R. van Gijn.

'I wish to take away that part of the bone, the support of the cheek and to show through the opening revealed the breadth and depth of the two cavities that hide behind it. In the cavity above is hidden the eye, the instrument of sight, and in that below is the humour which nourishes the roots of the teeth.'

(Leonardo da Vinci (1452–1519)—classical sections of the head)

Despite da Vinci's description of the maxillary sinus, it is customary to credit Nathanial Highmore (1613–1685) with the first description of the maxillary sinus—hence the 'antrum of Highmore'. Galen (130–201 AD) perhaps alluded to the paranasal sinuses (albeit in animals) when mentioning 'the porosity of bones'—although it was Emil Zuckerkandl's Normale und pathologische Anatomie der Nasenhöhle und ihrer pneumatischen Anhäge published in 1882 that provided a very complete description of the nasal cavity and paranasal sinuses (interestingly overlooking the ethmoidal and sphenoidal sinuses).

Maxillary tumours

Malignancy of the paranasal sinuses is uncommon, comprising 3% of all head and neck cancers. More than half are located in the maxillary antrum, and the majority are SCCs. Maxillary tumours may present late, and are first noted when local structures are invaded, producing symptoms. A knowledge of local anatomy indicates areas of invasion, which may initially be the thin anterior and posterior walls:

• Erosion through posterior wall into pterygopalatine fossa, with involvement of the maxillary artery causing epistaxis.
• Numbness of cheek—involvement of infraorbital nerve.
• Invasion into nose—obstruction, discharge, or pain.
• Dental symptoms—palpable mass, pain, fistula, or loose teeth.
• Orbital floor is more resistant to direct invasion, but involvement can cause pain, proptosis, epiphora, or impaired vision.

Sinusitis

Obstruction in the sinuses may lead to stasis of secretions, inflammation, and subsequent infection. Aetiology includes polyps, tumours, rhinitis, upper respiratory tract infections, and abnormal mucociliary function, such as cystic fibrosis. Sinusitis can be classified as acute, chronic, or fungal.

Acute sinusitis most commonly affects the maxillary sinus and presents as mid-facial pain and pyrexia, and pus may be seen at the middle meatus. Secondary infection with *Streptococcus pneumoniae* or *Haemophilus influenzae* may occur. Treatment with broad-spectrum antibiotics and a decongestant such as pseudo-ephedrine is first line. Chronic sinusitis persists for weeks to months and has similar first-line treatment. Granulation tissue, ulceration, and mucosal thickening may all develop. Intractable cases may necessitate functional endoscopic sinus surgery or open sinus surgery.

Allergic fungal sinusitis is associated with nasal polyps and asthma and is treated with steroids and itraconazole. Immunosuppressed patients may develop invasive fungal sinusitis requiring debridement, while chronic disease is most commonly secondary to aspergillosis and also necessitates debridement.

Intracranial extension of sinus infection is a life-threatening complication. Mechanisms of spread are:
- Direct spread (commonest).
- Haematogenous (insidious).
- Via cribriform plate of ethmoid bone.
- Perineural spread via cranial nerves.

The ear

Introduction

The delicate yet definitive deflections of the auricle (pinna) of the external ear contribute to the collection of sound. The external acoustic meatus is responsible for the transmission of sounds to the tympanic membrane, which in turn separates the external ear from the middle ear.

The middle ear is an air-filled, mucous membrane-lined space in the petrous temporal bone. It is separated from the inner ear by the medial wall of the tympanic cavity, bridged by the trio of ossicles.

The inner ear refers to the bony and membranous labyrinths and their respective contents. The osseous labyrinth lies within the petrous temporal bone. It consists of the cochlea anteriorly, semicircular canals posterosuperiorly, and intervening vestibule, the entrance hall to the inner ear, whose lateral wall bears the oval window occupied by the footplate of the stapes.

External ear

Auricle

The auricle is a predominantly cartilaginous projection on the side of the face, set at an angle of approximately 30°. Its elastic cartilage (0.5–2 mm) is continuous with the cartilage of the external acoustic meatus. The lobule of the ear is devoid of cartilage and is composed of fibrofatty tissue. The elevations on the cranial/posterior aspect of the auricle are named to correspond with depressions on their lateral surfaces, with the prefix 'eminentia'.

Features

See Fig. 14.1.

- The skin of the auricle is thin and firmly attached to the underlying cartilage. It contains minimal subcutaneous fat and numerous ceruminous glands (secrete cerumen or wax).
- *Helix*—posterior curved rim of auricle (free margin).
- *Antihelix*— ridge parallel to the antihelix. Leads to the forked crura superiorly that enclose the triangular fossa.
- *Triangular fossa*— depression between the two crura of the antihelix.
- *Scaphoid fossa*— depression between the helix and antihelix.
- *Concha (cymba and cavum)*—the deep 'shell' of the auricle. It is divided by the crus of the helix into the cymba conchae superiorly (overlying the suprameatal triangle of the temporal bone) and the cavum proper inferiorly.
- *Tragus*—the cartilaginous (often hairy) prominence that partly overlaps the meatus.
- *Antitragus*—tubercle on the lower antihelix, opposing the tragus.
- *Intertragic notch*—separates the tragus from the antitragus.
- *Lobule*—most inferior part of the auricle. Consists of fibro-fatty, soft, and non-cartilaginous tissue.
- *Ponticulus*—vertical ridge over the conchal eminence (cranial aspect). Attachment for auricularis posterior.
- *Fissures of Santorini*—inconsistent fatty-filled features of the tragal cartilage.

Etymology

- *Giovanni Domenico Santorini (1681–1737)*—Italian doctor and anatomist and author of *Observationes Anatomicae*. He lends his name to several other structures including *Santorini's vein* (prostatic venous plexus), *Santorini's duct* (accessory pancreatic duct), and *Santorini's cartilage* (corniculate cartilages, larynx).
- *Tragus*—from the Greek *tragos* meaning goat, in reference to the tuft of hair on a goat's chin and its resemblance to the ever-increasing hair that often grows on the tragus of older men.
- *Concha*—meaning large 'sea-shell'.
- *Cymba*—meaning 'cup' or 'bowl'.
- *Cavum*—meaning 'space'.

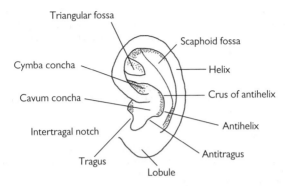

Fig. 14.1 Anatomy of the auricle.
Reproduced courtesy of Daniel R. van Gijn.

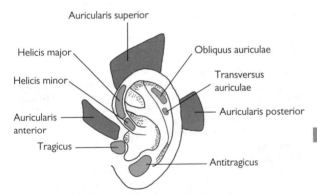

Fig. 14.2 The auricular muscles.
Reproduced courtesy of Daniel R. van Gijn.

Auricular muscles

The auricular muscles may be divided into extrinsic and intrinsic groups. The former connect the auricle to the scalp/skull and move the auricle as a whole. The latter connect the different parts of the auricle (Fig. 14.2). They receive a blood supply from the posterior auricular and superficial temporal arteries and they are innervated by temporal and posterior auricular branches of the facial nerve.

• *Extrinsic*—auricularis anterior, superior, and posterior.
• *Intrinsic*—helicis major and minor, tragicus, antitragicus, transversus auriculae, and obliquus auriculae.

Ligaments
Anterior, superior, and posterior ligaments connect the auricle to the zygo-matic process, external acoustic meatus, and mastoid process respectively.

Blood supply to auricle
See Fig. 14.3.
- *Posterior auricular artery* (ECA)—ascends between the auricular cartilage anteriorly and mastoid process posteriorly.
- *Superficial temporal artery*—provides anterior auricular branches to the lateral surface of the pinna.
- *Occipital artery branch.*

Nerve supply ('GALA')
The sensory innervation of the auricle is complicated, perhaps because the external ear represents an area where skin originally derived from a bran-chial region meets skin originally derived from a postbranchial region (Fig. 14.4). Nerves involved are:
- *Great auricular nerve*—supplies the cranial surface and posterior lateral surface of the helix, antihelix, and lobule.
- *Auricular branch of vagus nerve (Arnold's/Alderman's nerve)*—supplies the conchal bowl and posterior eminentia and communicates with cranial nerves VII and IX.
- *Lesser occipital nerve*—supplies the superior part of the cranial surface.
- *Auriculotemporal nerve*—supplies the tragus and the crus of the helix.

Great auricular nerve
The great auricular nerve originates from the cervical plexus (C2, C3) and provides sensation to the skin over the parotid gland, mastoid process, and outer ear. It is the most commonly injured nerve in facelift surgery and is encountered (and occasionally sacrificed/harvested) when raising subplatysmal flaps in neck dissection.

Surface markings
- Midpoint of the SCM.
- 6.5 cm below the external auditory meatus (McKinney's point, 1980).
- Parallel to the EJV which is 0.5 cm anterior at the same point.
- The *punctum nervosum* or nerve point of the neck is the point at the posterior border of the SCM where the four superficial branches of the cervical plexus emerge. Normally found at the junction of the upper and middle thirds of the SCM. It is erroneously used interchangeably with *Erb's point* (See 'Etymology and Erb's point' misnomer text box, Chapter 5)

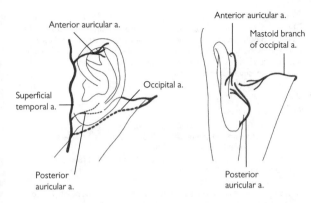

Fig. 14.3 Blood supply of the auricle (anterior and posterior).
Reproduced courtesy of Daniel R. van Gijn.

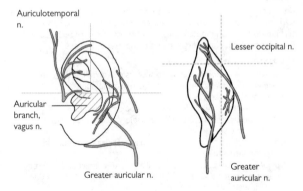

Fig. 14.4 Sensory nerve supply of the auricle (anterior and posterior).
Reproduced courtesy of Daniel R. van Gijn.

Microtia

There is a spectrum of ear deformities, from a small ear to complete absence (anotia), with or without atresia of the external auditory meatus and associated hearing deficit. Anomalies may occur in conjunction with other features of craniofacial macrosomia: deficiency in Orbital or Mandibular development (Ear anomaly), facial Nerve function or Soft tissue volume (OMENS classification scores the deformity in each of these five categories).

Management options

- *Prosthesis*—adhesive or osseointegrated.
- *Non-autologous reconstruction*—Medpor® implant as a single-stage reconstruction commonest.
- *Autologous reconstruction*—two-stage autologous technique using costal cartilage fixed to a base plate initially, with a second stage to release ear from the cranium for projection.
- In cases of atresia, hearing may be improved with a bone-anchored hearing aid; some centres offer ear canal reconstruction.

Prominent ears

Prevalence of 1–2%. Predominant deformities are an absent antihelical fold (conchoscaphal angle >90°) and/or a deep conchal bowl. Operative techniques focus on the deformity and consist of suture techniques, cartilage scoring, excisional surgery, or a combination of these.

Management options

- *Non-operative*—moulding may be successful within first 3 months of life when cartilage remains soft and malleable due to circulating maternal oestrogens.
- *Operative*—absent antihelical fold may be corrected by suture plication of cartilage or scoring; Gibson's principle states that cartilage folds away from the scored side.
- *Operative*—deep conchal bowl may have cartilage excised, with or without concha–mastoid sutures.
- *Operative*—prominent lobule is challenging to correct and may require an excisional technique from the lobule and mastoid skin to reduce its size, followed by plication to the cranium.

Pinnar haematoma and 'cauliflower ear'

An acute auricular (pinna) haematoma may follow blunt trauma to the external ear during contact sports such as rugby, boxing, and wrestling. Shearing of the perichondrium and associated vasculature causes separation from the underlying cartilage and results in a potential space for blood to accumulate. If left untreated, this can cause vascular compromise of the adjacent cartilage, resulting in the formation of neocartilage either side of the haematoma and the ensuing deformity known as 'cauliflower ear'.

Treatment options

- *Incision and drainage*—this involves making a linear incision through the skin overlying the haematoma to be drained, under local anaesthesia. The haematoma is evacuated and the space irrigated with normal saline.
- *Needle aspiration*—an 18-gauge needle or similar is used to aspirate the haematoma.

Following either incision and drainage or aspiration, a bolster needs to be placed (Fig. 14.5). This serves to close the dead space where the haematoma formed and ordinarily involves placing a dental roll parallel to the incision line either side of the ear, secured with mattress sutures. This can be removed 5–7 days following placement.

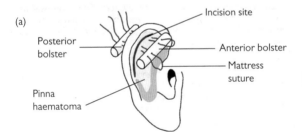

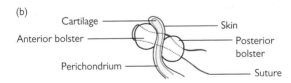

Fig. 14.5 (a) Drainage of a pinnar haematoma. (b) Cross-sectional view demonstrating 'through and through' bolster placement.

Reproduced courtesy of Daniel R. van Gijn.

External auditory canal

The external auditory canal is an S-shaped canal partly within the temporal bone, bridging the gap between the external auditory meatus and the tympanic membrane. It is short (approximately 2.5 cm from conchal floor to tympanic membrane). The lateral fibrocartilaginous one-third is continuous with the auricle while the medial two-thirds is formed by the bony margins of the temporal bone (Fig. 14.6).

Cartilaginous part

• Approximately 8 mm long.
• Continuous with auricular cartilage.
• Intimately related to the condylar process of the mandible, from which it is separated only by a slip of parotid tissue.

Osseous part

• 16 mm long.
• Formed by the squamous part of the temporal bone superiorly and the mastoid part of the temporal bone posteriorly.
• Anterior, inferior, and remaining posterior parts of the meatus are formed by the tympanic plate of the temporal bone.
• No subcutaneous tissue: the skin is directly opposed to periosteum and is continuous with the lateral surface of the tympanic membrane.
• Middle cranial fossa lies superiorly.
• *Foramen of Huschke*—dehiscence of the anteroinferior bony wall which is present in children younger than 4 years old and that may persist into adulthood. Provides a potential passage for the spread of infection from the meatus to parotid gland.

Blood supply

The principal blood supply is from branches of the ECA, including the:
• Posterior auricular artery.
• Deep auricular branch of the maxillary artery.
• Auricular branches of the superficial temporal artery.

Nerve supply (sensory)

• *Auriculotemporal branch of the mandibular nerve*—supplies the anterior and superior walls.
• *Auricular branch of vagus nerve*—supplies the posterior and inferior walls.

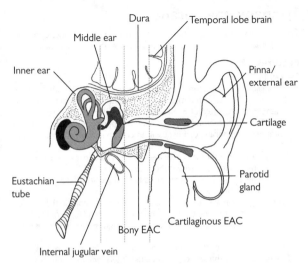

Fig. 14.6 The external, middle, and inner ear cavities and cartilaginous and bony ear canal, coronal section.

Reproduced courtesy of Daniel R. van Gijn.

Tympanic membrane

The tympanic membrane is the thin, semi-transparent, almost ovoid disc that separates the external acoustic meatus from the tympanic cavity.

Features

See Fig. 14.7.

* The anulus is the thickened edge of the pars tensa which is attached to the tympanic sulcus at the medial part of meatus. The anulus is deficient superiorly at the notch of Rivinus, where the pars flaccida is found.
* The tympanic membrane is divided into an upper (smaller) *pars flaccida* (Shrapnell's membrane or Rivinus' ligament) and a lower, larger and taut *pars tensa*.
* The tympanic membrane is concave laterally and convex medially. The point of maximum convexity is the *umbo*.
* The handle of the malleus is attached to the medial surface of the tympanic membrane.
* *Cone of light*—an area of reflected light seen in otoscopy in the antero-inferior quadrant of the tympanic membrane, extending from the umbo. It is generally a safe area for incisions and is 'lost' in middle ear infections.
* The tympanic membrane consists of an outer cuticular layer (continuous with the skin of the meatus), intermediate fibrous layer (the fibres radiate from the handle of the malleus), and an inner mucous layer.

Blood supply

The lateral aspect of the tympanic membrane is supplied by the vessels which supply the external auditory canal and are derived from the maxillary artery. The medial aspect is supplied by vessels bound for the middle ear.

* *Lateral surface*—deep auricular artery and its manubrial branch which runs along the handle of the malleus.
* *Medial surface*—anterior tympanic branch (maxillary artery); forms an inner peripheral vascular ring. *Stylomastoid branch* of the posterior auricular artery. (Fig. 14.8).

Nerve supply

See Fig. 14.9.

* *Lateral surface*—auriculotemporal branch (V_3), auricular branch of X (*Arnold's nerve*), and branches of VII, IX, and X.
* *Medial surface*—tympanic plexus (VII and IX) and branches of the chorda tympani nerve (VII).

Etymology

* *Augustus Quirinus Rivinus (1652–1723)*—German physician, botanist, and anatomist. Lends his name to the eponymous ducts of Rivinus, the collective name for the minor sublingual salivary ducts.
* *Umbo*—from the Latin for 'boss of shield' or knob/projection.
* *Henry James Shrapnell (1792–1834)*—English anatomist and first to describe the tympanic membrane. Not to be confused with Lieutenant General Henry Shrapnel (1761–1842), a British Army officer who lends his name to shrapnel, the fragmentation of artillery shells.

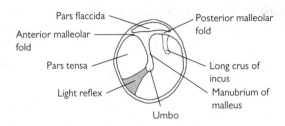

Fig. 14.7 Right tympanic membrane, lateral view.
Reproduced courtesy of Daniel R. van Gijn.

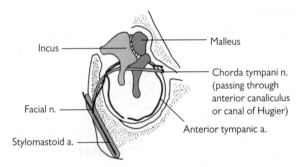

Fig. 14.8 Right tympanic membrane, internal aspect.
Reproduced courtesy of Daniel R. van Gijn.

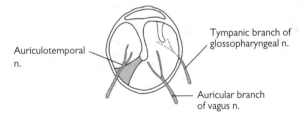

Fig. 14.9 Nerve supply to the tympanic membrane.
Reproduced courtesy of Daniel R. van Gijn.

Middle ear (tympanic cavity)

The complex anatomy of the middle ear can be conveniently considered as a narrow box with six walls, subdivided into the mesotympanum, epitympanum, and hypotympanum (Fig. 14.10).

- *Mesotympanum*—the main compartment of the tympanic cavity and the space directly medial to the tympanic membrane.
- *Epitympanum (attic/epitympanic recess)*—the space superior to the tympanic membrane, continuous with the mastoid air cells posteriorly via the aditus and antrum. It contains the head of the malleus and short process and body of the incus (Figs. 14.11 and Fig. 14.12). The *Prussak space* lies laterally (cholesteatoma typically begins here).
- *Hypotympanum*—a shallow depression below the membrane from which the pharyngotympanic (Eustachian) tube arises.

Boundaries

See Fig. 14.13 and Fig. 14.14.

- *Roof (tegmental)*—the thin tegmen tympani of the petrous temporal bone separates the dura of the middle cranial fossa from the middle ear.
- *Floor (jugular)*—thin, convex plate of bone which separates the middle ear from the superior bulb of the IJV (bony dehiscence possible). The tympanic branch of IX (Jacobsen's nerve) passes through the inferior tympanic canaliculus near the medial wall.
- *Lateral (membranous) wall*—principally the tympanic membrane. The lateral bony wall of the epitympanic recess contributes superiorly.
- *Medial (labyrinthine) wall*—separates the tympanic cavity from the inner ear. Features include the promontory (bulge) of the first turn of the cochlea, the oval (*fenestra ovalis/vestibuli*) and round (*fenestra rotunda*) windows, and the facial prominence.
- *Posterior (mastoid) wall*—features are the aditus (opening) of the mastoid antrum connecting the mastoid air cells and epitympanic recess. Medial to the aditus, the facial (nerve) canal descends between the posterior wall and antrum. The convex bulge of the lateral semicircular canal lies below the aditus on its medial wall.
- *Anterior (carotid) wall*—separates the tympanic cavity from the carotid canal. The opening of the osseous part of the pharyngotympanic (Eustachian) tube lies above and the canal for the tensor tympani below. Perforations are present for the caroticotympanic nerves and tympanic branch of the ICA.

Contents

The principal feature of the middle ear is the chain of three auditory ossicles, the malleus, incus, and stapes (Fig. 14.11 and Fig. 14.12). They transmit sound vibrations from the malleus at the tympanic membrane via the intervening incus, to the footplate of the stapes at the oval window. This delicate arrangement is intricately supported by five ossicular ligaments, with movement moderated by two intratympanic muscles, tensor tympani and stapedius.

- *Malleus (hammer)*—the largest ossicle, measuring 9 mm in length. It consists of a head which articulates with the incus at a cartilaginous facet, a neck, a manubrium, and anterior and lateral processes. The manubrium is attached to the upper part of the tympanic membrane and the tympanic sulcus.

- *Incus (anvil)*—consists of a cuboidal body (situated in the epitympanum) and long, short, and lenticular processes. Articulates at a saddle-shaped synovial joint with the head of the malleus and at a ball and socket synovial joint with the stapes.
- *Stapes (stirrup)*—consists of a head (articulates with the lenticular process of the incus), a neck (to which stapedius tendon is attached), two limbs (crura or processes) and a footplate which is attached to the margin of the fenestra vestibuli by an anular ligament.
- *Ligaments*—connect the ossicles to the tympanic walls: three for the malleus, one each for the incus and stapes.
- *Tensor tympani*—arises from the cartilaginous part of the pharyngotympanic tube, the greater wing of the sphenoid, and the petrous temporal bone. Attached to the handle of the malleus, where its tendon pulls the handle medially, tensing the tympanic membrane and damping (reducing) its oscillations. Innervated by the nerve to medial pterygoid (V_3).
- *Stapedius*—arises from the pyramidal eminence on the posterior wall of the tympanic cavity and inserts onto the posterior neck of the stapes. It acts to dampen vibrations passed to the cochlea via the fenestra vestibuli. Innervated by the stapedial branch of the facial nerve (paralysis leads to hyperacusis).

Chronic suppurative otitis media

Chronic inflammation of the middle ear and mastoid cavity, presenting with ear discharge and tympanic membrane perforation. The spread of infection will follow the path of least resistance and involve any of or a combination of walls of the tympanic cavity resulting in characteristic clinical signs:

- *Mastoiditis/mastoid abscess*—posterior wall spread via the aditus.
- *Temporal lobe abscess/meningitis*—if the thin tegmen tympani is breached superiorly.
- *Facial nerve palsy (lower motor neurone)*—if the thin facial canal medial to the aditus is breached.
- *Venous thrombosis (sigmoid or transverse)*—if infection spreads inferiorly through the convex plate of bone separating the middle ear from the superior bulb of the internal jugular vein.
- *Labyrinthitis*—if the infection spreads through the medial labyrinthine wall, resulting in vertigo and vomiting.

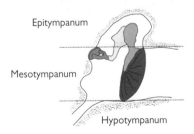

Fig. 14.10 The middle ear cavity, overview.
Reproduced courtesy of Daniel R. van Gijn.

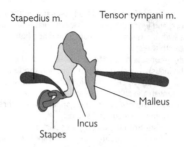

Fig. 14.11 The ossicles and muscles of the middle ear, overview.
Reproduced courtesy of Daniel R. van Gijn.

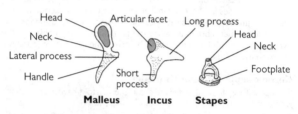

Fig. 14.12 The auditory ossicles.
Reproduced courtesy of Daniel R. van Gijn.

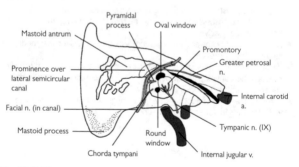

Fig. 14.13 The tympanic cavity, lateral view.
Reproduced courtesy of Daniel R. van Gijn.

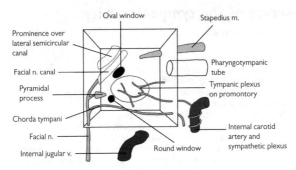

Fig. 14.14 The tympanic cavity, lateral view schematic.
Reproduced courtesy of Daniel R. van Gijn.

Nerves of the tympanic cavity

Tympanic plexus

See Fig. 14.15.

- The tympanic plexus of nerves is formed from the tympanic branch of the glossopharyngeal nerve and caroticotympanic nerves from the sympathetic plexus surrounding the ICA.
- Supplies the mucosa of the tympanic cavity, pharyngotympanic tube, and the mastoid air cells.
- Situated on the surface of the promontory.
- Branches are the lesser petrosal nerve (considered a continuation of the tympanic branch of the glossopharyngeal nerve), a deep branch that joins the greater petrosal nerve, and branches to the tympanic cavity.
- *Lesser petrosal nerve*—arises from the tympanic plexus and passes into the middle cranial fossa through the hiatus for the lesser petrosal nerve on the anterior surface of the petrous temporal bone. Exits the skull through the *canaliculus innominatus* to join the otic ganglion. Postganglionic parasympathetic secretomotor fibres travel with the auriculotemporal nerve to the parotid gland.

Facial nerve

The labyrinthine segment of the facial nerve runs from the fundus of the internal acoustic meatus to the geniculate ganglion, where the nerve makes its first bend/genu (knee). The shortest, narrowest part of the facial nerve, it lacks anastomosing arterial cascades, and so is susceptible to vascular compression. The tympanic segment curves around the oval window niche, then lies just anterior and inferior to the lateral semicircular canal. It bends at a second genu to become the mastoid segment which runs from the pyramidal process to the stylomastoid foramen. Its branches within the temporal bone arise from either the geniculate ganglion housed with the first genu, or from within the facial canal:

Branches from the geniculate ganglion

- *Greater (superficial) petrosal nerve*—a branch of the nervus intermedius containing parasympathetics destined for the pterygopalatine ganglion. It enters the middle cranial fossa through a hiatus on the anterior surface of the petrous temporal bone and is joined by the deep petrosal nerve (from the internal carotid sympathetic plexus) at the foramen lacerum to become the nerve of the pterygoid canal (vidian nerve).

Branches within the facial canal

- *Nerve to stapedius*—arises from behind the pyramidal eminence on the posterior wall of the tympanic cavity and supplies stapedius.
- *Chorda tympani*—enters the tympanic cavity through the posterior canaliculus; passes between the mucous and fibrous layers of the tympanic membrane, medial to the handle of the malleus, then along the anterior wall of the middle ear and through the anterior canaliculus before exiting the skull through the petrotympanic fissure.

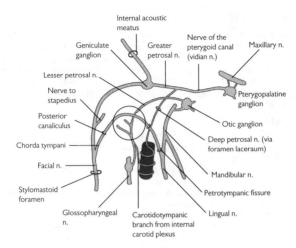

Fig. 14.15 Nerves of the tympanic cavity and contributions to the tympanic plexus (black circle).

Reproduced courtesy of Daniel R. van Gijn.

Etymology

- *Vidus Vidius (1509–1569)*—Italian surgeon and anatomist. Lends his name to the pterygoid canal (or vidian canal) inferomedial to the foramen rotundum and in turn the nerve that traverses it.

Tympanic neurectomy

The term 'tympanic neurectomy' was first coined by Golding-Wood in 1962 to describe the sectioning of the tympanic plexus for the treatment of aberrant/excessive saliva production (including Frey syndrome, crocodile tears, parotitis, salivary fistula, and drooling) and aural pain.

Inner ear

The inner ear refers to the bony and membranous labyrinths and their respective contents. The *osseous* labyrinth lies within the petrous temporal bone. It consists of the cochlea anteriorly, semicircular canals posterosuperiorly, and intervening vestibule. The *membranous* labyrinth is a closed system containing *endolymph* (surrounded by *perilymph*) which communicates with the subarachnoid space via the aqueduct of the cochlea (Fig. 14.16).

Cochlea

The anterior-most readily identifiable part of the osseous labyrinth—measuring 5 mm tall, 35 mm long, and 9 mm wide at its base. It consists of the following key features:

- *Modiolus*—the central axis of porous bone through which the canal of the cochlea spirals two and a half times around.
- *Osseous spiral lamina*—the bony ledge projecting from the modiolus into the canal, akin to a corkscrew.
- *Cochlear duct (scala media)*—membranous structure attached to the modiolus and inner cochlea wall. It is filled with endolymph and lies between the scala vestibuli above and scala tympani below.
- *Scala vestibuli*—perilymph-filled superior-most duct of the cochlea. It is separated from the cochlear duct by Reissner's vestibular membrane.
- *Scala tympani*—perilymph-filled inferior-most duct of the cochlea. It is separated from the cochlear duct by the spiral lamina.
- *Helicotrema*—the termination of the spiral lamina where the scala vestibuli and tympani meet.

Semicircular canals

The three interconnected semicircular canals lie in the petrous part of the temporal bone and are termed *superior*, *posterior*, and *lateral*. The former two are in the vertical plane while the latter is at 30° to the horizontal (Fig. 14.17).

- Each forms two-thirds of a circle lying approximately perpendicular to one another.
- Each contains the membranous endolymph-filled semicircular duct—forming approximately one-quarter of the diameter of the semicircular canal. Perilymph occupies the remainder.
- The lateral end of each canal dilates to form an ampulla.
- The ampulla houses an ampullary crest. Along the free edge of this lies the *cupula*—which detects endolymph movement via its stereocilia.
- Involved in detecting angular accelerations including head tilting and turning.

Vestibule

The central chamber of the bony labyrinth, measuring approximately 4 mm. It is the 'entrance hall' to the inner ear. Its lateral wall bears the oval window that is occupied by the footplate of the stapes. Its principal features are depressions and perforations that house/transmit the following features (Fig. 14.16 and Fig. 14.17):

- *Utricle (elliptical recess)*—lies on the medial wall in contact with the recessus ellipticus. It is paired with and communicates with the saccule via the utricosaccular duct. It bears the macula (a projection on its floor) which is the sensory organ of the utricle responsible for orientation, balance, and horizontal tilt. The utricle is supplied by the anterior vestibular artery (from the labyrinthine artery) and is innervated by the vestibulocochlear nerve.
- *Saccule (spherical recess)*—lies on the medial wall of the vestibule. It is a globular membranous sac, smaller than the utricle, vertically orientated. It communicates with the cochlea via the *ductus reuniens*. The saccular macula is sensitive to vertical acceleration. The saccule is supplied by anterior and posterior vestibular arteries and innervated by the inferior vestibular nerve (VIII).
- *Endolymphatic duct and sac*—formed from an extension of the utricular and saccular ducts. Runs within the osseous vestibular aqueduct, terminating as the blind-ending endolymphatic sac on the posterior aspect of the petrous temporal bone, where it is in contact with the dura.

Internal acoustic meatus

Overview

The internal acoustic meatus is a bony canal that runs 1 cm laterally within the petrous part of the temporal bone. It contains the facial nerve, nervus intermedius, vestibulocochlear nerve, vestibular ganglion, and labyrinthine artery (Fig. 14.18).

Features

- *Porus acusticus*—opening of the internal acoustic meatus found near the posterior surface of temporal bone.
- *Falciform crest*—a horizontal ridge that divides the internal acoustic meatus into superior and inferior portions.
- *Superior part*—facial nerve (anterior) and superior vestibular nerve (separated by *Bill's bar*).
- *Inferior part*—cochlear nerve (anterior trunk of VIII) and inferior vestibular nerve.

Etymology

- *Cochlea*—meaning 'snail' or 'screw'.
- *Vestibule*—meaning 'forecourt' or 'entrance'.
- *Scala*—meaning 'ladder' or 'staircase'.
- *Cupula*—the diminutive of cupa meaning 'cask' or 'barrel'.
- *William Fouts House (1923–2012)*—American otologist informally known as 'Dr Bill'.
- *Modiolus*—meaning 'hub of a wheel'.
- *Utricle*—Latin or French for '(little) leather bag'.
- *Saccule*—meaning 'small sac' or 'pouch'.
- *Falciform*—meaning 'like a sickle'.

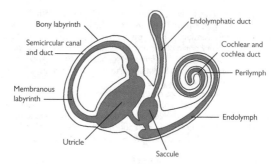

Fig. 14.16 Bony and membranous labyrinths.
Reproduced courtesy of Daniel R. van Gijn.

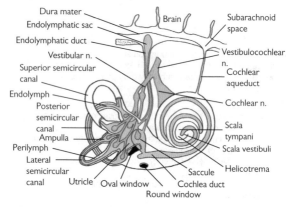

Fig. 14.17 Inner ear detail.
Reproduced courtesy of Daniel R. van Gijn.

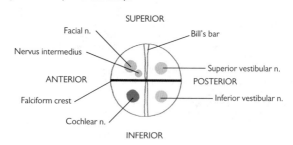

Fig. 14.18 The right internal acoustic meatus (internal view—within out).
Reproduced courtesy of Daniel R. van Gijn.

Embryology of the head and neck

Introduction

Development of the head is dominated by the changing shape of the brain and the formation of pharyngeal arches (Fig. 15.1) through which blood from the ventrally placed heart can pass to the dorsal aorta.

The origin of the cell population within the head and neck is important as it predicts the behaviour and attributes of the cells and their progeny. The nervous system in the head develops from:

- An epithelial neural plate which forms the CNS and motor nerves.
- Neural crest cells which form peripheral nervous system somatic sensory nerves and their nerve root ganglia containing first-order neurons; all the sympathetic and parasympathetic ganglia in the head and neck.
- Ectodermal placodes which invaginate later form specific ectodermal structures and contribute to the cranial nerve ganglia.

The neural crest also gives rise to an extensive mesenchymal population which contributes to the skull and enters and patterns the pharyngeal arches.

The *skull* (neurocranium) forms around the developing brain and its emerging nerves. The base of the skull forms initially in cartilage (endochondral ossification) and the vault forms from neural crest mesenchyme (intramembranous ossification).

The *face and jaws* (viscerocranium) form around the developing pharynx from a series of pharyngeal arches (numbered 1–6) which pass from the lateral sides of the pharynx to meet ventromedially (Table 15.1 and Figs. 15.2–15.5).

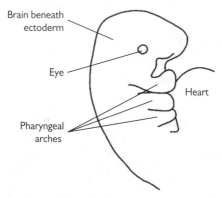

Fig. 15.1 Embryonic head showing pharyngeal arches touching heart, right lateral view.

Reproduced courtesy of Daniel R. van Gijn.

Table 15.1 Derivatives of the pharyngeal arches

No.	Arch name, named cartilage	Cartilage derivatives	Muscle derivatives	Nerve, associated foramina	Blood vessel
1	Mandibular Quadrate Meckel's	Incus Malleus Anterior ligament of malleus Spine of sphenoid Spheno mandibular ligament Genial tubercle of mandible	Tensor tympani Muscles of mastication Mylohyoid Anterior belly of digastric Tensor veli palatini	Trigeminal nerve (V_3) Foramen ovale	First arch artery (transitory)
2	Hyoid Reichert's	Stapes Styloid process Stylohyoid ligament Lesser horn Upper part of body of hyoid bone	Stapedius Stylohyoid 'Muscles of facial expression' Posterior belly of digastric Buccinator	Facial nerve (VII) Internal acoustic meatus Stylomastoid Foramen	Stapedial artery (transitory)
3	3rd arch	Greater horn Lower part of body of hyoid bone	Stylo pharyngeus	Glosso pharyngeal nerve (IX) Jugular foramen	CCA First part of ICA
4	4th arch	Thyroid cartilage Corniculate cartilage Cuneiform cartilage	Pharyngeal and extrinsic laryngeal muscles Levator veli palatine	Vagus nerve (X) pharyngeal branch Jugular foramen	Proximal subclavian artery—right Arch of aorta
6	6th arch	Arytenoid cartilages	Intrinsic laryngeal muscles	Vagus nerve (X) Recurrent laryngeal branch Jugular foramen	Disappears on right Ductus arteriosus on left

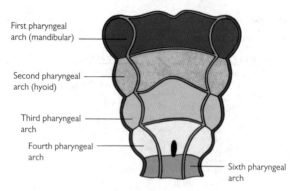

Fig. 15.2 Colour-coded pharyngeal arches.
Reproduced courtesy of Daniel R. van Gijn.

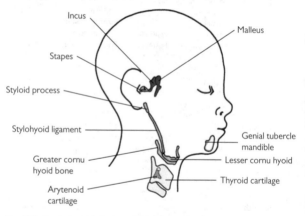

Fig. 15.3 Cartilaginous derivatives of the pharyngeal arches.
Reproduced courtesy of Daniel R. van Gijn.

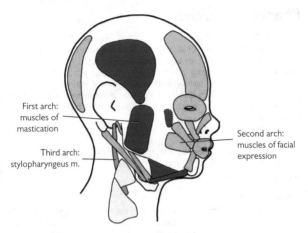

Fig. 15.4 Muscle derivatives of the pharyngeal arches.
Reproduced courtesy of Daniel R. van Gijn.

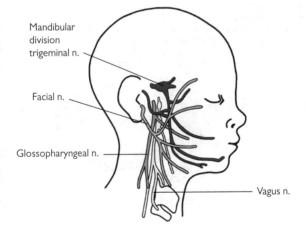

Fig. 15.5 Nervous derivatives of pharyngeal arches.
Reproduced courtesy of Daniel R. van Gijn.

Pharyngeal arches

Structure

Pharyngeal arches consist of an external epithelial ectoderm layer and an internal epithelial endoderm layer. They are separated by mesenchyme (primitive fibrocytes which make collagen, proteoglycans, and glycosaminoglycans). Between each arch the ectoderm and endoderm touch or are close—forming clefts externally and pouches internally (Table 15.2). Mesenchyme in each arch originates from neural crest which:

• Patterns the arch.
• Forms an arch cartilage.
• Forms the blood vessels.
• Provides connective tissue attachments for muscle and nerve which enters each arch.

See Figs. 15.6–15.8.

Development

Initially, the heart is immediately ventral to the first pharyngeal arches (➲ Fig. 15.1, p. 520). Vessels from the heart pass bilaterally through this arch to the dorsal aortae as the first arch arteries. As the more caudal arches develop, the heart descends and blood passes through relatively larger arch arteries; some arterial branches involute and do not retain a connection to the dorsal aorta.

• Third arch arteries form portions of the CCAs.
• Fourth arch arteries form the arch of the aorta on the left and the proximal part of the subclavian artery on the right.
• Sixth arch arteries form the ductus arteriosus on the left and involute on the right (pulmonary arteries remain on right and left).

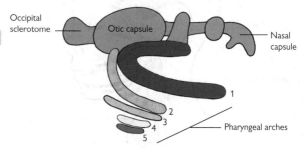

Fig. 15.6 Cartilaginous aspects of the base of the neurocranium and pharyngeal arches (lateral view).

Reproduced courtesy of Daniel R. van Gijn.

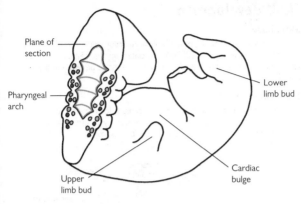

Fig. 15.7 Lateral view of embryo showing position of the pharyngeal arches.
Reproduced courtesy of Daniel R. van Gijn.

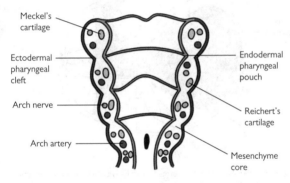

Fig. 15.8 Components of the pharyngeal arches, coronal section.
Reproduced courtesy of Daniel R. van Gijn.

Skull development

Skull base

Cranial nerves grow out from the brainstem accompanied by blood vessels. The relatively large nerves and their associated vessels create achondrogenic zones that form the skull base foramina between the developing skull bones (Fig. 15.9 and Fig. 15.10).

Skull calvaria

The roof and lateral walls of the neurocranium form by intramembranous ossification. The individual bones are separated by sutures that are foci for bone growth and that fuse at varying time points from the age of 3 months to 20 years of age.

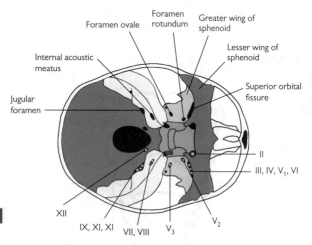

Fig. 15.9 Internal aspect of fully formed skull base with final positions of foramina and cranial nerves.

Reproduced courtesy of Daniel R. van Gijn.

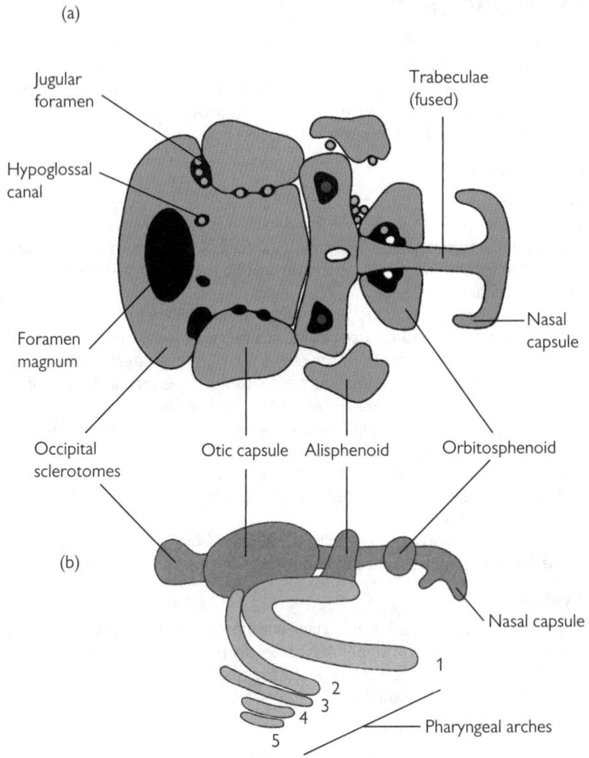

(a)

Jugular foramen

Trabeculae (fused)

Hypoglossal canal

Foramen magnum

Nasal capsule

Occipital sclerotomes

Otic capsule Alisphenoid Orbitosphenoid

(b)

Nasal capsule

1
2
3
4
5

Pharyngeal arches

Fig. 15.10 Elements of the cartilaginous skull base during development with cranial nerves between them (yellow). (b) Lateral view of the developing skull base and pharyngeal arches.

Reproduced courtesy of Daniel R. van Gijn.

Face, palate, and tongue

The face develops from the first pharyngeal arch and frontonasal process. The first arch is different from the other arches because it is C-shaped: it forms paired maxillary processes and paired mandibular processes (Fig. 15.11). The maxillary processes develop and grow medially beneath each eye to meet parts of the frontonasal process anteriorly.

Face proper

Contributions

- *Frontonasal process*—does not develop from a pharyngeal arch. Forms between ectoderm and forebrain. Olfactory placodes remain in contact with the forebrain and mesenchyme around them forms lateral and medial nasal processes.
- *Medial and lateral nasal processes*—fuse with maxillary processes in facial development. Failure to fuse results in a range of facial clefts.
- *Nasolacrimal duct*—maxillary processes fuse with the lateral nasal processes and a nasolacrimal duct extends from the medial border of each lower lid (lacrimal canaliculi) to the nasal cavity.
- *Nasal septum, nasal tip, and Cupid's bow*—formed by midline fusion of medial nasal processes.
- *Nasal alae*—formed by lateral nasal processes.
- *Mandible and lower lip*—paired mandibular processes grow medially, fusing in the midline.
- Progressive fusion of the maxillary and mandibular processes decreases the initial width of the mouth and forms the cheeks.

Eyelids

The eyelids form from folds of surface ectoderm containing a core of neural crest mesenchyme. The upper lids (from frontonasal process) and lower lids (from maxillary process) migrate together in the 3rd postmenstrual month and fuse at the tarsal plate.

Eyelashes and tarsal glands

- Develop from ectoderm/mesenchyme interactions.
- Lacrimal gland arises from a series of invaginations of ectoderm in the superior conjunctival fornix.
- Smooth muscle invades the upper eyelid together with striated muscle from the second arch.

Palate

See Fig. 15.12.

- *Primary palate and philtrum*—formed by medial nasal processes growing caudally and inserting between the lengthening maxillary processes. Failure of medial nasal processes to fuse with a maxillary process results in cleft lip.
- *Secondary palate*—medial portions of the maxillary processes form palatal shelves which grow towards the oropharyngeal floor. Initially vertically oriented, they demarcate the edges of the tongue.

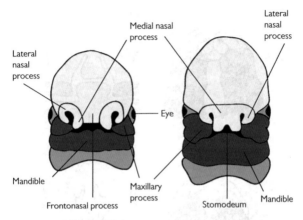

Fig. 15.11 Development of the face.
Reproduced courtesy of Daniel R. van Gijn.

- The edges of the palatal shelves later elevate and fuse across the midline from anterior to posterior to form the hard and soft palates. The process is delayed on the left side and in females, which may explain the higher incidence of isolated cleft palate on the left side and in females.
- Muscles from the first arch (tensor veli palatini) and fourth arch (levator veli palatini, palatoglossus, palatopharyngeus, musculus uvulae) migrate into the soft palate.

Tongue
See Fig. 15.13 and Fig. 15.14.
- When the edges of the palatal shelves extend to the floor of the oropharynx, they demarcate the surface of the tongue.
- The anterior two-thirds of the tongue form from the merging of two lateral lingual swellings and a median tongue bud (tuberculum impar), covered with ectodermal epithelium.
- Second arch endodermal epithelium forms the middle ear cavity and pharyngotympanic tube; it does not remain on the tongue surface.
- Third arch endodermal epithelium grows and joins with the first arch along a V-shaped line, the sulcus terminalis.
- Fourth arch forms the epiglottis.
- Intrinsic muscles of the tongue arise from occipital myotomes which migrate into the floor of the oropharynx together with their innervation from the hypoglossal nerve.

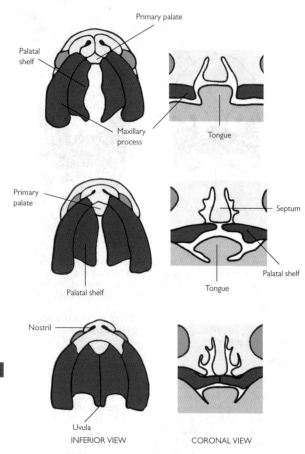

Fig. 15.12 Development of the palate at successive ages. Left column viewed from inferior aspect, right column coronal.

Reproduced courtesy of Daniel R. van Gijn.

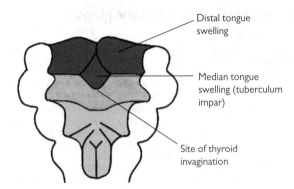

Fig. 15.13 Development of the pharyngeal floor and tongue.
Reproduced courtesy of Daniel R. van Gijn.

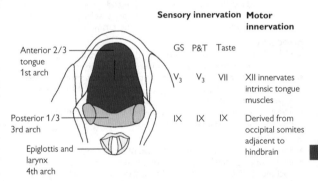

Fig. 15.14 Derivation and innervation of the tongue. Note that the second arch does not contribute to the surface of the tongue (GS: General sensation, P&T: Pain and temperature)
Reproduced courtesy of Daniel R. van Gijn.

Gums, teeth, and salivary glands

Gums and teeth

Initially, there is no distinction between the lip and gum in the upper and lower jaws. Mesenchymal swellings of the lower jaw form the gums and dental laminae, separated from the lip by a labiogingival sulcus and from the tongue by a linguogingival sulcus. For the upper jaw, the dental lamina remains attached to the palate and only a labiogingival sulcus forms.

Teeth form from ectodermal and mesenchymal interactions

- Locally, mesenchymal dental papillae induce the overlying ectoderm to form a series of enamel organs. Each forms a bell-shaped tooth bud.
- The dental papilla forms odontoblasts which produce dentine. The ectoderm forms ameloblasts which produce enamel.
- 20 tooth buds are formed (five in each jaw quadrant) with smaller precursor tooth buds for permanent teeth on the lingual side of the deciduous teeth.

Salivary glands

The salivary glands develop bilaterally from ectodermal and mesenchymal interactions in the oral cavity. Ectoderm forms solid diverticula which branch to form acini within the neural crest mesenchyme.

Parotid gland

- Forms from a groove and duct running dorsally from the angle of the mouth between the maxillary and mandibular processes.
- Connection to the oral cavity remains only at the ventral end (parotid duct), opening on the inside of the cheek at the level of the future upper second molar.
- The gland grows between the branches of the facial nerve; in the neonate it lies between the ear and masseter.

Submandibular gland

- Forms from the floor of the caudal part of the linguogingival groove.
- Initially opens at the lateral aspect of the tongue; the opening of the duct moves to become close to the median plane below the tip of the tongue.

Sublingual gland

- Forms from a number of small epithelial thickenings within and lateral to the linguogingival groove.
- Each thickening canalizes separately so multiple sublingual ducts open on the summit of the sublingual fold and some join the submandibular duct.

Thyroid gland

Overview

The thyroid gland arises as a midline thickening and invagination of epithelium in the floor of the pharynx, between the first and second pharyngeal pouches. A median thyroid diverticulum arises at the posterior part of the median tongue bud, the foramen caecum. It extends caudally as the thyroglossal duct, passing ventral to the developing hyoid bone. The thyroglossal duct bifurcates and the glandular tissue forms a medial isthmus and lateral lobes; the duct finally involutes (Fig. 15.15). Development of the thyroid gland is described in three chronological stages:

- 10–18 weeks—active formation of follicles and colloid accumulation.
- 19–29 weeks—gland is quiescent.
- 29 weeks onward—increase in epithelium/colloid ratio and decrease in follicle size.

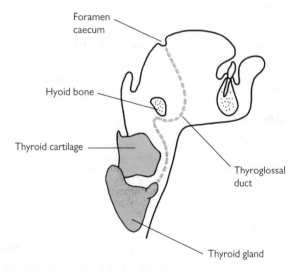

Fig. 15.15 Development of the thyroid gland.
Reproduced courtesy of Daniel R. van Gijn.

Thyroglossal duct cyst

- A fibrous cyst forms from a persistent thyroglossal duct.
- Generally midline, move upwards on protrusion of the tongue, explained by their developmental attachment to the tongue.
- Surgical treatment is by *Sistrunk's procedure*, which includes excision of the cyst and resection of the central part of the hyoid bone (Walter Sistrunk (1880–1933), American surgeon).

Development of the ear

Inner ear

Develops from an ectodermal otic placode adjacent to the second pharyngeal arch. See Fig. 15.16.

- Otic placode invaginates to form a fluid-filled otic vesicle.
- Outer cells become mechanosensory hair cells sensitive to the movement of the contained fluid.
- Sensitivity of the hair cells is modified by local addition of proteoglycan and glycosaminoglycans.
- Otic vesicle expands to form the membranous labyrinth (semicircular ducts, utricle, saccule, endolymphatic duct, and cochlea).
- Cochlea extends in a spiral fashion for 2.75 turns. The proximal connection to the saccule narrows to form the ductus reuniens.
- Otic vesicle is closely associated with branches of the vestibulocochlear nerve as it expands and changes shape to form the membranous labyrinth.

Labyrinth development

The entire membranous labyrinth becomes surrounded by an outer labyrinth of mesenchyme, which later differentiates into cartilage (otic capsule) and then bone (petrous part of temporal bone).

- Membranous labyrinth filled with endolymph (a fluid similar to CSF).
- Outer bony labyrinth contains perilymph (plasma filtrate with locally different electrolyte levels).

Middle ear

The cleft between the first and second arches stays close to the underlying first pouch. The tympanic membrane forms from the ectoderm and endoderm with an intervening layer of mesenchyme. See Fig. 15.16.

- Internally, the first pouch expands to form the tubotympanic recess which becomes the middle ear cavity.
- The connection to the nasopharynx narrows to form the pharyngotympanic (Eustachian, auditory) tube.
- The middle ear cavity expands around the developing ear ossicles.

External ear

The mesenchyme of the first and second arches proliferates around the first cleft; three auricular hillocks can be identified on each arch.

- *The first arch hillocks (1–3)*—give rise to the most medial part of the auricle: tragus, part of the concha, and crus of helix.
- *The second arch hillocks (4–6)*—form the majority of the auricle (the helix, lobule, anti-helix, and anti-tragus).
- The first cleft deepens, forming the external auditory meatus.

The caudal border of the second arch elongates, forming a flap of ectoderm and mesenchyme which grows caudally to attach to the pericardial bulge. It covers all of the lower pharyngeal clefts. Remaining spaces may enlarge as branchial cysts.

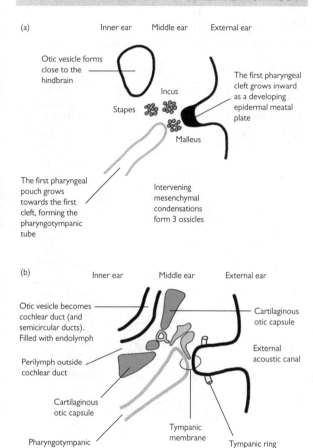

(a)

Inner ear   Middle ear   External ear

Otic vesicle forms close to the hindbrain

Incus

Stapes

Malleus

The first pharyngeal cleft grows inward as a developing epidermal meatal plate

The first pharyngeal pouch grows towards the first cleft, forming the pharyngotympanic tube

Intervening mesenchymal condensations form 3 ossicles

(b)

Inner ear   Middle ear   External ear

Otic vesicle becomes cochlear duct (and semicircular ducts). Filled with endolymph

Perilymph outside cochlear duct

Cartilaginous otic capsule

Pharyngotympanic (auditory) tube entrance

Cartilaginous otic capsule

External acoustic canal

Tympanic membrane

Tympanic ring around external acoustic canal

Fig. 15.16 (a) Early stage of ear development. (b) Later stage of ear development.
Reproduced courtesy of Daniel R. van Gijn.

Pharyngeal pouches

Table 15.2 lists the derivates of the pharyngeals pouches and clefts.

Table 15.2 Derivatives of the pharyngeal pouches and pharyngeal clefts

Between arches	Pouch	Develops into	Cleft	Develops into
1–2	First pouch	Tubotympanic recess forms tympanic cavity and pharyngotympanic tube invaded by lymphoid tissue (tubal tonsil) Lymphoid tissue also found on posterior part of tongue and in dorsal pharyngeal wall (adenoid or pharyngeal tonsil)	First cleft	Dorsal portion extends to form external acoustic meatus including outer surface of tympanic membrane and ceruminous glands
2–3	Second pouch	Palatine tonsil is invaded by lymphoid tissue		Second, third, and fourth pharyngeal clefts form part of cervical sinus Fusion of the caudal part of the hyoid arch with the hyoid elevation covers these clefts and the cervical sinus Platysma muscle migrates into the superficial fascia extending along the neck
3–4	Third pouch Dorsal and ventral parts	Ventral part forms thymus. Grows caudally to enter anterior mediastinum Dorsal part forms inferior parathyroid gland (parathyroid III) Joined to thymus initially and taken caudally as thymus descends		
4	Fourth pouch Dorsal and ventral parts	Dorsal part forms superior parathyroid gland (parathyroid IV) Contacts the lateral lobe of the thyroid gland Remains cranial to parathyroid III Caudal pharyngeal complex		

Glossary

Accessory From the Latin *accessio* meaning 'an approach'. Given as the name of the cranial part of the 11th cranial nerve by Thomas Willis in his *Cerebri Anatomie* (1664) owing to it being 'accessory' to the vagus nerve.

Alveolus From the Latin meaning 'a small tray or basin'. It was applied to a board game involving small engraved depressions to hold game markers such as pebbles and thus leant itself to mean any small compartment or cavity. Vesalius was the first to use it in the context of the socket of a tooth and, in turn, the alveolar components of the mandible and maxilla. Its reference to the alveoli of the lungs wasn't established until 300 years later.

Angina From the Latin verb *angere* meaning 'to choke or throttle', *angina* literally means 'sore throat'. A brawny, bilateral submandibular and sublingual cellulitis is Ludwig's angina (after the German surgeon Wilhelm von Ludwig, 1790–1865). *Angina pectoris* is perhaps its most well-known use, in reference to the crushing central chest pain characteristic of myocardial ischaemia.

Annulus A misspelling (according to the latest *Nomina Anatomica*) of the Latin *anulus* meaning 'a little ring', and diminutive of *anus*, which refers to a more substantially sized ring. The Latin *annus* refers to a calendar year, also a cyclical/circular event.

Aponeurosis In ancient Greek, there was no distinction between nervous structures and tendons. *Neuros* therefore collectively referred to all dense white strands with *apo-neurosis* meaning 'from a tendon' (in this case).

Arachnoid From the Greek meaning 'spider-like' referring to (in the context of this book) the delicate layer surrounding the brain and spinal cord. *Arachne* was a mythological maiden of Lydia, adept at weaving. On challenging the Goddess Athena, she was ultimately turned into a spider and hanged in her own web (details of this process differ according to source)—ultimately lending her name to all things spider related.

Arytenoid From the Greek meaning 'like a pitcher'—with its pyramidal shape resembling a ladle or cup.

Atlas Referring to the mythical titan condemned to carry the weight of the earth and celestial heavens on his shoulders. The atlas bone—or first cervical vertebra—bears the weight of the head in similar fashion. A 'compilation of maps' also owes its etymological origin to the adornment of the figure of Atlas bearing the globe on maps.

Autonomic From the Greek *auto-* and *nomos* literally meaning 'a law unto itself'. The autonomic nervous system was initially thought to function independently from higher control from the brain.

Buccal Of presumed dual origin: from the Hebrew *bukkah* meaning 'hollow' or empty' and the Latin *bucca* meaning both the physical/anatomical cheek and descriptive term for a 'loud-mouthed individual'. The Latin *buccina* means 'trumpet'. The buccinator muscle, integral to the blowing action required to play the trumpet, owes its name to this origin. Other associations include the word *buckle* which refers to the fastening of a helmet chin strap against one's cheek.

Bulbar In reference to the eye (as in *retrobulbar*), refers to *bulbus* meaning 'bulb shaped', especially resembling a medium-sized onion.

Calculus From the Latin for 'pebble' and possibly the diminutive of *calx* meaning 'limestone'. Salivary (among other) ducts may be blocked by pebble-like stones. The mathematical sense of the word (along with *calculate*) relates to the historic use of pebbles and stones in counting.

Capillary An amalgamation of the Latin *caput* (head) and *pilus* (hair), together meaning 'a hair of the head', referring to the extremely fine nature of capillary blood vessels. The use of *capillary* to describe the comparison is attributed to Leonardo da Vinci.

Caverna From the Latin for 'cavern' or 'cave'. With more specific regard to the cavernous sinuses, refers to the multiple venous caverns or channels that drain blood from the cranium.

Chyle From the Greek *chylos* meaning 'juice or fluid' referring to the milky consistency of the bodily fluid formed from lymph and emulsified fats from the digestion of fats in the small bowel.

Circulation From the Latin *circulare* meaning 'to make a circle'. The capillary link between the venous and arterial circulations was made by William Harvey (1578–1657) in *De Motu Cordis* (1628)—completing Galen's (131–201) initial work on the circulation of blood.

Clinic From the French *clinique* meaning 'at the bedside', itself from the Latin *kline* meaning 'a couch or bed'—principally referring to the medical management of patients conducted at the bedside. Derivations include *clinician* (a medically trained person tasked with the care of patients at the bedside) and the *clinoid processes*, that refer to the bony projections defining the pituitary fossa that resemble a four-poster bed.

Corrugator From the Latin *corrugare* meaning 'to wrinkle'. *Nares corrugare* was a term used by the Romans to describe the wrinkling of the nose in either distaste or disgust. In subtle contrast, the corrugator supercilii muscles, a common target of botulinum toxin injection, act to pull the eyebrows inferomedially, causing vertical wrinkles in the glabella region—in turn, making it less smooth than the word *glabella* suggests.

Debridement From the French word, consisting of *de* meaning 'not' and *brider* meaning 'bridle', together literally meaning 'unbridling'. Principally referring to its initial use in the process of cutting and dividing bands of tissue, debridement is now used more generally in the removal of injured or necrotic tissue.

Epiglottis Initially thought to be an extension or appendage of the tongue, hence its name *epi-* meaning 'upon' or 'in addition to' and *glotta* meaning 'tongue'.

Epistaxis From the Greek *stazein* meaning 'to let fall, drop by drop' or more specifically 'a dripping' (in this case, of blood from the nose).

Eye From the Teutonic *auge* referring to the organ of vision. Interestingly, the Norse *vindauga* (meaning 'wind-eye') became our 'window'.

Fascia From the Latin meaning 'a band or bandage' or 'a wisp of cloud'. Both likenesses may be seen anatomically, depending on location.

Fontanelle From the diminutive of the Latin *fontana* meaning 'a spring or fountain', perhaps referring to the pulsations felt at the fontanelles prior to their closure.

Frenulum From the diminutive of the Latine *frenum* meaning 'a bridle'. The lingual and labial frenum restrain their respective structures, acting as and resembling a bridle.

Ganglion From the Greek *ga[n]gglion* which was initially used for any small subcutaneous nodule and persists today in the description tendinous cysts of the wrist. Its most common current usage refers to nerve complexes— an association initially described by Galen owing to their appearance of 'small nodes'.

Gargle An onomatopoeic word along with the Greek *gargarizein* meaning 'to wash the throat'. 'Jargon' is a related word, initially from the French *jargon* meaning 'the chattering of birds' referring to the unintelligible sound arising from the throat.

Geniculate The diminutive of the Latin *genu* meaning 'knee'. The appearance of a 'little knee' has been applied to knotted or nodal structures with an acute bend, such as the geniculate ganglion of the facial nerve. *Genuflect*, meaning 'to bend the knee' or 'bow down' shares a common origin.

Gingiva From the Latin meaning 'gum of jaws', but perhaps derived from *gignere* meaning 'to bear or to produce' owing to the appearance of the teeth seemingly erupting from the gums.

Glabella From the Latin *glaber* meaning 'hairless or bald' referring to either/ both the bony smooth area of the frontal bone between the superciliary arches or to the (not always) smooth skin between the eyebrows. *Glaber* was an affectionate Roman nickname for a prepubescent slave. *Glabrous*, referring to skin devoid of hair such as the soles of the feet and palms of the hand, shares a common stem.

Gland From the Latin *glans* meaning 'a nut or acorn', which shares an association with *glans penis*. The Greek *adenos* was used in specific reference to lymph glands, derived from the word *adēn*, also meaning 'acorn'. Adeno- is now the common prefix used for glandular or gland-like containing structures, such as in *adenocarcinoma*.

Glenoid From the Greek *glēnēs* meaning 'eyeball' and *eidos*/*oid* meaning 'like'—possibly owing to the similarities between the bony concavity of the glenoid fossa and the orbit.

Incise/incisor/incisure From the Latin *incidere* meaning 'to carve or cut into'. An *incisor* is a tooth capable of achieving this and *incisura* describes a notch or cleft, as if the consequence of a cut.

Infection (bacteria/virus) From the Latin *inficere* meaning 'to dye or stain' or 'to corrupt or spoil', owing to the original (ancient) belief that disease could spread by the invasion of the body by invisible agents.

Integument From the Latin *integumentum* meaning 'a covering', and in this instance the organ of the skin. Related words include *tegmen* and *tectum* meaning 'to shelter to hide' such as the *tegman tympani*, the roof of the middle ear. The word *detective* derives from a common stem, describing someone who uncovers mysteries and problems.

Lagophthalmos From the Greek *lagōs* meaning 'hare', in reference to hares being born with their eyes open and in turn corresponding to the meaning of lagophthalmos being an inability to completely close the eyelids.

Lens From the Latin *lentis* referring to what we know as the lentil and describing the similarity in size and shape of the lentil bean to the lens of the eye. The Greek for the lentil bean is *phakos* which also lends itself to words pertaining to the lens, such as *aphakia* (the absence of the lens) and ophthalmological procedures such as *phacoemulsification*, a method used in modern cataract surgery.

Ligate From the Latine *ligare* meaning 'to bind or tie'. Associated words include *ligament* (integral in the binding together of two structures), *ligature* (a suture used as a tie), *obligation* (a course of action where one is morally or legally bound), and perhaps most interestingly, *religion*, which may also be view as a bond or pledge.

Lumen From the Latin meaning 'light', referring to the perception of light when viewing through a hollow viscus, opened space, or tubular structure—with the word ultimately describing that space rather than light itself.

Lymph From the Latin *lympha* meaning 'clear water', especially that from flowing springs. It is related to and influenced by the Greek *nymphē* meaning a bride. A nymph was thought to be a 'goddess of a spring', presiding over springs, lakes, and forests. The association with lymphatic vessels was the assumption that these presumed veins carried a watery fluid rather than blood.

Malar From the Latin meaning 'the cheekbone' or possibly related to *malum* meaning 'an apple', perhaps in reference to the similarity of a rosy, pronounced cheekbone to an apple.

Malignant From the Latin *malignus* meaning 'spiteful, mean, or malicious' or more literally, 'born to be bad' (from *mal-* meaning 'bad' and *gnatus sum* meaning 'to be born').

Masticate From the Greek *mastazein* meaning 'to chew or to gnash the teeth'. From this, comes *mastiche* which is the name for the resinous 'chewing' gum produced by the Mastic tree, traditionally found on the island of Chios. These 'tears of Chios' were first mentioned by Hippocrates. The Romans used *masticare* to specifically describe the chewing of this gum rather than *mandere* (also meaning to chew and the origin of 'mandible').

Mediastinum From the Latin *medius* meaning 'middle' and *stare* 'to stand' describing the position of the mediastinum 'standing in the middle' of the thorax. *Mediastinus* literally means 'a servant or drudge' perhaps owing the idea of a servant acting as an intermediary, standing in the middle.

Mental Refers to either 'the mind' from the Latin *mens* or from the Latin *mentum* meaning 'the chin'.

Migraine Derived originally from the Greek *hemi* meaning 'half' and *kranion* meaning 'the skull' referring to the characteristic of migraine (occasionally) producing a unilateral severe pain in the head. The Latin *hemicrania* was subsequently shortened to *migraena*.

Mucus From the Latin meaning 'a slimy discharge from the nose', with the Greek *mukter* meaning 'the nose or snout' (the colloquial 'snot', incidentally comes from 'snout' in direct association). 'Mucus' and 'mucous' are incorrectly used interchangeably—with the former more correctly being the noun and the latter, the adjective.

Mumps From the Icelandic *mumpa* meaning 'to eat greedily, to fill the mouth full' relating to the appearance of bilateral preauricular region parotid swelling mimicking a large mouthful. Interestingly, the word 'mumble' shares a common origin, possibly relating to the sound one would make were they to have a full mouth.

Nausea From the Greek *nausia* meaning 'seasickness', via the Greek *naus* meaning 'ship'. Related words include 'nautical' and 'navy'—the latter from the Latin *navis*.

Node/nodule From the Latin *nodus* meaning 'a knot or knob' referring to the characteristics of s subcutaneous lump or lymph node. The diminutive form *nodule* means 'little knot'.

Occlusion From the Latin *occludere* meaning 'to close or shut up' in reference to either the meeting of the mandibular and maxillary dental arches or the closure/blockage of a path.

Palpebral From the Latin *palpebra* which the Romans used to refer to the eyelid, itself from the Latin *palpitare* meaning 'to quiver', owing to the tendency of eyelids to flutter. A related word is 'palpitation'—the abnormality felt by a patient when the heart beats or flutters irregularly or strongly.

Papilla Latin for 'nipple or teat', derived from *pappare* meaning 'to consume pap in the manner of an infant'. While initially constrained to the description of the nipple of the female breast, the term *papilla* is now applied to all manner of nipple-like projections.

Patient From the Latin *patior* meaning 'to suffer'. The two principal uses of the term are as a noun ('a person who suffers') and an adjective ('to bear') and share a common origin.

Pedicle From the Latin *pediculus* (the diminutive of *pes or pedis*) meaning 'a little foot'—used to describe a stalk or stem and in turn, the attachment of organs. *Pediculus* was also used to describe the louse due to its many legs, and lends its name to the word *pediculosis* to describe a lice infestation.

Phrenic From the Greek *phrēn* meaning 'the mind or seat of reason' perhaps under the assumption that the diaphragm was the seat of all emotions given its proximity to the revered organs of the heart, liver, and spleen. *Phrenic* now refers to structures pertaining to the diaphragm such as the phrenic nerve. Words such as *frenetic*, *frenzy*, and *frantic* arise from a common stem.

Pinna Latin meaning 'feather or wing'.

Pituitary From the Latin *pituita* meaning 'phlegm' which refers to the ancient assumption that the brain secreted a mucoid substance through the nose—a process thought by Aristotle necessary to cool a hot temper. The attachment of the pituitary gland to the brain, termed the *infundibulum* by Vesalius, means 'funnel' and strengthens the aforementioned initial notions.

Ptosis Meaning 'falling' and relates to the Greek *piptein* meaning 'to fall down'. The term was (much) later applied to the drooping of the upper eyelid as a result of an oculomotor (third cranial nerve) palsy among other causes.

Pupil From the Latin *pupa* meaning 'a doll' presumably (and perhaps tenuously) in reference to the observation that when one looks closely enough into the pupil of another, one can see a miniature doll-like image of oneself. The Greek *korē* also means doll and lends itself to related words such as *anisocoria*—a condition in which the pupils are of different sizes.

Ranula The diminutive of the Latin *rana* meaning 'a frog' in reference to a swelling in the floor of the mouth (related to a mucus extravasation cyst of the sublingual glands) resembling the throat of a croaking frog.

Scalp From the Old Norse *skalp* meaning 'a sheath or husk' perhaps in reference to ability to peel the skin of the scalp (most freely in the subgaleal plane) from the underlying skull below. An opportunity most frequently utilized by the American Indians.

Scapula From the Greek *skaptein* meaning 'to dig' due to the resemblance of the broad, flat, and inferiorly pointed scapula to a trowel or spade.

Skeleton From the Greek *skeletos* meaning 'dried up, parched, or withered'. The term was probably initially applied to a mummy or withered corpse rather than referring specifically to the bony skeleton.

Skull Relates to the Nordic words *skal* or *skul* meaning 'bowl or shell' (given a presumed use of the skull as a receptacle) and shares a common origin with the Nordic toast *Skoal*.

Sphincter From the Greek *sphinktēr* meaning 'that which constricts'. The mythical Sphinx had the body of a lion, the head and breasts of a woman, and the wings of an eagle. The Sphinx would stand on top of a rock outside the city of Thebes and pose unanswerable riddles to travellers. Those who answered incorrectly were strangled, lending the name of the Sphinx to all things that constrict. The Sphinx was ultimately defeated by Oedipus and killed itself in anger, leaving Oedipus to take the throne of the dead king of Thebes.

Squamous From the Latin *squama* meaning 'the scale of the fish or serpent'. The squamous cells of the epidermis are thin, flat, and stratified in layers, resembling scales. Associated words include the *squamal* parts of the frontal, temporal, and occipital bones owing to their flat shape. *Desquamation* or shedding of the skin from *desquamare* was what the Romans used for 'scraping the scales of a fish'.

Stent A supporting device to either hold something in place or in the case of tubular stents, keep open stenotic lumens of tubular structures. Generally felt to originate from the English dentist Charles Thomas Stent (1807–1885), who made a plastic substance (later known as Stent's mass) used to take an impression of teeth to fabricate a dental prosthesis from when set. Stent's mass was used for various other purposes in maxillofacial surgery and beyond, with the term ultimately taking on its current usage.

Syringe From the Greek *syringx* meaning 'a shepherd' pipe', named after the Greek nymph, Syrinx. Syrinx was chased down to the river Ladon by Pan, the god of flocks, herds, and nature (and also, for similar reason lends his name to *panic*). Upon reaching the river, Syrinx transformed into a bunch of reeds. Pan, clutching the reeds in dismay, let out a great sigh creating a tone across the reeds, acting as a pipe. Syrinx, in turn and as a consequence of her transformation into reeds, lent her name to all things tubular.

Temple The origins of the word *temple* are unclear. One possibility is from the Greek *temnein* meaning to 'wound or maim in battle'—owing to the vulnerability of the region to injury due to the thinness of the bones in the region and the underling middle meningeal artery at the *pterion*. Another suggestion is that the appearance of visible, pulsating (superficial temporal) vessels in the region provides an indication of one's *temperament*.

Trachea From the Greek *traxus* meaning 'rough'. All major conduits in the body were initially considered by the ancient anatomists to conduct air. The Greek *artēria* (meaning 'to carry air') was the windpipe, and was more specifically called the *artēria traxeia* meaning 'the rough artery' given its corrugations and cartilaginous rings. The *artēria* was dropped in approximately the fifteenth century and the windpipe became known as the trachea.

Tragus From the Greel *tragos* meaning 'he-goat'—referring to the resemblance of the tuft of hair hanging from a goat's neck with the tuft of hairs sprouting from the tragus of predominantly, older men.

Trismus From the Greek *trismos* meaning 'a scream, grinding, gnashing, or rasping'—perhaps describing the only manageable actions and sounds a patient suffering with trismus can manage. Trismus describes the restriction in mouth opening classically (but no longer commonly) due to tetanus or 'lockjaw'.

Tympanum From the Latin *tympanum* meaning 'a drum', describing the resemblance of the tympanic membrane with that of a taut drum.

Uvula The diminutive of the Latin *uva* meaning 'grape'. The word was initially attached to what we now refer to as the uvula by the French surgeon Guy de Chauliac (1300–1368). Despite only referring to it as the *uvula* in its swollen state, the term has remained regardless of pathology. A related word is *uvea*, the collective word for the iris, ciliary body, and choroid. On removing the stem of a grape, the stemless end of the grape was thought to resemble the eyeball with its central pupil.

Vaccine From the Latin *vacca* meaning 'a cow', with *vaccinia* referring to cowpox, a viral disease of cattle. The English physician Edward Jenner (1749–1823) recognized that milkmaids who caught cowpox seemed to experience a reduced risk of subsequently getting smallpox. He (rather bravely) inoculated an 8-year-old boy with the contents of a pustule from the hand of a local milkmaid. The same boy on being inoculated with smallpox, suffered no ill effect.

Velum The Latin word meaning 'a sail, curtain, or an awning'. The tensor and levator veli palatini are paired muscles of the soft palate, which itself hangs rather like an awning at the back of the bony palate. Related words include *veil* and *reveal*.

Vertex From the Latin *vertere* meaning 'to turn'. Literal translations of *vertex* range from 'a whirlpool, whirlwind, or tornado', 'the summit of a mountain', and 'the top of the head'. The latter refers to the whorl of hairs that form at the crown of the scalp in the region of the vertex.

Index

For the benefit of digital users, indexed terms that span two pages (e.g., 52–53) may, on occasion, appear on only one of those pages.